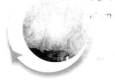

Clinical
Cases In Basic
Biomedical Science

Core Clinical Cases

Titles in the series include:

Core Clinical Cases in Basic Biomedical Science
Author: Samy A. Azer

Core Clinical Cases in Obstetrics & Gynaecology 2nd Edition
Authors: Janesh K. Gupta, Gary Mires & Khalid S. Khan

Core Clinical Cases in Paediatrics
Authors: Andrew Ewer, Timothy G. Barrett & Vin Diwakar

Core Clinical Cases in Psychiatry
Authors: Tom Clark, Ed Day & Emma C. Fergusson

Coming soon…

Core Clinical Cases in the Medical and Surgical Specialities
Edited by Steve Bain & Janesh K. Gupta

Core Clinical Cases in Medicine & Surgery
Edited by Steve Bain & Janesh K. Gupta

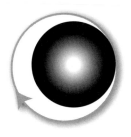

Core
Clinical
Cases In Basic
Biomedical Science

A problem-based learning approach

Samy A. Azer MB BCh MSc Medicine PhD (Syd) MEd MPH (NSW) FACG
Senior Lecturer in Medical Education, Faculty of Medicine,
Dentistry and Health Sciences, University of Melbourne,
Australia

Core Clinical Cases series edited by

Janesh K. Gupta MSc MD FRCOG
Clinical Senior Lecturer/ Honorary Consultant in
Obstetrics and Gynaecology, University of Birmingham,
Birmingham Women's Hospital, Birmingham, UK

Hodder Arnold

A MEMBER OF THE HODDER HEADLINE GROUP

First published in Great Britain in 2006 by
Hodder Education, a member of the Hodder Headline Group,
338 Euston Road, London NW1 3BH

http://www.hoddereducation.co.uk

Distributed in the United States of America by
Oxford University Press Inc.,
198 Madison Avenue, New York, NY10016
Oxford is a registered trademark of Oxford University Press

Whilst the advice and information in this book are believed to be true and
accurate at the date of going to press, neither the author[s] nor the publisher
can accept any legal responsibility or liability for any errors or omissions
that may be made. In particular, (but without limiting the generality of the
preceding disclaimer) every effort has been made to check drug dosages;
however it is still possible that errors have been missed. Furthermore,
dosage schedules are constantly being revised and new side-effects
recognized. For these reasons the reader is strongly urged to consult the
drug companies' printed instructions before administering any of the drugs
recommended in this book.

British Library Cataloguing in Publication Data
A catalogue record for this book is available from the British Library

Library of Congress Cataloging-in-Publication Data
A catalog record for this book is available from the Library of Congress

ISBN-10: 0 340 816716
ISBN-13: 978 0 340 81671 4

1 2 3 4 5 6 7 8 9 10

Commissioning Editor: Georgina Bentliff
Project Editor: Heather Smith
Production Controller: Jane Lawrence
Cover Design: Georgina Hewitt

Typeset in 9 on 12 pt Frutiger Light Condensed by Phoenix Photosetting, Chatham, Kent
Printed and bound in Malta

What do you think about this book? Or any other Hodder Arnold title?
Please visit our website at www.hoddereducation.co.uk

This book is dedicated to my parents and my family.
Mary, Sarah and Diana have given me the love and support necessary to write this book. I also dedicate this book to my students who have inspired me to create this work.

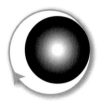

Contents

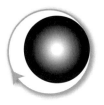

Foreword

The introduction of integrated case-based or problem-based learning to health professional courses has revolutionized how health professional students learn basic sciences. They now learn the requisite science in a way that is contextually rich, relevant and imparts the vitality of real patient problems. Evidence shows that students find this approach more stimulating and engaging than traditiional courses. However, one challenge these students face is finding textbooks that approach basic sciences in a similar integrated fashion.

This book provides students with a contextually rich, evidence-based and integrated approach to learning the basic sciences relevant to many health professions, including medicine. Using carefully crafted realistic patient scenarios the learner learns to apply their developing basic science knowledge to make relevant clinical decisions. The range of cases is broad stretching from the cranial nerves to the gastrointestinal system and the questions embedded in the cases stimulate the learner to reflect on their own knowledge base, to seek further knowledge and to apply that knowledge and get timely, explicit and specific feedback.

It is a pleasure to commend this book to you. It displays the author's broad knowledge of education, basic science and clinical medicine, and is highly deserving of a place on each medical student's desk.

Associate Professor Susan Elliott
MBBS MD FRACP
Associate Dean (Academic Programs)
Director, Faculty Education Unit
Faculty of Medicine, Dentistry and Health Sciences
The University of Melbourne
Victoria, Australia

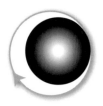

Series preface

'A History Lesson'

Between about 1916 and 1927 a puzzling illness appeared and swept around the world. Dr von Economo first described encephalitis lethargica (EL), which simply meant 'inflammation of the brain that makes you tired'. Younger people, especially women, seemed to be more vulnerable but the disease affected people of all ages. People with EL developed a 'sleep disorder', fever, headache and weakness, which led to a prolonged state of unconsciousness. The EL epidemic occurred during the same time period as the 1918 influenza pandemic, and the two outbreaks have been linked ever since in the medical literature. Some confused it with the epidemic of Spanish flu at that time while others blamed weapons used in World War I.

Encephalitis lethargica (EL) was dramatised by the film Awakenings (book written by Oliver Sacks who is an eminent Neurologist from New York), starring Robin Williams and Robert De Niro. Professor Sacks treated his patients with L-dopa, which temporarily awoke his patients giving rise to the belief that the condition was related to Parkinson's disease.

Since the 1916–1927 epidemic, only sporadic cases have been described. Pathological studies have revealed an encephalitis of the midbrain and basal ganglia, with lymphocyte (predominantly plasma cell) infiltration. Recent examination of archived EL brain material has failed to demonstrate influenza RNA, adding to the evidence that EL was not an invasive influenza encephalitis. Further investigations found no evidence of viral encephalitis or other recognised causes of rapid-onset parkinsonism. MRI of the brain was normal in 60% but showed inflammatory changes localised to the deep grey matter in 40% of patients.

As late as the end of the 20th century, it seemed that the possible answers lay in the clinical presentation of the patients in the 1916–1927 epidemic. It had been noted by the clinicians at that time that the CNS disorder had presented with pharyngitis. This led to the possibility of a post-infectious autoimmune CNS disorder similar to Sydenham's chorea, in which group A beta-hemolytic streptococcal antibodies cross-react with the basal ganglia and result in abnormal behaviour and involuntary movements. Anti-streptolysin-O titres have subsequently been found to be elevated in the majority of these patients. It seemed possible that autoimmune antibodies may cause remitting parkinsonian signs subsequent to streptococcal tonsillitis as part of the spectrum of post-streptococcal CNS disease.

Could it be that the 80-year mystery of EL has been solved relying on the patient's clinical history of presentation, rather than focusing on expensive investigations? More research in this area will give us the definitive answer. This scenario is not dissimilar to the controversy about the idea that streptococcal infections were aetiologically related to rheumatic fever.

With this example of a truly fascinating history lesson, we hope that you will endeavour to use the patient's clinical history as your most powerful diagnostic tool to make the correct diagnosis. If you do you are likely to be right 80 to 90% of the time. This is the basis of all the Core Clinical Cases series, which will make you systematically explore clinical problems through the clinical history of presentation, followed by examination and then the performance of appropriate investigations. Never break that rule.

Janesh Gupta
2005

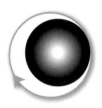

Preface

Most of the medical and health professional schools in the UK, North America, Middle East, South East Asia and Australia are moving to new courses, which are systems-based. In addition, many of these schools are implementing integrated problem-based learning or case-based approaches in their curricula. These new approaches aim at enhancing students' understanding, critical thinking, reasoning and communication skills rather than rote or didactic learning.

This book has been designed with these changes in mind, and with the aim to help students review knowledge learnt in basic sciences and practice clinical scenario-based questions. The questions in the book test a number of cognitive skills including hypotheses generation, collection of more information by asking history questions, interpretation of clinical findings and laboratory results, construction of mechanisms and refining their hypothesis on the basis of evidence available from history, clinical examination and investigatioins. It provides revision for basic sciences needed in these courses and allows for the discussion of 45 clinical scenarios addressing important principles related to different body systems. This approach is intended to emphasize the importance of knowledge of basic sciences for the understanding of medicine. It also aims at enhancing students' skills and motivates them at an early stage of their course.

The clinical cases chosen are those that enable students to discuss the relevance of many aspects of basic sciences in relation to specific clinical problems and demonstrate the role of basic sciences in understanding pathophysiology, differential diagnoses, laboratory and radiological changes and management options related to the cases.

This book is not aimed at replacing standard textbooks recommended to students and other resources. A list of these resources, has been included at the end of the book as well as a list of useful reviews related to the principles discussed in the cases have been included at the end of each chaper. This book should be used in conjunction with your recommended textbooks; I would recommend using it as a review resource when you complete the study of a body system. It will also be useful for your study throughout the year and before summative examinations.

Samy A. Azer
MB BCh MSc Medicine Med (NSW) PhD (Syd) FACG MPH (NSW)
Australia, 2005

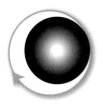

Acknowledgements

Several colleagues and students have made an invaluable contribution to the revision of this book. Among those who have helped me, I would like to convey special thanks to these students Sarah Azer, Rebecca Barton, Liew Kwee Chin, Cheng He, Lindy Washington, and Sarah Wongseelashote.

I would also like to thank and acknowledge the significant contribution of a number of staff at Hodder Arnold Publishers, particularly Ms Georgina Bentliff, for her continuous support and encouragement during the preparation of the manuscript, Ms Heather Smith, the manager of the project, for her editorial support and enthusiastic follow-up of the project and Ms Liz Weaver for her excellent proof reading.

I am also grateful to my medical and physiotherapy students, from whom I continue to learn how to create teaching and learning material and assessment questions that match with the curriculum structure and allow them to apply knowledge learnt from a wide range of basic sciences in the first three years of their course.

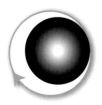

Abbreviations

17-OHP	17-hydroxyprogesterone
A&E	accident and emergency
A/C	alveo-capillary
ACE	angiotensin-converting enzyme
ACh	acetylcholine
ACTH	adrenocorticotrophic hormone
ADH	antidiuretic hormone
AF	atrial fibrillation
AIDS	acquired immune deficiency syndrome
ALT	alanine aminotransferase
ALP	alkaline phosphatase
ANA	antinuclear antibody
ANS	autonomic nervous system
APTT	activated partial thromboplastin time
APUD	amine precursor uptake and decarboxylation
AST	aspartate aminotransferase
A-V	atrioventricular
BCP	basic calcium phosphate
BMI	body mass index
CAH	congenital adrenal hyperplasia
cDNA	complementary DNA
CF	cystic fibrosis
CFTR	CF transmembrane conductance regulator
CH50	total haemolytic complement
CK	creatine kinase
CK-MB	creatine kinase MB

CNS	central nervous system
cMOAT	canalicular multispecific organic anion transporter
COPD	chronic obstructive pulmonary disease
COX	cyclo-oxygenase
CPPD	calcium pyrophosphate dehydrate
CRH	corticotrophin- releasing hormone
CRP	C-reactive protein
CSF	cerebrospinal fluid
CT	computed tomography
DHA	dehydroepiandrosterone
DIC	disseminated intravascular coagulation
DPG	2,3-diphosphoglycerate
DVT	deep venous thrombosis
ECF	extracellular fluid
ECG	electrocardiogram
ECl	enterochromaffin-like
EMG	electromyography
ERCP	endoscopic retrograde cholangiopancreatography
ESR	erythrocyte sedimentation rate
FEV_1	forced expiratory volume in 1 s
FT_4	free thyroxine
FSH	follicle-stimulating hormone
FVC	forced vital capacity
G-6-PD	glucose-6-phosphate dehydrogenase
GABA	γ-aminobutyric acid
GFR	glomerular filtration rate
GGT	γ-glutamyl transferase
GH	growth hormone
GHRH	GH-releasing hormone
GnRH	gonadotrophin-releasing hormone

GRP	gastrin-releasing peptide.
HAART	combination antiretroviral therapy
HAV	hepatitis A virus
Hb	haemoglobin
HBV	hepatitis B virus
HBcA	hepatitis B core antibody
HBsA	hepatitis B surface antigen
HCV	hepatitis C virus
HDL	high-density lipoprotein
HIV	human immunodeficiency virus
HMG-CoA	hydroxymethylglutaryl coenzyme A
HRCT	high-resolution computed tomography
ICF	intracellular fluid
IF	intrinsic factor
Ig	immunoglobulin
IGF-I	insulin-like growth factor I
IL	interleukin
INR	international normalized ratio
ITP	idiopathic thrombocytopenic purpura
JG	juxtaglomerular
JVP	jugular venous pressure
LDH	lactate dehydrogenase
LDL	low-density lipoprotein
LH	luteinizing hormone
LMNL	lower motor neuron lesion
LMW	low molecular weight
LT	leukotriene
LV	left ventricular
MAC	*Mycobacterium avium* complex
MCV	mean corpuscular volume

MRA	magnetic resonance angiography
MRI	magnetic resonance imaging
MRP2	multidrug resistance-associated protein 2
MS	mitral stenosis
MSUM	monosodium urate monohydrate
NK	natural killer
NSAIDs	non-steroidal anti-inflammatory drugs
PA	posteroanterior
PAF	platelet-activating factor
PCP	*Pneumocystis carinii* pneumonia
PCR	polymerase chain reaction
PCV	packed cell volume
PRL	prolactin
PT	prothrombin time
PP	pancreatic polypeptide
PTH	parathyroid hormone
PWI	perfusion-weighted image
RDW	red cell distribution width
RER	rough endoplasmic reticulum
RT-PCR	reverse transcription polymerase chain reaction
SA	sinoatrial
SHBG	sex hormone-binding globulin
SLE	systemic lupus erythematosus
T_3	triiodothyronine
T_4	thyroxine
TB	tuberculosis
TG	triglyceride
Th2	T-helper 2
TIA	transient ischaemic attack
TRH	thyroid-releasing hormone

TSH	thyroid-stimulating hormone
TT	thrombin time
UMNL	upper motor neuron lesion
UV	ultraviolet
VLDL	very-low-density lipoprotein
WBC	white blood cell
WCC	white blood cell count
ZN	Ziehl–Neelsen

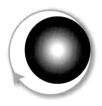

About the author

Dr Azer is a Senior Lecturer in Medical Education in the Faculty of Medicine, Dentistry and Health Sciences, the University of Melbourne. He is a gastroenterologist/hepatologist by training and was awarded Fellowship of the American College of Gastroenterology in 1998. He has national and international input in the use of problem-based learning in medical and health professional education. Dr Azer has coordinated the delivery of Problem-based learning (PBL) at the University of Melbourne in its first two and half years. He is the director of the PBL training programmes and has trained over 500 PBL tutors since 1999. He has led the Faculty in amending the style of assessment and has a major input in writing PBL style of questions. Dr Azer was the Chair of the Faculty Excellence in Teaching Awards Subcommittee in 2003–2004.

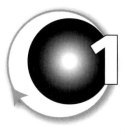

Biliary system and pancreas

? Questions for each of the case scenarios given

Q1: What are the possible causes (hypotheses) for the presenting problem?
Q2: What further questions would you like to ask to help you differentiate between your hypotheses?
Q3: What investigations would be most helpful to you and why?
Q4: In the light of the clinical presentation, how would you interpret the laboratory test results?
Q5: What is your final hypothesis?
Q6: What issues in the given history, examination and laboratory tests support your final hypothesis?

Clinical cases

● CASE 1.1 – I have severe pain in my tummy.

You are working with Dr Samantha McLean in her clinic. Lydia Greenwood, a 20-year-old shop assistant, comes in complaining of sudden right upper quadrant pain for the last 5 hours. Her pain started half an hour after having dinner. She describes the pain as 7 out of 10 and moving to her right scapula. She has severe nausea and vomited twice over the last 3 hours. She gives no history of chronic disorders, intravenous drug use or travel overseas. On examination, she is in pain and her vital signs are as shown in Table 1.1.

Table 1.1 Vital signs of Case 1.1

Vital signs	Lydia's results	Normal range
Blood pressure (mmHg)	120/80	100/60–135/85
Pulse rate (/min)	110	60–100
Respiratory rate (/min)	18	12–16
Temperature (°C)	38.3	36.6–37.2

Abdominal examination

- Abdominal guarding and tenderness below the right costal margin on palpation. She halts her inspiration during palpation

- Normal bowel sounds.

● CASE 1.2 – I have developed yellowish eyes.

Michael May, a 68-year-old pensioner, is admitted to a local hospital because of progressive jaundice, weakness and upper abdominal pain over the last 4 weeks. The pain is constant and radiates to his back. Michael has also lost about 5 kg in weight over the last 2 months. He worked in a chemical factory for over 25 years. He drinks a glass of wine every day. He smoked 25 cigarettes per day for over 30 years but ceased smoking 2 years ago. On examination, Michael is jaundiced. He has no spider naevi or palmar erythema. His vital signs are normal.

Abdominal examination:

- A non-tender mass is felt below his right costal margin (most probably the gallbladder)
- No palpable spleen
- No shifting dullness
- Digital rectal examination: stools are pale
- Urinalysis: bilirubin +++.

Cardiovascular and respiratory examinations are normal.

● CASE 1.3 – I have recurrent abdominal pain and loose bowel motions.

Ms Lisa Johnson, a 45-year-old businesswoman, presents with sudden upper abdominal pain during a business dinner in Japan. She is brought by ambulance to the emergency department of a local hospital. Lisa has had recurrent abdominal pain and loose bowel motions for over 2 years. Her stools are pale, bulky and offensive in odour. Her abdominal pain is sometimes severe and requires pain-killers. She admits that she drinks one to two glasses of red wine per day and has increased her drinking pattern despite her GP's advice to decrease drinking. On examination, she looks anxious. Her vital signs are all normal. There is tenderness in the upper part of her abdomen. The liver and spleen are not palpable. Urinalysis: glucose +.

Cardiovascular and respiratory examinations are normal.

Integrated medical sciences questions

CASE 1.1 – Discuss the role of bile salt metabolism in the formation and treatment of gallstones (cholelithiasis).

CASE 1.2 – Discuss the mechanisms underlying Michael's jaundice.

CASE 1.3 – Discuss the pathophysiological and pathological changes responsible for Lisa's abdominal pain and loose bowel motions.

Key concepts

In order to work through the core clinical cases in this chapter, you will need to understand the following key concepts.

The main functions of the pancreas

- Pancreatic secretion contains enzymes for digestion of proteins, carbohydrates and fats.

- Pancreatic secretion contains large amounts of bicarbonate ions (important in neutralizing the acid chyme that comes from the stomach into the duodenum).

- Secretion of trypsin inhibitor, which prevents digestion of the pancreas itself by its proteolytic enzymes.

- The endocrine part of the pancreas, the islets of Langerhans, secretes insulin and glucagon directly into the bloodstream. These hormones are important in regulation of the blood sugar levels.

- The pancreas secretes other hormones such as amylin, somatostatin and pancreatic polypeptide. Their functions are not well established.

The role of the pancreas in digestion: the digestive enzymes secreted by the pancreas and their function

The pancreatic secretions are important in the digestion of proteins, carbohydrates and fats (Table 1.2).

Table 1.2 Functions of pancreatic digestive enzymes

Pancreatic digestive enzymes	Functions[a]
Trypsin	Digests proteins into peptides of various sizes but does not release individual amino acids. Trypsinogen is the inactive form secreted by the pancreatic cells. It is activated to trypsin in the intestine via the effect of an enzyme called enterokinase (secreted by intestinal mucosa)
Chymotrypsin	Digests proteins into peptides of various sizes but does not release individual amino acids
Carboxypolypeptidase A and B	These are exopeptidases that remove amino acids from the C terminals of polypeptides
Elastases and nucleases	Their function is not known
Pancreatic amylase	Hydrolyses starches, glycogen and most carbohydrates (except cellulose) to disaccharides
Pancreatic lipase	Important for fat digestion
Cholesterol esterase	Hydrolyses cholesterol esters
Phospholipase	Splits fatty acids from phospholipids

[a]The majority of pancreatic enzymes are secreted as inactive precursors and undergo activation in the duodenum. This mechanism protects the pancreas from autodigestion.

The hormones secreted by the pancreas and their functions

Table 1.3 Functions of hormones secreted by the pancreas

Pancreatic hormones	Cell of the islet of Langerhans	Function
Insulin	β	Anabolic hormone; plays important role in carbohydrate, fat and protein metabolism, regulates blood glucose levels, facilitates store of excess energy, and promotes the uptake of amino acids by cells and conversion of amino acids into protein
Glucagon	α	Regulates blood glucose level, opposes the actions of insulin, increases blood glucose concentration and causes glycogenolysis, and increases gluconeogenesis Other effects: – activates adipose cell lipase. – inhibits the storage of triglycerides by the liver – prevents the liver removing fatty acids from blood
Somatostatin	δ	Inhibits glucagon and insulin secretion Decreases the motility of the stomach, duodenum and gallbladder Decreases the absorption process in the gastrointestinal tract
Amylin	β	Secreted along with insulin. We are not aware of its function
Pancreatic polypeptide	PP cell	Uncertain function

The main functions of the gallbladder

● Storage of bile until needed for digestion in the duodenum

● Concentration of bile up to 15-fold its normal concentration.

The main stimulus for gallbladder contraction

Cholecystokinin (CCK) is the most potent stimulus for gallbladder contraction. CCK, a hormone secreted by special cells in the duodenal mucosa, is secreted in response to the presence of fatty foods in the duodenum. CCK also causes relaxation of the sphincter of Oddi, resulting in the passage of bile into the duodenum.

The composition of bile

Water, bile salts (mainly glycine- or taurine-conjugated cholic and chenodeoxycholic acids), bilirubin, cholesterol, phospholipids (lecithin), and electrolytes such as Na^+, K^+, Ca^{2+}, Cl^- and bicarbonates. Drug metabolites can also be excreted into bile.

The role of bile salts in digestion

● Bile salts play an important role in digestion and absorption of fats.

● Bile salts help to emulsify the large fat particles of food into small particles.

● Bile salts prepare fats for the action of pancreatic lipase.

● Bile salts help in the absorption of fat-soluble vitamins (A, D, E and K).

Answers

● CASE 1.1 – I have severe pain in my tummy.

Q1: What are the possible causes (hypotheses) for the presenting problem?

A1

Possible causes (hypotheses) for Lydia's abdominal pain and fever are:

- Acute cholecystitis
- Acute appendicitis
- Perforated peptic ulcer
- Acute pancreatitis
- Right lower lobe pneumonia
- Acute pyelonephritis of the right kidney
- Acute hepatitis.

Q2: What further questions would you like to ask to help you differentiate between your hypotheses?

A2

Further history questions are shown in Table 1.4.

Table 1.4 Further history questions for Case 1.1

History questions	In what way answers can help
Have you noticed any colour changes in your urine? Do you have any pain on passing urine? Ask about sex preference, practice of safe sex, tattooing, travel overseas, intravenous drug use, contact with patients with hepatitis	Dark urine may suggest presence of blood (renal stones) or conjugated bilirubin (hepatitis). These factors increase the risk for hepatitis
Alcohol intake and medications	Excessive alcohol intake can produce alcoholic hepatitis and pancreatitis. Some drugs may cause hepatocellular damage (e.g. chlorpropamide, erythromycin, thiazide diuretics, paracetamol, p-aminosalicylic acid, isoniazid) or increase the tendency for biliary calculi formation
Last menstrual period	Lydia might be pregnant (nausea and vomiting may occur in early pregnancy)

Past history, family history and social history

It is important to find out if she has had any trouble with her urinary tract, liver, biliary system or blood disease. Also some haemolytic diseases are inherited (e.g. thalassaemia) and increase the risk of developing gallstones

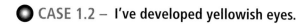

Q3: What investigations would be most helpful to you and why?

A3

Further investigations

- Full blood examination

- Liver function tests: serum total bilirubin, alanine aminotransferase (ALT), aspartate aminotransferase (AST), alkaline phosphatase (ALP), γ-glutamyl transferase (GGT), serum albumin and prothrombin time

- Serum amylase

- Erect chest radiograph

- Ultrasound examination of the upper abdomen.

 CASE 1.2 – I've developed yellowish eyes.

Q1: What are the possible causes (hypotheses) for the presenting problem?

A1

The picture does not suggest chronic liver disease (no spider naevi, palmar erythema, splenomegaly or ascites). The presentation of progressive jaundice, weight loss, palpable gallbladder and increased bilirubin in urine support the diagnosis of obstructive jaundice caused by cancer of the head of pancreas or of the ampulla of Vater or bile duct (cholangiocarcinoma), or metastatic cancer (e.g. enlarged lymph nodes obstructing the common bile duct). The possibility that biliary obstruction is caused by a stone (choledocholithiasis) is less likely because the patient's pain is constant and his jaundice progressive, and there is no history of biliary colic.

Most likely causes

- Cancer of head of pancreas

- Cancer of the common bile duct

- Cancer of the ampulla of Vater

- Metastatic cancer (enlarged lymph nodes obstructing the biliary system)

- Intrahepatic metastasis.

Q2: What further questions would you like to ask to help you differentiate between your hypotheses?

A2

Past history of biliary colic, jaundice, fever, rigors and liver problems. Details of medications and any past investigations. Any changes in bowel habits, bleeding per rectum or bowel problems, or surgery.

 Q3: What investigations would be most helpful to you and why?

A3

Further investigations

- Full blood examination
- Liver function tests
- Full blood examination
- Tumour markers (e.g. CA19-9)
- Abdominal computed tomography (CT)
- Chest radiograph
- Endoscopic retrograde cholangiopancreatography (ERCP).

● CASE 1.3 – I have recurrent abdominal pain and loose bowel motions.

 Q1: What are the possible causes (hypotheses) for the presenting problem?

A1

Possible causes (hypotheses) for Lisa's presentation are:

- Chronic pancreatitis
- Acute pancreatitis complicating chronic pancreatitis
- Acute cholecystitis (choledocholithiasis) – less likely
- Acute hepatitis.

The presence of chronic recurrent abdominal pain, steatorrhoea (excessive loss of fat in stools causing the patient's stools to become pale, bulky and with offensive odour) and impairment of her blood glucose metabolism (diabetes) are supportive of chronic pancreatitis. She might also have attacks of acute pancreatitis complicating chronic pancreatitis.

Chronic pancreatitis is characterized by irreversible morphological changes in the pancreas, resulting in pain and loss of function. Chronic alcoholism is one of the most common causes of non-obstructive pancreatitis. Other causes include: (1) malnutrition, (2) idiopathic causes in about 20 per cent of cases, (3) trauma, (4) metabolic causes, e.g. hypertriglyceridaemia and hypercalcaemia, and (5) inherited, e.g. cystic fibrosis.

Obstructive causes of chronic pancreatitis are: (1) benign obstruction of sphincter of Oddi or papillary stenosis and (2) obstruction of the ampulla of Vater or ductal system by a tumour.

Q2: What further questions would you like to ask to help you differentiate between your hypotheses?

A2

More details about her abdominal pain including type of pain, severity, location, radiation, aggravating factors and methods of relief. History of body weight loss, medications and any previous investigations.

 Q3: What investigations would be most helpful to you and why?

A3

Further investigations

- Full blood examination
- CT of upper abdomen
- Liver function tests
- Serum amylase, serum trypsinogen
- 72-hour faecal fat determination
- Blood glucose, urea, creatinine, sodium and potassium
- Faecal chymotrypsin or elastase.

Further progress

 CASE 1.1 – I have severe pain in my tummy.

Dr McLean arranges for some blood tests for Lydia. The results are shown in Table 1.5.

Table 1.5 Blood text results for Case 1.1

Blood test	Lydia's results	Normal range
Haemoglobin (Hb) (g/L)	130	115–160
White blood cell count (WCC) ($\times 10^9$/L)	15 000	4.0–11.0
Packed cell volume (PCV)	0.55	0.39–0.63
Platelet count ($\times 10^9$/L)	420	150–400
Serum bilirubin (total) (μmol/L)	35	0–19
Serum ALP (IU/L)	160	0–120
Serum AST (IU/L)	42	0–40
Serum ALT (IU/L)	55	0–55
Serum GGT (IU/L)	95	0–50
Serum albumin (g/L)	45	35–50
Prothrombin time (s)	20	18–22
Serum amylase (U/L)	45	25–125

Erect chest radiograph: both lungs are clear; no free subdiaphragmatic gas.

Ultrasound examination of the upper abdomen: the gallbladder wall is slightly thickened and some fluid is seen around the gallbladder. Three 'acoustic shadows' are seen, indicating the presence of gallstones. The liver and pancreas are normal.

CASE 1.2 – I've developed yellowish eyes.

The registrar arranges for some blood tests. The results of blood tests are shown in Table 1.6.

Table 1.6 Blood test results for Case 1.2

Blood test	Michael's results	Normal range
Hb (g/L)	95	115–160
WCC ($\times 10^9$/L)	4	4.0–11.0
PCV	0.42	0.39–0.63
Platelet count ($\times 10^9$/L)	295	150–400
Serum bilirubin (total) (μmol/L)	95	0–19
Serum albumin (g/L)	42	35–50
Serum AST (IU/L)	44	0–40
Serum ALT (IU/L)	59	0–55
Serum ALP (IU/L)	850	0–120
Serum GGT (IU/L)	434	0–50
Prothrombin time (s)	23	18–22

Chest radiograph: both lungs are clear.

Tumour marker, Ca19.9: 960 units/mL (normal range: 0–37 U/mL).

Abdominal CT: a large mass occupying the head of the pancreas. Dilated common bile duct and intrahepatic ducts, indicating extrahepatic biliary obstruction. No liver metastases and normal spleen.

ERCP: evidence of cancer of the head of the pancreas. Common bile duct and intrahepatic ducts are dilated. No evidence of cancer of the ampulla of Vater or bile duct (cholangiocarcinoma).

CASE 1.3 – I have recurrent abdominal pain and loose bowel motions.

The hospital registrar arranges for some tests. The results of her lab tests are shown in Table 1.7.

Table 1.7 Blood test results for Case 1.3

Test	Lisa's results	Normal range
Hb (g/L)	135	115–160
WCC (× 10⁹/L)	4.5	4.0–11.0
PCV	0.47	0.39–0.63
Platelet count (× 10⁹/L)	320	150–400
Serum sodium (mmol/L)	141	135–145
Serum potassium (mmol/L)	3.5	3.5–5.0
Blood urea (mmol/L)	5.5	2.5–8.3
Serum creatinine (mmol/L)	0.08	0.05–0.11
Serum albumin (g/L)	32	35–50
Serum total bilirubin (μmol/L)	78	0–19
Serum ALT (IU/L)	37	0–55
Serum AST (IU/L)	39	0–40
Serum ALP (IU/L)	120	0–120
Serum GGT (IU/L)	310	0–50
Serum amylase (U/L)	110	25–125
Total serum calcium (mmol/L)	2.4	2.1–2.55
Fasting blood glucose (mmol/L)	9	3.9–5.8

72-h faecal fat: 9.5 g/24 h (normal range: <7 g/24 h).

Plain radiograph of the abdomen: evidence of calcification in the upper abdomen.

CT of the abdomen: small atrophic pancreas, calcification seen in the pancreas. Liver, gallbladder and spleen normal.

Further questions

● CASE 1.1 – I have severe pain in my tummy.

 Q4: In the light of the clinical presentation, how would you interpret the laboratory test results?

A4

Table 1.8 Interpretation of lab test results for Case 1.1

Test	Changes	Interpretation
Hb	Normal	Haemolysis is less likely to be the cause of Lydia's jaundice
WCC	Raised	Raised WCC + fever + sudden abdominal pain suggest an acute inflammatory process (e.g. acute cholecystitis, acute pancreatitis, acute appendicitis)
Serum bilirubin (total)	Raised	The presence of abdominal pain and fever suggests acute cholecystitis and pancreatitis
Serum ALP	Mildly raised	Raised ALP may occur in partial biliary obstruction, cholestasis and bone disorders
Serum AST	Upper limit of normal	The results do not match with haemolysis or acute hepatitis
Serum ALT	Upper limit of normal	The results do not match with acute hepatitis
Serum GGT	Mildly raised	The mild rise in GGT together with raised ALP support the diagnosis of biliary obstruction
Serum amylase	Normal	Acute pancreatitis is less likely
Erect chest radiograph	Both lungs are clear. No free subdiaphragmatic gas	This excludes right lower pneumonia and perforated duodenal ulcer (perforated duodenal ulcer is associated with free subdiaphragmatic gas in 70 per cent of patients)
Ultrasound examination of the upper abdomen	The gallbladder wall is slightly thickened and some fluid is seen around the gallbladder. Three 'acoustic shadows' are seen, indicating the presence of gallstones. The liver and pancreas are normal	These findings together with the biochemical changes support the diagnosis of acute cholecystitis

Q5: What is your final hypothesis?

A5

The clinical picture and the laboratory results are suggestive of acute cholecystitis.

 Q6: What issues in the given history, examination and laboratory tests support your final hypothesis?

A6

Supportive evidence

History

- Acute right upper quadrant abdominal pain
- Pain is referred to her right scapula
- Severe nausea and vomited twice
- No history of travel overseas.

Examination

- Abdominal guarding and tenderness below the right costal margin on palpation
- She halts her inspiration during palpation
- Tachycardia and fever: 38.3°C.

Investigations

- Raised WCC and serum bilirubin
- Mildly raised ALP and GGT
- Upper limit of normal AST and ALT
- Normal serum amylase
- Erect chest radiograph: both lungs are clear; no free subdiaphragmatic gas
- Ultrasound examination of her upper abdomen: the gallbladder wall is slightly thickened and some fluid around the gallbladder is seen. Three 'acoustic shadows' are seen indicating the presence of gallstones. The liver and pancreas are normal.

● CASE 1.2 – I've developed yellowish eyes.

Q4: In the light of the clinical presentation, how would you interpret the laboratory test results?

A4

Table 1.9 Interpretation of lab test results for Case 1.2

Test	Changes	Interpretation
Hb	Below the lower normal limit	Blood loss from a cancer, decreased appetite, malnutrition, shortened life span of red blood cells, bone marrow suppression
WCC	Lower normal limit	White blood cells (WBCs) are expected to be raised in the presence of infection. Possibly there is some suppression of his immune system
Serum bilirubin (total)	Raised	In the light of raised bilirubin in urine (+++), the raised total serum bilirubin is most probably caused by conjugated bilirubin
Serum albumin	Normal range	This matches with the clinical findings and the absence of clinical findings suggestive of chronic liver disease
Serum AST	Just above the upper limit of normal	Hepatitis is less likely
Serum ALT	Just above the upper limit of normal	Hepatitis is less likely
Serum ALP	Raised +++	Together with jaundice and the appearance of bilirubin in urine (+++), obstruction is the most common cause
Serum GGT	Raised +++	Suggests obstruction of biliary system/alcohol effect
Prothrombin time	Just above the upper limit of normal	The presence of obstructive jaundice and the lack of bile salt in the intestine → interference with the absorption of fat-soluble vitamins (A, D, E and K). In the liver, vitamin K participates in carboxylation of glutamic acid residues of some proteins involved in blood coagulation, explaining the slight increase in the prothrombin time
Chest radiograph	Both lungs are clear	No evidence of metastases to the lungs
Tumour marker CA19-9	Raised	The sensitivity of this test ranges from 81 to 85 per cent and its specificity from 81 to 90 per cent. This test cannot replace fine-needle aspiration biopsy of the pancreas under CT or endoscopic ultrasound guidance. However, it is useful in monitoring the response to treatment

Abdominal CT	A large mass occupying the head of the pancreas. Dilated common bile duct and intrahepatic ducts, indicating extrahepatic biliary obstruction. No liver metastases and normal spleen	The CT is able to detect cancer of the head of the pancreas in > 82 per cent of patients. In approximately 5–15 per cent of patients with proven cancer pancreas, the CT shows generalized enlargement of the pancreas and no conclusive evidence of carcinoma. In these patients, other investigations such as ERCP, selective angiography, radionuclide pancreatic scintigraphy and tumour markers are indicated Sometimes, it is very difficult to differentiate cancer of the pancreas from chronic pancreatitis and even laparotomy, and percutaneous aspiration biopsy of the pancreas under CT guidance are of limited help in some cases
ERCP	Evidence of cancer of the head of the pancreas. Common bile duct and intrahepatic ducts are dilated. No evidence of cancer of the ampulla of Vater or bile duct (cholangiocarcinoma)	Ampullatory carcinomas and distal cholangiocarcinomas may manifest with biliary obstruction, fever, weight loss and jaundice. The ERCP is very helpful in excluding or confirming these causes

Q5: What is your final hypothesis?

A5

The clinical findings and the investigations support the diagnosis of cancer of the head of the pancreas.

Q6: What issues in the given history, examination and laboratory tests support your final hypothesis?

A6

Supportive evidence

History

- Progressive jaundice, weakness

- Upper abdominal pain over the last 4 weeks

- Weight loss

- ? occupational exposure to chemicals (e.g. benzidine and β-naphthylamine are risk factors).

Examination

- Jaundiced

- No signs of chronic liver disease (e.g. spider naevi or palmar erythema)

- Enlarged tender gallbladder

- No splenomegaly.

- Urine: bilirubin +++.

Investigations

- Low Hb

- Raised serum bilirubin +++

- Raised serum ALP and GGT +++

- Little rise in transaminases (AST and ALT)

- Chest radiograph: both lungs are clear

- Tumour markers, Ca19.9: 960 U/mL (very raised)

- Abdominal CT: a large mass occupying the head of the pancreas. Dilated common bile duct and intrahepatic ducts, indicating extrahepatic biliary obstruction. No liver metastases and normal spleen.

- ERCP: evidence of cancer of the head of the pancreas. Common bile duct and intrahepatic ducts are dilated. No evidence of cancer of the ampulla of Vater or bile duct (cholangiocarcinoma).

Cancer of the head of the pancreas is the fourth leading cause of cancer in adults. Contributing factors include age, gender (more in males), exposure to carcinogens, cigarette smoking, chronic pancreatitis, a high-fat diet and occupational exposure to chemicals such as benzidine and β-naphthylamine. Neither alcohol nor coffee consumption is a risk factor.

● CASE 1.3 – I have recurrent abdominal pain and loose bowel motions.

> **Q4: In the light of the clinical presentation, how would you interpret the laboratory test results?**

A4

Table 1.10 Interpretation of lab test results for Case 1.3

Test	Changes	Interpretation
72-h faecal fat	Raised	Fats require bile salts and pancreatic lipase for digestion and absorption. Excessive loss of fat in her stools (steatorrhoea) is most probably caused by pancreatic damage (e.g. chronic pancreatitis) and a lack of pancreatic lipase
Plain radiograph of the abdomen	Evidence of calcification in the upper abdomen	20–50 per cent of patients with alcoholic pancreatitis will show pancreatic calcification on plain radiograph of the abdomen. Calcifications not detected on plain films may be detected by CT of the upper abdomen. The mechanisms responsible for pancreatic calcification in alcohol-associated chronic pancreatitis are:
CT of the abdomen	Small pancreas, calcification	

		– increased secretion of ionized calcium by pancreatic ductules – decreased solubility of secretory protein (GP2) – decreased secretion of lithostatin – formation of calcium–protein complex → intraductal protein precipitates → obstruction of ductules → progressive damage of pancreas → necrosis + fibrosis and calcium deposition
Serum amylase	Normal	Acute pancreatitis is usually diagnosed on the basis of compatible clinical findings and a serum amylase > 500 IU/l. Serum amylase is elevated in approximately 75 per cent of patients with acute pancreatitis. The level of serum amylase usually reaches a peak within 24 h of the onset of the illness and remains high for 1–3 days. Usually serum amylase returns to normal range within 3–5 days unless complications occur (e.g. pancreatic cyst) The results do not match with acute pancreatitis. The presence of low levels of circulating pancreatic amylase or trypsin-like immunoreactivity in the presence of upper abdominal pain and steatorrhoea are suggestive of the diagnosis of chronic pancreatitis. However, serum amylase is of no use in the diagnosis of chronic pancreatitis
Serum GGT	Raised	This is most probably related to her alcohol drinking (enzyme induction of GGT by alcohol)
Total serum calcium	Normal	In some cases serum calcium may be raised. Normal levels of serum calcium do not exclude the diagnosis of chronic pancreatitis
Fasting blood glucose	Raised	Damage of the islet of Langerhans is a late complication of chronic pancreatitis; 80–90 per cent of the gland must be severely damaged before the appearance of clinical diabetes

Q5: What is your final hypothesis?

A5

The clinical presentation and investigations are supportive of the diagnosis of chronic pancreatitis, most probably caused by chronic alcohol intake.

> **Q6:** What issues in the given history, examination and laboratory tests support your final hypothesis?

A6

Supportive evidence

History

- Chronic alcohol intake
- Recurrent abdominal pain for a few years
- Steatorrhoea (stools are loose, pale, bulky and offensive).

Examination

- Tenderness of her upper abdomen
- Liver and spleen are not palpable
- Vital signs normal
- Urinalysis: glucose +.

Investigations

- Increased 72-hour faecal fat
- Plain radiograph/CT of abdomen: calcification and a small stone in the pancreatic duct
- Serum amylase normal in the presence of abdominal pain and steatorrhoea
- Raised blood glucose levels.

ii Integrated medical sciences questions

● CASE 1.1 – Discuss the role of bile salt metabolism in the formation and treatment of gallstones (cholelithiasis).

Biliary cholesterol is solubilized by bile salts and lecithin present in the bile. Any excess in cholesterol concentration in bile, together with decreased bile salts and lecithin concentrations → bile becomes supersaturated with cholesterol → increased tendency for cholesterol gallbladder stones.

Changes in the hepatic activities of two key enzymes, hydroxymethylglutaryl coenzme A (HMG-CoA) reductase and 7α-hydroxylase, could result in increased cholesterol synthesis and inhibition of hepatic bile salt synthesis, respectively. These changes disturb the balance between cholesterol and bile salts in bile and result in lithogenic bile and gallstone formation.

Any disorder of the terminal ileum (e.g. Crohn's disease) or resection of the terminal ileum → impaired absorption of bile acids → interruption of the enterohepatic circulation of bile salts → depletion of bile acid pool → increased tendency for gallbladder stones.

Pharmacological agents that increase the secretion of cholesterol into bile and interfere with hepatic uptake of bile salts (e.g. ciclosporin, ethinylestradiol, oestrogen and oral contraceptives) → interruption of the enterohepatic circulation of bile salts → formation of gallstones.

Pharmacological agents that interfere with the intestinal absorption of bile acids (e.g. cholestyramine) → disturbance of the balance of cholesterol:bile salt in bile → increased gallstones.

Oral treatment with bile salts (e.g. ursodeoxycholic acid and chenodeoxycholic acid) has been effectively used in solubilization of gallstones and their treatment. The mechanism underlying this treatment is: ursodeoxycholic acid will enrich the bile acid pool and inhibit the hepatic enzyme HMG-CoA reductase activity → decreased cholesterol levels and increased bile acid to cholesterol ratio in bile → solubilization of gallbladder stones.

● CASE 1.2 – Discuss the mechanisms underlying Michael's jaundice.

Mechanism

The presence of risk factors such as ageing, male gender, smoking, and possibly exposure to chemicals at the chemical factory such as benzidine and β-naphthylamine (neither alcohol nor coffee consumption is a risk factor) → gradual changes in the duct epithelial cells (over-expression of *Her-2/neu* and point mutations in the *k-ras* gene, inactivation of *p16* gene, inactivation of *p53*, *DPC4* and *BRCA2* gene (late)) → progressive invasion of intraductal epithelial cells of the pancreas, mainly in the region of the head of pancreas → ductal adenocarcinoma mass → invasion of the common bile duct and ampulla of Vater → obstruction of bile flow into the duodenum → regurgitation of bile and conjugated bilirubin to the hepatic canaliculi, liver cells (hepatocytes), intercellular spaces → passage of conjugated bilirubin into the hepatic sinusoids → conjugated bilirubin appears in systemic blood (it is water soluble) → appears in urine (dark urine) + precipitation of conjugated bilirubin in the sclerae of the eye (jaundice).

● CASE 1.3 – Discuss the pathophysiological and pathological changes responsible for Lisa's abdominal pain and loose bowel motions.

Pathogenesis

Chronic alcoholism → increase in basal secretion of pancreatic proteins + inhibition of trypsin inhibitors → precipitation of protein plugs → blockage of small ductules of pancreas → activation of pancreatic enzymes before their release from the pancreas → inflammation of the pancreas (recurrent episodes of acute pancreatitis) → calcium mixes with precipitated protein plugs → more structural damage + more blockage of pancreatic ductules + gradual deterioration of pancreatic function + local infiltration of inflammatory cells → acinar atrophy + progressive fibrosis of exocrine pancreas + irritation of nerve endings in the pancreas → sensory pain impulses perceived by the brain.

Gradual impairment of the exocrine function of the pancreas → failure of pancreas to secrete pancreatic lipase → interference with fat digestion and absorption → loss of fat in stool (steatorrhoea) → stools are loose, pale, bulky and with an offensive odour.

Main pathological changes in chronic pancreatitis

● Extensive atrophy of the exocrine glands of the pancreas

● Extensive fibrosis of the pancreas is usually present

● Infiltration of inflammatory cells around pancreatic lobules and ducts

● Obstruction of pancreatic ductules by protein plugs

● Calcification of the pancreatic tissues

● Pseudocysts may be present.

Further reading

American College of Obstetricians and Gynecologists Women's Health Care Physicians. Cholecystitis, biliary tract surgery and pancreatitis. *Obstetrics and Gynecology* 2004;**104**(suppl 4):17S–24S.

Cohen SA, Siegel JH. Endoscopic retrograde cholangiopancreatography and the pancreas: when and why? *Surgical Clinics of North America* 2001;**81**:321–328.

DiMagno EP, Rober HA, Tempero MA. AGA technical review on the epidemiology, diagnosis and treatment of pancreatic ductal adenocarcinoma. *Gastroenterology* 1999;**117**:1464–1484.

Fletcher ND, Wise PE, Sharp KW. Common bile duct papillary adenoma causing obstructive jaundice: case report and review of the literature. *American Surgeon* 2004;**70**:448–452.

Ginsberg GG. New developments in pancreatic cancer. *Seminars in Gastrointestinal Disease* 2000;**11**:162–167.

Hruban RH, Goggins M, Parsons J, Kern SE. Progression model for pancreatic cancer. *Clinical Cancer Research* 2000;**6**:2969–2972.

Palazzo L, O'Toole D. Biliary stones: including acute biliary pancreatitis. *Gastrointestinal Endoscopy Clinics of North America* 2005;**15**:62–82.

Paumgartner G, Sauerbruch T. Gallstones: Pathogenesis. *Lancet* 1991;**338**:1117.

Raraty MG, Counor S, Criddle DN, Sutton R, Neoptolemos JP. Acute pancreatitis and organ failure: pathophysiology, natural history, and management strategies. *Current Gastroenterology Reports* 2004;**6**:99–103.

Rescorla FJ. Cholelithiasis, cholecystitis, and common bile duct stones. *Current Opinion in Pediatrics* 1997;**9**:276–282.

Rocha Lima CM, Centeno B. Update on pancreatic cancer. *Current Opinion in Oncology* 2002;**14**:424–430.

Shah K, Wolfe RE. Hepatobiliary ultrasound. *Emergency Medicine Clinics of North America* 2004;**22**:661–673.

Taylor B. Carcinoma of the head of the pancreas versus chronic pancreatitis: diagnostic dilemma with significant consequences. *World Journal of Surgery* 2003;**27**:1249–1257.

Trauner M, Meier PJ, Boyer JL. Molecular pathogenesis of cholestasis. *Mechanisms of Disease* 1998;**339**:1217.

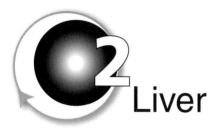

Liver

Questions

Clinical cases

Key concepts

Answers

Q1: What are the possible causes for the presenting problem?
Q2: What further questions would you like to ask to help you differentiate between your hypotheses?
Q3: What investigations would be most helpful to you and why?
Q4: In the light of the clinical presentation, how would you interpret the laboratory test results?
Q5: What is your final hypothesis?
Q6: What issues in the given history, examination and laboratory tests support your final hypothesis?

Clinical cases

● CASE 2.1 – I felt very frustrated and kept taking paracetamol.

Vivien Ray, a 22-year-old secretary, is brought by ambulance to the accident and emergency (A&E) department of a local hospital because of anorexia, right upper quadrant abdominal pain, nausea and recurrent vomiting. She has no history of loose bowel motions, fever or rigor. Vivien has no significant past medical history and has always been in good health. She had a sexual partner but they are no longer together. Yesterday, she accidentally discovered that he has married her best friend. She was very upset by the news and felt very frustrated and down. She admits that she has increased her alcohol drinking over the last few months. As a result of her frustration, she kept taking paracetamol tablets; about 20 hours ago she swallowed a total of 18 tablets. Her last menstrual period is over 2 months late and she is afraid she might be pregnant. On examination, Vivien looks pale and jaundiced. Her vital signs are shown in Table 2.1.

Table 2.1 Vital signs for Case 2.1

Vital signs	Vivien's results	Normal range
Blood pressure (mmHg)	90/70	100/60–135/85
Pulse rate (/min)	95	60–100
Respiratory rate (/min)	18	12–16
Temperature (°C)	37.1	36.6–37.2

- There are no spider naevi or palmar erythema.

- Abdominal examination: her liver is not palpable; the liver span is 11 cm. Her spleen is not palpable. No shifting dullness on percussion of her abdomen.

- Neurological examination: she is a little bit drowsy. No evidence of a focal lesion.

● CASE 2.2 – I have vomited blood.

Miriam Lue, a 48-year-old businesswoman, is brought by ambulance to the A&E department of a local hospital after vomiting blood twice (about 800 mL). She also complains of enlargement of her abdomen, which has come on rapidly over the last fortnight. In response to further questions from the A&E registrar, Dr Raj Kumar, she says, 'Over the last few months, I have always felt tired and have lost my appetite.' Her hospital file shows that she received counselling for her alcohol problem 12 months ago. No records since then. On examination, she is jaundiced and looks unwell. Numerous spider naevi are noted on her face, arms and shoulders. Her vital signs are shown in Table 2.2.

Table 2.2 Vital signs for Case 2.2

Vital signs	Miriam's results	Normal range
Blood pressure (mmHg)	90/60	100/60–135/85
Pulse rate (/min)	130	60–100
Respiratory rate (/min)	22	12–16
Temperature (°C)	36.9	36.6–37.2

- She has bilateral ankle oedema.
- It is difficult to palpate the liver.
- The spleen is felt 2 cm below the left costal margin.
- Percussion of the abdomen reveals shifting dullness.

⬤ CASE 2.3 – My urine is as dark as tea.

You are working with Dr Sam MacLeod in his clinic. Graham Doniash, a 35-year-old nurse, comes in because of generalized fatigue. For the last 2 days, he has noticed that his urine has become as dark as tea. Yesterday, his girlfriend noticed that his eyes were yellowish. He also has mild discomfort in the right upper quadrant of his abdomen. Further questions reveal that, about 6 weeks ago, he was working with an international aid organization in Eritrea as a volunteer nurse. He is not on any medications apart from the anti-malarial drugs that he received for his travel overseas. He used to drink an Eritrean herbal drink three times daily. He denies intravenous drug use. He had sexual intercourse with two girls while over there. On examination, both his sclerae are yellowish in colour. He has no spider naevi or palmar erythema. His vital signs are shown in Table 2.3.

Table 2.3 Vital signs for Case 2.3

Vital signs	Graham's results	Normal range
Blood pressure (mmHg)	110/80	100/60–135/85
Pulse rate (/min)	95	60–100
Respiratory rate (/min)	19	12–16
Temperature (°C)	38	36.6–37.2

Abdominal examination

- The liver is tender and the liver span measures 18 cm.
- The spleen is not palpable.

Integrated medical sciences questions

CASE 2.1 – Discuss the different mechanisms by which paracetamol overdose may cause hepatic injury/dysfunction.

CASE 2.2 – The level of several hormones may have changed in Miriam's blood because of her condition. List two hormones that you believe may have undergone a change in level in Miriam's blood. State the changes that have occurred (raised or decreased), the possible physiological or pathological mechanisms by which the changes occur, and the outcomes of these changes.

CASE 2.3 – Explain how ethanol intake could affect the normal metabolism of fatty acids in the liver cells (hepatocytes). What are the consequences of these biochemical/physiological changes?

🔑 Key concepts

In order to work through the core clinical cases in this chapter, you will need to understand the following key concepts.

The main functions of the liver

- Production of glucose (gluconeogenesis and glycogenolysis)

- Glucose consumption (glycogen synthesis, glycolysis, fatty acid synthesis)

- Cholesterol and triglyceride (TG) synthesis

- Secretion of cholesterol and TG in the very-low-density lipoprotein (VLDL) particles

- Synthesis and secretion of pre-high-density lipoprotein (pre-HDL) particles

- Bile salt (cholic acid and chenodeoxycholic acid) synthesis and conjugation

- Uptake, conjugation and secretion of bilirubin

- Detoxification of ammonia to urea (urea cycle)

- Detoxification of drugs (through phase I and II biotransformation)

- Excretion of drug metabolites in bile

- Synthesis of binding proteins (e.g. ceruloplasmin, albumin, transferrin, metallothionein)

- Uptake and storage of vitamins (vitamins A, D and B_{12} and folate)

- Synthesis of plasma proteins (e.g. albumin, clotting factors, apolipoproteins, angiotensinogen, insulin-like growth factor I)

- Synthesis of glutathione

- Kupffer cells and natural killer (NK) cells which help in clearance of bacteria and foreign antigens in the portal circulation.

The main cells of the liver and the functions of each cell

Table 2.4 summarizes the different types of liver cells and their functions.

Table 2.4 Functions of different liver cells

Liver cells	Functions
Liver cells (hepatocytes)	Hepatocytes are highly specialized and metabolically active. They are arranged into cords and characterized by the presence of two domains: the sinusoidal and canalicular domains. They perform most of the functions of the liver
Stellate cells (Ito cells)	Present between hepatocytes Store small amounts of fat and vitamin A Play a role in the development of liver diseases Other functions have not yet been explored
Kupffer cells (liver macrophages)	Present in the sinusoidal spaces. They can engulf bacteria and secrete cytokines that can modulate other elements of the immune system
Natural killer (NK) cells	These cells are located in the liver sinusoids and are exposed to the portal blood. They are in close contact with endothelial cells (forming the walls of the liver sinusoids) and Kupffer cells. NK cells are anchored in the endothelial lining, allowing perfusion of the liver without losing them
Endothelial cells	Make up the walls of the sinusoids. Secrete powerful vasoactive peptides, such as endothelins

The metabolism of bilirubin

● Seventy to ninety per cent of bilirubin is derived from haemoglobin of red blood cells.

● About 10 per cent of bilirubin is derived from myoglobin, P-450 cytochromes and liver peroxidase.

● Normally, the half-life of red blood cells is approximately 120 days. Old red blood cells are destroyed by mononuclear phagocytic cells of the liver, spleen and bone marrow.

● Opening of the haem molecule at its α-bridge carbon by microsomal enzymes results in tetrapyrrole biliverdin (a green pigment) and carbon monoxide.

● Through the action of biliverdin reductase, biliverdin is reduced to bilirubin.

● Bilirubin is kept as a soluble compound in blood by tight binding to albumin.

● The hepatic translocation of bilirubin involves **four** processes:

(1) uptake of bilirubin at the sinusoidal domain of liver cells mainly by facilitated transport and to a less extent by diffusion; bilirubin leaves albumin before being taken up by liver cells

(2) intracellular binding of bilirubin to a cytosolic protein (member of the glutathione-S-transferase family)

(3) conjugation of bilirubin by conversion to mono- and diglucuronides; conjugation occurs in the smooth endoplasmic reticulum

(4) secretion of bilirubin mono- and diglucuronides into the bile via a canalicular ATP-dependent transporter; the two transporters responsible for this process are: the multidrug resistance-associated protein 2 (MRP2) and the canalicular multispecific organic anion transporter (cMOAT).

- Conjugation of bilirubin to bilirubin mono- and diglucuronides has the following physiological effects:
  - increased solubility of bilirubin
  - enhancement of the elimination of bilirubin from the body
  - reduction in the ability of bilirubin to diffuse across the blood–brain barrier.

The main mechanisms responsible for the development of hyperbilirubinaemia

Unconjugated hyperbilirubinaemia

- Increased production of bilirubin (haemolysis, blood transfusion)

- Decreased sinusoidal uptake

- Decreased intrahepatic conjugation (physiological jaundice, breast milk jaundice, Gilbert's syndrome, Crigler–Najjar syndromes).

Conjugated hyperbilirubinaemia (and mixed)

- Acute hepatocellular injury (hepatitis A, B and C, ethanol, acute fatty liver of pregnancy, drugs)

- Chronic hepatocellular injury (hepatitis B and C, ethanol, haemochromatosis)

- Familial cholestatic disorders

- Inflammation of intrahepatic bile ductules

- Defective canalicular transport (Dubin–Johnson syndrome)

- Obstruction of bile duct (gallstones, inflammation, metastatic lymph nodes, pancreatic carcinoma).

Cirrhosis

Cirrhosis is among the top causes of death in Australia, the USA and western countries. The main causes of cirrhosis in the western environment are alcoholic liver disease (about 70 per cent), viral hepatitis (10 per cent), biliary disease (8 per cent), haemochromatosis (5 per cent), cryptogenic cirrhosis and other causes (10 per cent).

Main histological changes in cirrhosis

- Disturbance of the liver architecture and loss of liver cells

- The presence of regenerative nodules surrounded by dense connective tissues

- Liver cells may show fatty changes (caused by increased deposition of fatty acids and triglycerides in hepatocytes and failure of their excretion); intracytoplasmic fat appears as empty vacuoles in the cytoplasm of hepatocytes

- Mallory's hyaline body in the cytoplasm of injured hepatocytes: acetaldehyde produced as a result of ethanol metabolism is responsible for liver injury and possibly the formation of Mallory's hyaline body

- Increased collagen synthesis by fibroblasts and the peri-sinusoidal cells of Ito

- Inflammatory infiltrate: increased neutrophils and polymorphs.

The role of alcohol in the development of fatty liver

Ethanol plays a significant role in the development of fatty liver. The mechanisms by which ethanol may cause this change are summarized as follows:

- Ethanol alters the rate of hepatic synthesis and removal of fatty acids from liver cells.

- Ethanol inhibits the oxidation of fatty acids in hepatocytes to CO_2.

- Ethanol enhances the esterification of fatty acids.

- Ethanol alters the capacity of liver mitochondria to oxidize acetyl-CoA.

- Ethanol increases the ratio $NADH^+:NAD^+$, which, when elevated, inhibits several enzymes of the tricarboxylic acid cycle.

- Ethanol causes inhibition of VLDL synthesis.

- Ethanol interferes with VLDL secretion (VLDLs are responsible for the removal of TGs and cholesterol from the liver).

The mechanisms underlying the development of portal hypertension

The portal vein is formed by the union of the superior mesenteric and splenic veins. The normal pressure in the portal vein is 5–8 mmHg. The following are the mechanisms underlying portal hypertension:

- Prehepatic: blockage of the portal vein before it enters the liver (e.g. portal vein thrombosis)

- Intrahepatic: intrahepatic disturbance of the normal architecture of the liver (e.g. cirrhosis)

- Posthepatic: hepatic venous blockage outside the liver (e.g. the Budd–Chiari syndrome).

Chronic liver damage → activation of stellate cells → transformation into myofibroblasts → contraction of these myofibroblasts (stimulated by mediators such as nitric oxide, prostaglandins and endothelin) → interference with the intrahepatic blood flow patterns + increased resistance to intrahepatic blood flow. Also the activation of stellate cells → activation of fibrinogenesis and progressive fibrosis and formation of small hepatic nodules → portal hypertension (resistance to blood flow) → stimulation of portosystemic anastomosis (portosystemic shunt) to overcome the portal hypertension and the resistance to intrahepatic blood flow.

The consequences of portal hypertension and cirrhosis

- Oesophageal varices

- Oesophageal haemorrhage

- Ascites

- Portosystemic encephalopathy

- Renal failure

- Bacteraemia/infection of ascitic fluid

- Malnutrition

- Hepatocellular carcinoma.

Answers

 CASE 2.1 – I felt very frustrated and kept taking paracetamol.

 Q1: What are the possible causes for the presenting problem?

A1

- Acute liver failure (widespread hepatocellular necrosis)
- Acute paracetamol toxicity
- Acute fatty liver of pregnancy
- Alcoholic hepatitis
- Acute viral hepatitis (less likely)

 Q2: What further questions would you like to ask to help you differentiate between your hypotheses?

A2

Table 2.5 Further history questions for Case 2.1

History questions	In what way answers can help
Approximate number of paracetamol tablets she swallowed	The severity of paracetamol poisoning is dose related
Any pre-existing liver disease or nutritional problems (anorexia nervosa)	The damage caused by paracetamol will be enhanced if there is a prior liver condition or anorexia nervosa
Whether she had swallowed any other medications (names of these medications and number of tablets, and when she swallowed them)	Enzyme-inducing drugs and alcohol increase the damage caused by paracetamol
More details about her periods: regularity, use of any contraception and symptoms suggesting early pregnancy (e.g. breast changes; she has already complained of nausea and vomiting)	To assess whether she is pregnant and whether acute fatty liver of pregnancy is a possible cause
Other risk factors for viral hepatitis (e.g. intravenous drug use, unprotected sex with multiple partners, tattooing, travel overseas)	To assess other possible causes for her presentation

Q3: What investigations would be most helpful to you and why?

A3

- Liver function tests.
- Plasma paracetamol concentration
- Prothrombin time
- Blood glucose level
- Blood urea, creatinine, sodium and potassium
- Pregnancy test.

⬤ CASE 2.2 – I've vomited blood.

 Q1: What are the possible causes for the presenting problem?

A1

- Bleeding oesophageal varices.
- Bleeding from oesophageal tear
- Bleeding gastric ulcer (e.g. aspirin-associated bleeding ulcers)
- Bleeding duodenal ulcer.

 Q2: What further questions would you like to ask to help you differentiate between your hypotheses?

A2

Table 2.6 Further history questions for Case 2.2

History questions	In what way answers can help
Amount of blood vomited and any precipitant	This might be useful in the assessment of the haemodynamic changes of the patient
Past history of vomiting blood or bleeding from anywhere (date, amount, hospital management and whether endoscopic examination was undertaken)	Re-bleeding from oesophageal varices after initial bleed may occur within 2–3 months in 30 per cent of patients. Factors that may increase the risk of bleeding from oesophageal varices are: age > 60 years old; coagulopathy; presence of associated medical conditions, e.g. chronic renal failure, chronic chest problem, recent myocardial infarction); and history of re-bleeding after initial bleed

| Recent ingestion of aspirin, or NSAIDs, warfarin, corticosteroids | The presence of jaundice, signs of chronic liver disease (e.g. spider naevi on her face, arms and shoulders) and signs suggestive of portal hypertension (splenomegaly, ascites and ankle oedema), raise the possibility of bleeding from oesophageal varices (dilated submucosal veins). We might, however, be dealing with a different pathological cause on this occasion. It might be useful to ask about intake of drugs such as aspirin and NSAIDs which may cause bleeding from gastric ulcers |
| Past investigations for her liver problem (liver function tests, screening for hepatitis, INR, ultrasound and laboratory examination of ascitic fluid) | These results may provide you with a baseline information about the status of her liver, complications, current treatment and the cause of her liver problem (cirrhosis) |

INR, international normalized ratio; NSAIDs, non-steroidal anti-inflammatory drugs.

 Q3: What investigations would be most helpful to you and why?

A3

- Blood group and cross-matching
- Full blood examination
- Liver function tests
- Blood urea, creatinine and electrolytes
- Upper gastrointestinal endoscopy
- Prothromin time or international normalized ratio (INR).

When Miriam's condition improves and the acute bleeding problem has been solved, we may ask for:

- Screen for hepatitis
- Ultrasound examination of upper abdomen
- α-Fetoprotein
- Liver biopsy (be sure that there is no active bleeding and the INR is normal before undertaking this procedure).

 CASE 2.3 – **My urine is as dark as tea.**

 Q1: What are the possible causes (hypotheses) for the presenting problem?

A1

- Viral hepatitis (exposure to several risk factors: contact with patients, accidental pin prick, travel overseas and unprotected sex)

- Herbally induced hepatitis.

- Drug-induced hepatocellular damage

- Obstruction of bile duct (tumour, metastatic lymph node, gallstones, cholangiocarcinoma)

- Haemolysis (antimalarial-induced glucose-6-phosphate [G-6-PD] deficiency) – less likely.

 Q2: What further questions would you like to ask to help you differentiate between your hypotheses?

A2

Table 2.7 Further history questions for Case 2.3

History questions	In what way answers can help
Any history of contact with hepatitis patients while overseas? Any history of accidental pin prick or blood transfusion overseas?	Hepatitis can be caused by hepatitis viruses A, B, C, D or E. In children, infection with hepatitis A virus may be asymptomatic in 70–80 per cent of patients. In adults, infection is more likely to produce symptoms, although only 30–40 per cent of patients are jaundiced. Infection with hepatitis B and C viruses is also usually asymptomatic except in intravenous drug users where > 90 per cent of patients are jaundiced
Any history of fever, anorexia, skin rash, joint pains (arthralgia), urinary changes?	Approximately 5–10 per cent of patients with acute hepatitis A or B infection have non-specific symptoms such as arthralgia (pain affecting the wrist, elbows, knees or ankles as a result of formation of immune complexes), and a maculopapular rash. General symptoms such as fever, muscle aches, nausea, vomiting, change in the sense of smell, headache, loose bowel motions and tiredness are usually present
	Patients with acute hepatitis A infection may present with a profound cholestatic illness, dark urine, jaundice and itching
Any past history of hepatitis, hepatobiliary disorders or blood disorders?	Hepatitis D infection may occur in a carrier of hepatitis B virus
Medications, allergy and details about the herbal drink he used to drink while overseas	Herbal drinks, medication and chemicals may cause acute hepatitis

Q3: What investigations would be most helpful to you and why?

A3

- Full blood examination

- Liver function tests

- Screen for hepatitis
- Ultrasound of upper abdomen
- Blood assay for toxic metabolites
- Prothrombin time or INR
- Urinalysis for bilirubin.

Further progress

● CASE 2.1 – I felt very frustrated and kept taking paracetamol.

The results of the patient's blood tests are shown in Table 2.8.

Table 2.8 Blood test results for Case 2.1

Laboratory test	Vivien's results	Normal range
Haemoglobin (Hb) (g/L)	120	115–160
Packed cell volume (PCV)	0.46	0.37–0.46
White cell count (WCC) ($\times 10^9$/L)	10	4.0–11.0
Platelet count ($\times 10^9$/L)	210	150–400
Serum bilirubin (μmol/L)	35	0–19
Serum aspartate aminotransferase (AST) (IU/L)	2070	0–40
Serum alanine aminotransferase (ALT) (IU/L)	3600	0–55
Serum alkaline phosphatase (ALP) (IU/L)	110	0–120
Serum γ-glutamyltransferase (GGT) (IU/L)	58	0–50
Prothrombin time (s)	29	18–22
Serum albumin (g/L)	41	35–50
Blood urea (mmol/L)	15	2.5–8.3
Serum creatinine (mmol/L)	1.4	0.05–0.11
Serum sodium (mmol/L)	132	135–145
Serum potassium (mmol/L)	3.2	3.5–5.0
Fasting blood glucose (mmol/L)	2.5	3.6–5.3

- Screening for hepatitis: negative
- Paracetamol blood level: 55 μg/mL at 20 h
- Pregnancy test: negative.

● CASE 2.2 – I've vomited blood.

Dr Kumar arranges for some blood tests for Miriam. The results of her blood tests are shown in Table 2.9.

Table 2.9 Blood test results for Case 2.2

Blood test	Miriam's results	Normal range
Hb (g/L)	75	115–160
PCV	49	0.37–0.46
WCC ($\times 10^9$/L)	3	4.0 – 11.0
Platelet count ($\times 10^9$/L)	100	150–400
Serum bilirubin (total) (μmol/L)	95	0–19
Serum ALP (IU/L)	165	0–120
Serum AST (IU/L)	155	0–40
Serum ALT (IU/L)	65	0–55
Serum GGT (IU/L)	460	0–50
Serum albumin (g/L)	27	35–50
Prothrombin time (s)	26	18–22
Blood urea (mmol/L)	1.7	2.5–8.3
Serum creatinine (mmol/L)	0.06	0.05–0.11
Serum sodium (mmol/L)	133	135–145
Serum potassium (mmol/L)	3.5	3.5–5.0

Upper gastrointestinal tract endoscopy: evidence of fresh bleeding from oesophageal varices. No evidence of oesophageal tear or peptic ulcer.

Ultrasound examination of the upper abdomen: the liver is shrunken and its surface irregular and nodular. There is no focal lesion/mass found in the liver. The biliary tree is normal. The pancreas is normal in size and texture. The spleen is enlarged and there is evidence of free fluid in the peritoneal cavity (ascites). Both kidneys are normal in shape and size.

α-Fetoprotein: normal range.

Liver biopsy report: there is evidence of distortion of the lobular architecture of the liver. The liver is studded with regeneration nodules surrounded with dense fibrous tissues. The liver cells are variable in size and some cells show evidence of fatty change (steatosis) where the cytoplasm displays fat globules and as a result the nucleus is pushed to one side. There are also Mallory's hyaline bodies (accumulation of filaments and cytoskeleton of damaged cells) in the cytoplasm of some liver cells. A few neutrophils infiltrating the injured liver cells are seen.

● CASE 2.3 – My urine is as dark as tea.

Dr MacLeod arranges for some blood and urine tests for Graham. The results are shown in Table 2.10.

Table 2.10 Test results for Case 2.3

Test	Graham's results	Normal range
Hb (g/L)	125	115–160
WCC ($\times 10^9$/L)	3000	4.0–11.0
Serum bilirubin (total) (μmol/L)	100	0–19
Serum ALP (IU/L)	180	0–120
Serum AST (IU/L)	4707	0–40
Serum ALT (IU/L)	4855	0–55
Serum albumin (g/L)	37	35–50
Prothrombin time (s)	26	18–22

Screening for hepatitis

- Hepatitis C virus (HCV) antibody: negative
- HCV RNA polymerase chain reaction (PCR): negative
- Hepatitis B surface antigen (HBsA): negative
- Hepatitis B core antibody (HBcA): negative
- Serum IgM anti-HBV: negative
- Serum IgM anti-hepatitis A virus (anti-HAV): ++++
- Serum IgG anti-HAV: +.

Further questions

● CASE 2.1 – I felt very frustrated and kept taking paracetamol.

Q4: In the light of the clinical presentation, how would you interpret the laboratory test results?

A4

Table 2.11 Interpretation of lab test results for Case 2.1

Test	Results	Interpretation
Serum bilirubin	Raised	The rise in transaminases is disproportionate to the rise of total serum bilirubin. This is typical in acute paracetamol overdose. This might help to differentiate paracetamol (acetaminophen)-induced hepatotoxicity from viral hepatitis, biliary obstruction or cholestatic disease
Serum AST and serum ALT	Raised	Raised serum AST and ALT activities reflect massive damage of hepatocytes (e.g. acute widespread hepatocellular necrosis). The mechanisms of hepatocyte death are poorly understood. Necrosis is recognized as the mode of cell death and apoptosis has been ruled out The possible causes of liver cell damage in paracetamol overdose are: ● Production of large amounts of a toxic metabolite known as *N*-acetyl-*p*-benzoquinonimine → depletion of intracellular glutathione required for detoxification of this metabolite ● Formation of intracellular protein adducts ● Protein adducts target mitochondrial proteins → mitochondrial damage, loss of energy production and impairment of cellular functions ● Alteration of plasma membrane ATPase activity ● Loss of mitochondrial or nuclear ion balance and increased cytosolic Ca^{2+} concentrations, mitochondrial Ca^{2+} cycling activation of proteases and endonucleases and DNA strand breaks ● Activation of Kupffer cells → release of hydrolytic enzymes, eicosanoid, nitric oxide, superoxide and inflammatory cytokines → hepatic cellular damage
Serum ALP	Normal	Serum ALP is raised in conditions associated with cholestasis and biliary obstruction. None of these changes occurs in paracetamol overdose
Serum GGT	Raised	In alcohol-associated liver injury, the half-life of GGT is about 28 days (normal 7–10 days) → increased serum GGT activity Cholestasis and impairment of canalicular function also cause increased serum GGT activity, and it is induced by alcohol and some drugs (e.g. phenytoin)

Prothrombin time	Raised	Raised INR or prolonged prothrombin time is the result of: (1) lack of vitamin K or (2) the inability of the failing liver cells to use vitamin K to produce the coagulation factors II, VII, IX and X. The most likely cause of the patient's coagulopathy is the failure of the liver cells to use vitamin K, which is a fat-soluble vitamin produced by intestinal bacteria and essential for the γ-carboxylation of certain glutamate residues in coagulation factors II, VII, IX and X
		Coagulopathy is commonly seen in acute liver failure such as paracetamol overdose and may be associated with a tendency to bleed
Serum albumin	Normal	A normal serum albumin does not exclude acute massive liver damage. Serum albumin concentration may remain within normal range in acute liver disorders because of the prolonged half-life of albumin (about 3 weeks)
Serum sodium and potassium	Low	Hyponatraemia and hypokalaemia are commonly seen in acute liver failure
Blood glucose	Low	Hypoglycaemia usually occurs in acute liver failure
Blood urea and creatinine	Raised	Might occur as a result of paracetamol-induced acute tubular necrosis. Rarely occurs in the absence of fulminant hepatic failure
Screening for hepatitis	Negative	The possibility that her acute liver problem is caused by hepatitis is less likely. A number of viruses are able to cause acute/subacute liver failure including: hepatitis A, B, D and E virus; cytomegalovirus; Epstein–Barr virus; and herpes simplex virus
Paracetamol blood level	55 µg/mL at 20 h	Intake of about 7.5–10 g paracetamol (acetaminophen) is toxic in healthy adults. Approximately 4–6 g may be enough to induce acute liver failure in chronic alcohol users. After oral ingestion, paracetamol is rapidly absorbed and a serum peak level is achieved in < 1 h. Paracetamol is mainly metabolized in the liver via the cytochrome P-450 mixed function oxidase enzyme system. Ninety-five per cent of the metabolites produced are non-toxic conjugates of glucuronide and sulphate. Paracetamol toxicity is caused by a metabolite, which constitutes only 5 per cent of paracetamol metabolites. This metabolite is known as N-acetyl-p-benzoquinonimine and when it is produced in large amounts it binds to glutathione (GSH) to form a GSH conjugate. After a toxic dose of paracetamol, total hepatic GSH is depleted by as much as 90 per cent and, as a result, the metabolite covalently binds to cysteine groups on intracellular protein, forming paracetamol–protein adducts. It is believed that these protein adducts play a central role in centrilobular hepatic necrosis observed in paracetamol overdose
		At the usual therapeutic doses, this metabolite (N-acetyl-p-benzoquinonimine) is detoxified in the liver by conjugating with sulphhydryl group of glutathione and excreted in urine as mercapturic acid and cysteine conjugates

A plasma paracetamol concentration of 55 µg/ml at 20 h after ingestion indicates high probability of hepatic injury and the need to start treatment with *N*-acetylcysteine. The Rumack–Matthew nomogram helps in the assessment of patients with paracetamol overdose

Pregnancy test	Negative	This helps in exclusion of pregnancy and the possibility of acute fatty liver of pregnancy

 Q5: What is your final hypothesis?

A5

The clinical picture and laboratory results are supportive of the diagnosis of acute liver failure caused by paracetamol (acetaminophen) overdose.

 Q6: What issues in the given history, examination and laboratory tests support your final hypothesis?

A6

Supportive evidence

History

- She presents with anorexia, right upper quadrant abdominal pain, nausea and recurrent vomiting. She has no history of loose bowel motions, fever or rigor.

- No significant past medical history and has always been in good health.

- She had a sexual partner but they are no longer together.

- Yesterday, she accidentally discovered that he has married her best friend. She was very upset by the news and felt very frustrated and down.

- She has increased her alcohol drinking over the last few months.

- She swallowed about 18 tablets 20 h ago.

- Her last menstrual period is over 2 months late and she is afraid that she might be pregnant.

Examination

- She looks pale and jaundiced.

- Her blood pressure is 90/70 mmHg, her pulse 95/min and her respiratory rate 18/min.

- She is afebrile.

- There are no spider naevi or palmar erythema.

- Abdominal examination: her liver is not palpable; the liver span is 11 cm.

- Her spleen is not palpable.

- No shifting dullness on percussion of her abdomen.

- Neurological examination: she is a little bit drowsy.

- No evidence of a focal neurological lesion.

Investigations

- Serum bilirubin: raised

- Serum AST and ALT: raised ++++

- ALP: normal

- GGT: raised +

- Serum albumin: normal range

- Prothrombin time: prolonged

- Serum sodium and potassium: low

- Blood glucose level: low

- Blood urea and creatinine: raised

- Screening for hepatitis: negative

- Paracetamol blood concentration: 55 µg/mL at 20 h

- Pregnancy test: negative.

CASE 2.2 – I've vomited blood.

Q4: In the light of the clinical presentation, how would you interpret the laboratory test results?

A4

Table 2.12 Interpretation of lab test results for Case 2.2

Test	Changes	Interpretation
Hb	Low	Acute blood loss from oesophageal varices. Other factors that might have contributed to low Hb (anaemia) are: malnutrition; malabsorption; bone marrow suppression; hypersplenism (destruction of red blood cells in spleen); and blood loss from the gastrointestinal system
WCC	Low	Possibly as part of hypersplenism (a peripheral blood cytopenia caused by hyperactive spleen)

Platelet count	Low	Possibly as part of hypersplenism (a peripheral blood cytopenia resulting from a hyperactive spleen)
Serum bilirubin (total)	Raised	Mainly caused by cholestasis and interference with canalicular secretion of conjugated bilirubin
Serum ALP	Raised	Mainly caused by cholestasis and interference with canalicular functions
Serum AST	Raised	Alcohol increases mitochondrial AST activity in plasma (other causes of hepatitis do not); alcohol produces a decrease of only the cytosolic AST activity; and pyridoxine deficiency is common in people with alcohol problems and decreases hepatic ALT activity. These effects might explain why the AST:ALT ratio of this patient is 2:1
Serum ALT	Slightly raised	ALT is found mostly in the liver cells. Its level in the blood is not raised possibly because of loss of liver cells and their replacement with fibrous tissues. Pyridoxine deficiency is common in people with alcohol problems and decreases hepatic ALT activity
		With disease progression, ALT blood levels may gradually decrease to below the lower limit of normal range. This does not imply an improvement in liver function but rather more loss of liver cells and the inability of liver cells to produce ALT
Serum GGT	Raised	The half-life of GGT is about 28 days in alcohol-associated liver injury (normally 7–10 days)
		Cholestasis and impairment of canalicular function have also contributed
Serum albumin	Low	Low serum albumin (hypoalbuminaemia) as a result of decreased synthetic abilities of the liver, malnutrition and malabsorption
Prothrombin time	Prolonged	Prolonged prothrombin time (coagulopathy) as a result of lack of vitamin K
		Vitamin K is a fat-soluble vitamin produced by intestinal bacteria. This vitamin is essential for the γ-carboxylation of certain glutamate residues in coagulation factors II, VII, IX and X. Deficiency of vitamin K caused by intrahepatic cholestasis and fat malabsorption (lack of bile) results in prolonged prothrombin time
		The failure of the liver cells to use vitamin K to synthesize the coagulation factors has also contributed to this problem
Blood urea	Low	Despite the patient's blood loss (haematemesis) and decreased renal perfusion, her blood urea is below the lower limit of normal range, and the reason for this is related to the failure of her liver cells to synthesize urea (urea cycle).

		Normally, the liver cells are able to synthesize urea from ammonia, carbon dioxide and aspartate. With the development of liver failure, large amounts of ammonia appear in the blood as the liver cannot use them to synthesize urea
Upper gastrointestinal endoscopy	Evidence of fresh bleeding from oesophageal varices. No evidence of oesophageal tear or peptic ulcer	At the lower third of the oesophagus, the oesophageal tributaries of the left gastric vein (which drains into the portal vein) anastomose with the oesophageal tributaries of the azygos (systemic) veins. With the development of cirrhosis and portal hypertension, the portosystemic anastomoses veins at the lower end of the oesophagus become dilated and prominent. Rupture of these veins, as in this case, results in haematemesis
Ultrasound examination of the upper abdomen	The liver is shrunken; its surface is irregular and nodular. There is no focal lesion/mass found in the liver. The biliary tree is normal. The pancreas is normal in size and texture. The spleen is enlarged and there is evidence of free fluid in the peritoneal cavity (ascites). Both kidneys are normal in shape and size	Cirrhosis of the liver is characterized by fibrosis and regeneration of the hepatic parenchyma in a nodular formation. The nodular formation in cirrhosis has been classified into: micronodular (nodules < 3 mm in size are predominantly present) and macronodular (nodules > 3 mm)
α-Fetoprotein	Normal range	One of the complications of cirrhosis is the development of hepatocellular carcinoma. Both α-Fetoprotein and ultrasound are useful in follow-up of patients with cirrhosis and help in early detection of hepatocellular carcinoma
Liver biopsy	There is evidence of distortion of the lobular architecture of the liver. The liver is studded with regeneration nodules surrounded with dense fibrous tissues. The liver cells are variable in size and some cells show evidence of fatty change (steatosis) where the cytoplasm displays fat globules and the nucleus as a result is pushed to one side. There are also Mallory's hyaline bodies (accumulation of filaments and cytoskeleton of damaged cells) in the cytoplasm of some liver cells. A few neutrophils infiltrating the injured liver cells are seen	These histological findings are consistent with cirrhosis

Q5: What is your final hypothesis?

A5

The clinical picture and laboratory results are supportive of the diagnosis of bleeding from oesophageal varices. As a result of her liver cirrhosis and progressive resistance to blood flow in the liver, the pressure in the portal tract (flow rate × resistance – Ohm's law) is increased. When the portal pressure is > 10 mmHg the condition is called portal hypertension. The increased portal pressure has also resulted in (1) splenomegaly, (2) ascites formation and (3) oesophageal varices.

Q6: What issues in the given history, examination and laboratory tests support your final hypothesis?

A6

Supportive evidence

History

- The patient presents with vomiting blood twice (about 800 mL).

- She complains of enlargement of her abdomen, which has come on rapidly over the last fortnight. She has always felt tired and lost her appetite.

- Her hospital file shows that she received counselling for her alcohol problem 12 months ago. No records since then.

Examination

- The patient is jaundiced and looks unwell.

- Numerous spider naevi are noted on her face, arms and shoulders.

- Her blood pressure is 90/60 mmHg, pulse rate 130/min, respiratory rate 22/min.

- She is afebrile.

- She has bilateral ankle oedema.

- It is difficult to palpate the liver.

- The spleen is felt 2 cm below the left costal margin.

- Percussion of the abdomen reveals shifting dullness.

Investigations

- Hb, white blood cells (WBCs), platelets: low.

- Serum bilirubin: raised.

- Liver function tests: raised.

- Prothrombin time: prolonged.

- Serum albumin: low.

- Upper gastrointestinal endoscopy: evidence of fresh bleeding from oesophageal varices. No evidence of oesophageal tear or peptic ulcer.

- Ultrasound of upper abdomen: the liver is shrunken, its surface irregular and nodular. There is no focal lesion/mass found in the liver. The biliary tree is normal. The pancreas is normal in size and texture. The spleen is enlarged and there is evidence of free fluid in the peritoneal cavity (ascites). Both kidneys are normal in shape and size.

- α-Fetoprotein: normal range.

- Liver biopsy (performed a few days later, after the correction of coagulopathy and control of haematemesis): there is evidence of distortion of the lobular architecture of the liver. The liver is studded with regeneration nodules surrounded with dense fibrous tissues. The liver cells are variable in size and some cells show evidence of fatty change (steatosis), where the cytoplasm displays fat globules and the nucleus, as a result, is pushed to one side. There are also Mallory's hyaline bodies (accumulation of filaments and cytoskeleton of damaged cells) in the cytoplasm of some liver cells. A few neutrophils infiltrating the injured liver cells are seen.

CASE 2.3 – My urine is as dark as tea.

 Q4: In the light of the clinical presentation, how would you interpret the laboratory test results?

A4

Table 2.13 Interpretation of lab test results for Case 2.3

Test	Results	Interpretation
WBC	Low	Low WBCs may occur with acute viral infections
Serum bilirubin (total)	Raised	The raised serum bilirubin may be caused by: cholestasis; decreased hepatic uptake; and regurgitation to the sinusoidal domain of conjugated bilirubin. It is less likely to be caused by haemolysis
Serum ALP	Raised	The rise of ALP is usually mild and reflects the intrahepatic cholestasis produced by the viral infection
Serum AST and ALT	Both raised	In acute hepatitis A, the rise in serum ALT and AST activities can be substantially higher than that observed in acute hepatitis B or C. In general, the degree of aminotransferase elevation roughly correlates with the severity of the acute hepatitis A
		The overall severity of the infection is, however, demonstrated by the bilirubin blood level and the prothrombin time
Serum albumin	Normal	The ability of the liver cells to synthesize albumin may have been compromised and gradually the serum albumin value will drop. The long half-life of albumin (about 3 weeks) may have masked this pathological change

Prothrombin time	Prolonged	This test results together with serum bilirubin level reflect the severity of the disease
		Prolonged prothrombin time indicates the inability of the liver cells to synthesize vitamin K-dependent coagulation factors II, VII, IX and X
Screening for hepatitis	Serum IgM anti-HAV: ++++	The incubation period of hepatitis A ranges from 15 to 50 days (mean 30 days)
	Serum IgG anti-HAV: + Screening for hepatitis B and C is negative	The sensitivity of IgM anti-HAV measurement for acute hepatitis is 100 per cent, the specificity is 99 per cent and the positive predictive value is 88 per cent
		The length of time that the IgM anti-HAV test remains positive varies, but it is usually about 5–10 months after onset. In most patients, the biochemical evidence of hepatitis resolves either before or by the time of the disappearance of IgM anti-HAV
		The IgG response to HAV is delayed compared with IgM and is long-lived. It accounts for resistance to reinfection

 Q5: What is your final hypothesis?

A5

The clinical picture and laboratory results are supportive of the diagnosis of acute hepatitis A infection.

 Q6: What issues in the given history, examination and laboratory tests support your final hypothesis?

A6

Supportive evidence

History

- The patient comes in because of generalized fatigue all over his body. His urine is dark as tea.

- His eyes are yellowish.

- He has mild discomfort in the right upper quadrant of his abdomen.

- He recently worked for an international aid organization in Eritrea as a volunteer nurse.

- He is not on any medications apart from the anti-malarial drugs.

- He used to drink an Eritrean herbal drink three times daily.

- He denies intravenous drug use.

- He had sexual intercourse with two girls while over there.

Examination

- The patient's sclerae are yellowish in colour.

- He has no spider naevi or palmar erythema.

- His blood pressure is 110/80 mmHg.

- His pulse rate is 95/min and respiratory rate 19/min.

- His temperature is 38°C.

- The liver is tender, the liver span measures 18 cm and the spleen is not palpable.

Investigations

- Hb: normal

- WBCs: decreased

- Serum total bilirubin: raised

- Serum transaminases AST and ALT: raised ++++

- Serum ALP: mildly raised

- Serum albumin: normal

- Prothrombin time: prolonged

- Screening for hepatitis: serum IgM anti-HAV: ++++; serum IgG anti-HAV: +; screening for hepatitis B and C is negative.

👥 Integrated medical sciences questions

⬤ CASE 2.1 – Discuss the different mechanisms by which paracetamol overdose may cause hepatic injury/dysfunction.

- Hepatotoxicity may occur after the ingestion of a single dose of 10–15 g paracetamol (20–30 tablets).

- Doses of 20–25 g or more (over 40 tablets) are particularly fatal.

- Paracetamol is metabolized in the liver via the P-450 cytochromes, producing an intermediate compound, *N*-acetyl-*p*-benzoquinonimine, which is very electrophilic.

- *N*-Acetyl-*p*-benzoquinonimine is normally eliminated by conjugation with GSH → metabolization to a mercapturic acid → excretion into the urine.

- The large amounts of *N*-acetyl-*p*-benzoquinonimine formed in the body by paracetamol overdose → depletion of glutathione → loss of antioxidant defence → hepatocytes susceptible to oxidant injury + dysfunction of cellular organelles and massive damage of liver cells in the centrilobular region.

- Paracetamol hepatotoxicity spares the periportal region and results in high serum AST and ALT levels (because of massive liver cell damage in the centrilobular region).

⬤ CASE 2.2 – The level of several hormones may have changed in Miriam's blood because of her condition. List two hormones that you believe may have undergone a change in level in Miriam's blood. State the changes that have occurred (raised or decreased), the possible physiological or pathological mechanisms by which the changes occur and the outcomes of these changes.

Table 2.14 Changes in hormones in Case 2.2

Hormone	Change	Physiological/pathological causes	Outcomes
Aldosterone (an adrenal steroid secreted by the cells of the zona glomerulosa)	Increased serum levels	The secretion of aldosterone is controlled by angiotensin II (angiotensin II is an octapeptide formed in blood by proteolytic cleavage of a precursor produced by the liver known as angiotensinogen)	Replenishing blood volume and conservation of sodium
		The cleavage of angiotensinogen is catalysed by the enzyme renin, resulting in the release of angiotensin I	
		Angiotensin I is biologically inactive and is rapidly converted to angiotensin II by angiotensin-converting enzyme (ACE)	
		Angiotensin II has a very short half-life and may be further metabolized to angiotensin III and angiotensin IV	
		Renin is synthesized and secreted by the juxtaglomerular cells	
		The stimuli for the release of renin in her condition are:	
		– the juxtaglomerular cells are richly innervated by sympathetic nerve fibres → reflex activation by drop in blood pressure and hypovolaemia	
		– blood pressure is sensed as tension exerted on the smooth muscles of the afferent glomerular arterioles (part of the juxtaglomerular apparatus)	
		– drop of blood pressure is also sensed by decreased glomerular filtration rate	
Antidiuretic hormone (ADH)	Increased serum level	The stimuli for the release of ADH are: (1) decreased blood pressure, (2) increased angiotensin II in the blood	Thirst and water conservation
		It is of limited value because little urine reaches the collecting ducts	

● CASE 2.3 – **Explain how ethanol intake could affect the normal metabolism of fatty acids in the liver cells (hepatocytes). What are the consequences of these biochemical/physiological changes?**

Table 2.15 Biochemical/phsiological changes in Case 2.3

Normal biochemical/physiological process	Effects of ethanol	Outcomes
Synthesis of fatty acids by liver cells, oxidation of fatty acids and their secretion as VLDLs. Normally the amount of fatty acids in the liver depends on the balance of the processes of delivery, synthesis and removal	Ethanol alters the rate of synthesis and removal of fatty acids	Deposition of fatty acids in the liver
Utilization of metabolites via the tricarboxylic acid cycle in hepatocytes	Ethanol metabolism in the liver spares the utilization of other oxidizable fuels. It has a direct inhibitory effect on the tricarboxylic acid cycle in hepatocytes	Deposition of fatty acids in the liver
Oxidation of fatty acids in hepatocytes to CO_2	Ethanol inhibits the oxidation of fatty acids in hepatocytes to CO_2 Ethanol enhances the esterification of fatty acids Ethanol alters the capacity of liver mitochondria to oxidize acetyl-CoA Ethanol increases the ratio NADH:NAD, which when elevated inhibits several enzymes of the tricarboxylic acid cycle	Deposition of fatty acids in the liver
Incorporation of hepatic triglycerides into VLDLs followed by its secretion into the sinusoidal blood	Ethanol causes inhibition of VLDL synthesis Ethanol interferes with VLDL secretion	Deposition of fatty acids in the liver

Further reading

Allison ME. Fatty liver. *Hospital Medicine* 2004;**65**:609–612.

Arroyo V. Pathophysiology, diagnosis and treatment of ascites in cirrhosis. *Annals of Hepatology* 2002;**1**:72–79.

Azer SA. Esophageal varices. In: Qureshi WA, Talavera F, Bank S, Mechaber AJ, Katz J (eds), *Medicine, Ob/Gyn, Psychiatry and Surgery, Gastroenterology. eMedicine*, USA, 2001. www.emedicine.com/med/topic745.htm (accessed 28 March 2005).

Butterworth RF. Molecular neurobiology of acute liver failure. *Seminars in Liver Disease* 2003;**23**:251–258.

Dufour DR, Lott JA, Nolte FS, Gretch DR, Koff RS, Seeff LB. Diagnosis and monitoring of hepatic injury. I. Performance characteristics of laboratory tests. *Clinical Chemistry* 2000;**46**:2027–2049.

Dufour DR, Lott JA, Nolte FS, Gretch DR, Koff RS, Seeff LB. Diagnosis and monitoring of hepatic injury. II. Recommendations for use of laboratory tests in screening, diagnosis and monitoring. *Clinical Chemistry* 2000;**46**:2050–2068.

Garcia-Tsao G. Portal hypertension. *Current Opinion in Gastroenterology* 2004;**20**:254–263.

Gines P, Arroyo V, Rodes J. Pathophysiology, complications and treatment of ascites. *Clinics in Liver Disease* 1997;**1**:129–155.

Kamisako T, Kobayashi Y, Takenchi K, Ishihara T, Higuchi K, Tanaka Y *et al*. Recent advances in bilirubin metabolism research: the molecular mechanism of hepatocyte bilirubin transport and its clinical relevance. *Journal of Gastroenterology* 2000;**35**:659–664.

Lauterburg BH. Analgesics and glutathione. *American Journal of Therapeutics* 2002;**9**:225–233.

Lee WM. Acute liver failure in the United States. *Seminars in Liver Disease* 2003;**23**:217–226.

Maher JJ. Alcoholic steatosis and steatohepatitis. *Seminars in Gastrointestinal Disease* 2002;**13**:31–39.

Marsano LS, Mendez C, Hill D, Barve S, McClain CJ. Diagnosis and treatment of alcoholic liver disease and its complications. *Alcohol Research and Health* 2003;**27**:247–256.

Mendez-Sanchez N, Almeda-Valdes P, Uribe M. Alcoholic liver disease. An update. *Annals of Hepatology* 2005;**4**:32–42.

Nebert DW, Russell. Clinical importance of the cytochromes P450. *Lancet* 2002;**360**:1155–1162.

Nelson DR. Cytochrome P450 gene superfamily. Available at http://drnelson.utmem.edu/cytochromeP450.html (accessed 28 March 2005).

Poynard T, Yuen M-F, Ratziu V, Lai CL. Viral hepatitis C. *Lancet* 2003;**362**;2095–2100.

Riordan SM, Williams R. Alcohol exposure and paracetamol-induced hepatotoxicity. *Addiction Biology* 2002;**7**:191–206.

Riordan SM, Williams R. Mechanisms of hepatocyte injury, multiorgan failure and prognostic criteria in acute liver failure. *Seminars in Liver Disease* 2003;**23**:203–215.

Rumack BH. Acetaminophen poisoning. *American Journal of Medicine* 1983;**75**:104–112.

Schwarz KB, Balistreri W. Viral hepatitis. *Journal of Pediatric Gastroenterology and Nutrition* 2002;**35**(suppl 1):S29–S32.

Scottocasa GL, Passamonti S, Battistou L, Pascolo L, Tiribelli C. Molecular aspects of organic anion uptake in liver. *Journal of Hepatology* 1996;**24**(suppl 1):36–41.

Shaffer EA. Cholestasis: The ABCs of cellular mechanisms for impaired bile secretion-transporters and genes. *Canadian Journal of Gastroenterology* 2002;**16**:380–389.

Thomson BJ, Finch RG. Hepatitis C virus infection. *Clinical Microbiology and Infection* 2005;**11**:86–94.

Trauner M, Fickert P, Stauber RF. Hepatocellular bile salt transport: lessons from cholestasis. *Canadian Journal of Gastroenterology* 2000;**14** (suppl 1D):99D–104D.

Vaquero J, Chung C, Cahill ME, Blei AT. Pathogenesis of hepatic encephalopathy in acute liver failure. *Seminars in Liver Disease* 2003;**23**:259–269.

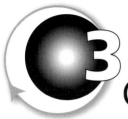

Gastrointestinal system

| ? | Questions for each of the case scenarios given |

Q1: What are the possible causes for the presenting problem?
Q2: What further questions would you like to ask to help you differentiate between your hypotheses?
Q3: What investigations would be most helpful to you and why?
Q4: In the light of the clinical presentation, how would you interpret the laboratory test results?
Q5: What is your final hypothesis?
Q6: What issues in the given history, examination and laboratory tests support your final hypothesis?

Clinical cases

● CASE 3.1 – I've taken aspirin tablets because of my shoulder pain.

Ms Linda Hart, a 62-year-old retired nurse, is brought to the accident and emergency (A&E) department at a local hospital by ambulance at 4am. She is pale and vomiting fresh blood. Although drowsy, she is oriented and able to answer questions. Ms Hart gives a history of vomiting large amounts of fresh blood at her house, before arriving at the hospital. Last night she started vomiting repetitively. Thirty minutes later, the vomitus became bloody. Ms Hart gives a history of recurrent pain in her right shoulder, for which she takes aspirin tablets. Further questions reveal that Ms Hart has been taking antacids containing magnesium hydroxide and aluminium hydroxide for heartburn for some time and has recently experienced abdominal pain and indigestion. She has been drinking for the last few years and has increased her consumption recently. On examination, she looks pale but is not jaundiced and there are no spider naevi or palmar erythema. Her vital signs are shown in Table 3.1.

Table 3.1 Vital signs for Case 3.1

Vital signs	Linda's results	Normal range
Blood pressure (mmHg)	100/60 (lying flat)	100/60–135/85
Pulse rate (/min)	105	60–100
Respiratory rate (/min)	20	12–16
Temperature (°C)	36.5	36.6–37.2

● Abdominal examination: mild tenderness of the epigastrium. The liver and spleen are not palpable.

● Per rectum examination: melaena stool on the gloved examining finger.

● Cardiovascular and respiratory examinations are normal.

The A&E registrar inserts a large intravenous line in her forearm and she is started on Hartmann's solution intravenously (replacement therapy of extracellular fluid [ECF] losses).

● CASE 3.2 – It was not my appendix.

Nicole Brown, a 25-year-old primary school teacher, comes in to see her GP because of generalized ill health and abdominal pain of about 1 month's duration. Her pains are intermittent and are mainly located in her right lower abdomen. The pain is not related to meals or menstruation. Sometimes the pain wakens her from sleep and on two occasions she was unable to go to work because of it. Nicole hates being ill so she did not seek medical advice. Last week Nicole noticed a skin rash over her shins (erythema nodosum). She also noticed that her stools have become looser than they used to be. She gives no history of rectal bleeding. She has lost 3 kg in body weight over the last 2 months. Nicole is not on any medications and has no history of allergies. She does not drink or smoke. On examination, she has tenderness and guarding of the right iliac fossa. Her GP suspects that Nicole might need an operation. He prepares a reference letter to the local hospital and arranges an ambulance to transfer her. The surgeon, who operates on Nicole a few hours later, finds that Nicole's terminal ileum is acutely inflamed and her appendix is normal.

● CASE 3.3 – I always feel tired and fatigued.

John Laurence, a 58-year-old taxi driver, comes in to see his local GP, Dr Sarah Goodman, because of progressive tiredness and fatigue for over 8 months. He also feels short of breath when he does a little exercise. He has no history of cough, chest pain or palpitations, and has always been fit. He has recently lost his appetite and has lost 4 kg in body weight over the last 6 months. He had initially attributed his loss of body weight to his depression after hearing about the death of two of his brothers in a motor car accident overseas. He also gives a history of recent changes in his bowel motions; he used to move his bowels once daily, but now he has constipation for 3–4 days followed by one or two loose bowel motions. He has no bleeding per rectum. He has a long history of abdominal discomfort and dyspepsia, and was diagnosed with irritable colon about 8 years ago. About that time, he had a colonoscopy and it was normal. On examination, he looks pale. His vital signs are shown in Table 3.2.

Table 3.2 Vital signs for Case 3.3

Vital signs	John's results	Normal range
Blood pressure (mmHg)	115/80	100/60–135/85
Pulse rate (/min)	90	60–100
Respiratory rate (/min)	15	12–16
Temperature (°C)	36.9	36.6–37.2

- Abdominal examination: no tenderness or rigidity. No organomegaly or palpable masses. Per rectum examination showed no melaena or rectal bleeding.
- No finger clubbing.
- Cardiovascular and respiratory examinations are normal.

👥 Integrated medical sciences questions

● CASE 3.1 – Discuss the role of parietal cells in the secretion of hydrochloric acid (HCl) and the different mechanisms by which pharmacological agents may control HCl secreted by parietal cells.

● CASE 3.2 – What are the long-term consequences of the surgical removal of the terminal ileum? Discuss the role of the terminal ileum in absorption.

● CASE 3.3 – Discuss the risk factors for the development of colon cancer. Include in your answer the role of genetics in the pathogenesis of colorectal cancer.

🔑 Key concepts

In order to work through the core clinical cases in this chapter, you will need to understand the following key concepts:

The functions of the main cells in the stomach

Table 3.3 Characteristics and functions of main cells in the stomach

Cell	Main characteristics	Functions
Mucus neck cells	Columnar cells Resemble the surface lining cells Have short microvilli Nuclei are basally located Well-developed Golgi apparatus and rough endoplasmic reticulum	Produce soluble mucus that helps lubricate the chyme
Stem cells	Relatively few Do not have many organelles but rich in ribosomes	Proliferate to replace all the specialized cells lining the fundic glands
Parietal (oxyntic) cells	Pyramidal cells Located in the upper half of fundic glands	Produce HCl and the gastric intrinsic factor (IF), which is essential for the absorption of vitamin B_{12}, mainly in the terminal ileum
Peptic cells (also known as chief cells)	Mostly found in the base of fundic glands They are small cells, displaying a basophilic cytoplasm	Secrete pepsinogen
Enteroendocrine cells (APUD cell)	A group of small cells; they stain with silver stains (also called argyrophilic cells)	Secrete hormone-like substance

APUD, amine precursor uptake and decarboxylation.

Differences between cyclo-oxygenase 1 and cyclo-oxygenase 2

Table 3.4 Differences between the enzymes COX-1 and COX-2

Characteristic	COX-1	COX-2
COX genes	Expressed constitutively in most cells	Upregulated by cytokines, stress, tumour promoters
Function of COX	Prostaglandin production that subserves housekeeping functions, e.g. gastric epithelial cytoprotection and haemostasis	Prostaglandin formation in inflammation and cancer

Example of COX inhibitors	Aspirin, NSAIDs (non-specific inhibition of both COX-1 and COX-2)	Celecoxib, rofecoxib, valdecoxib (selective COX-2 inhibitors)
Effects of COX inhibitors	May produce gastrointestinal bleeding, gastric irritation, gastritis, peptic ulcer	Less likely to produce gastrointestinal side effects
	Inhibits platelet aggregation	Does not inhibit platelet aggregation
		Prothrombotic, enhancing atherosclerosis and increasing the risk of cardiovascular diseases

COX, cyclo-oxygenase; NSAIDs, non-steroidal anti-inflammatory drugs.

The main causes of peptic ulcer

- Non-steroidal anti-inflammatory drugs (NSAIDs)

- *Helicobacter pylori* infection

- Exposure of the body to severe stress, e.g. massive burn, operation.

The mechanisms by which *H. pylori* may cause peptic ulcer

- Stimulation of the release of cytokines such as interleukins 6 and 8 (IL-6 and IL-8)

- Stimulation of gastric acid secretion (possible that IL-6 and IL-8 act locally and stimulate parietal cells to produce more HCl)

- Antagonizing gastric acid inhibition (possibly *H. pylori* interferes with the function of somatostatin-producing cells in the antrum)

- Production of toxins (e.g. vacuolating toxin and urease), contributing to the pathogenesis of duodenal ulcer

- Activation of inflammatory infiltration/reaction in the lamina propria of the stomach

- Interference with normal production of mucus.

The functions of the large bowel

- Absorption of most of the water in the chyme, leaving about 100 mL of fluids to be excreted in the faeces

- Absorption of electrolytes, mainly sodium and chloride, leaving about 1–5 mmol to be lost in the faeces

- Storage of faeces, mainly in the distal half of the colon

- The bacteria in the colon aid in the synthesis of vitamins K and B_{12} and thiamine.

Table 3.5 Main pathological differences between Crohn's disease and ulcerative colitis

Characteristic	Crohn's disease	Ulcerative colitis
Predominant area involved	Terminal ileum and ascending colon	The descending colon
Distribution of the lesion	Patchy with skipped areas	Diffuse lesions, no skipped areas
Intestinal walls	All layers are involved → thickened and rigid walls	Affected intestinal walls remain thin
Intestinal lumen	Narrowed, irregular, stenosed	Dilated – megacolon may occur
Mucosa	Deep linear ulcerations – 'cobblestone appearance'	Friable 'superficial ulcers'
Serosa	Involved in inflammation	Not involved in the disease
Inflammatory process	Transmural	Limited to the mucosa
Granuloma formation	Present	No
Adhesions	Present	No
Fistulae	Present	No
Perianal abscess and fistulae	Present (> 50 per cent)	Rarely present (1–3 per cent)
Other extraintestinal signs (percentage patients):		
– uveitis	5	50
– peripheral arthritis	20	10
– erythema nodosum	20	5
– pyoderma gangrenosum	1	2–5
Development of colon cancer in the future	Less common (< 1 per cent)	Occur in about 10–12 per cent of patients (about 10 years after diagnosis)
Development of liver complications (percentage patients):		
– fatty liver	About 30–40	About 30–40
– cirrhosis	< 1	Rare
– sclerosing cholangitis	About 30	About 30
– gallstones	About 15	Rare

Table 3.6 The mechanisms by which diarrhoea may occur

Mechanism	Example
Inflammatory exudation (diarrhoea secondary to inflammation of the intestinal walls)	Inflammatory bowel disease (ulcerative colitis)
Motility disorder (short transit time)	Autonomic disorders, e.g. diabetes mellitus
	Thyrotoxicosis
Secretory diarrhoea (excessive secretion of water secondary to disturbance of cellular transporters by bacteria or its toxins)	Excessive use of laxatives
	Gastrointestinal infection (enterotoxins)
Osmotic diarrhoea	Lactose therapy
	Disaccharidase deficiency (lactase deficiency)
Malabsorption (interference with the normal absorptive processes in the small intestine)	Pancreatic enzyme deficiency (e.g. chronic pancreatitis)
	Bacterial overgrowth
	Interruption of the enterohepatic circulation of bile salts (e.g. as a consequence of surgical removal of the terminal ileum)
	Loss of enterocytes (radiation of intra-abdominal cancer)
	Lymphatic obstruction

What are the nutritional deficiencies that may occur as a result of these gastrointestinal disorders?

- Partial gastrectomy (stomach resection)
- Coeliac disease
- Chronic pancreatitis
- Surgical resection of the terminal ileum
- Biliary atresia
- Primary lactase deficiency.

Table 3.7 Nutritional deficiencies and disease

Disease/condition	Structures/organs affected	Nutritional deficiencies that may occur
Partial gastrectomy (stomach resection)	Loss of parietal cells Parietal cells produce HCl and gastric intrinsic factor	Interference with duodenal absorption of iron and microcytic anaemia may result. Rarely, sufficient loss of intrinsic factor occurs, resulting in macrocytic anaemia (vitamin B_{12} deficiency)
Coeliac disease	Mucosal lining of the duodenum and jejunum	Malabsorption of fat and iron
Chronic pancreatitis	Mainly the exocrine function of the pancreas	Fat digestion
Crohn's disease affecting the terminal ileum/surgical resection of the terminal ileum	Loss of the absorptive surface of terminal ileum	Interference with the enterohepatic circulation of bile salts and malabsorption of vitamin B_{12}
Biliary atresia	Congenital absence of the extrahepatic biliary duct system	Malabsorption of fat and fat-soluble vitamins (A, D, E and K)
Primary lactase deficiency	Small intestine	Lactose hydrolysis resulting in osmotic diarrhoea
Primary or secondary sclerosing cholangitis	Stenosis of the intrahepatic and extrahepatic biliary system	Lack of bile salts essential for the absorption of fat and fat-soluble vitamins (A, D, E and K)

Answers

 CASE 3.1 – I've taken aspirin tablets because of my shoulder pain.

Q1: What are the possible causes for the presenting problem?

A1

Possible causes (hypotheses) for Linda's haematemesis (vomiting blood) are bleeding from:

- a stomach ulcer (possibly caused by aspirin)

- a duodenal ulcer

- oesophageal varices: this hypothesis is less likely because there are no signs of chronic liver disease (spider naevi or palmar erythema) and none suggestive of portal hypertension (ascites, or hepatosplenomegaly)

- a tear in the oesophagus (caused by repeated vomiting)

- a cancer in her oesophagus/stomach (cancers may ulcerate and bleed); this is also less likely.

Q2: What further questions would you like to ask to help you differentiate between your hypotheses?

A2

Table 3.8 Further history questions for Case 3.1

History questions	In what way answers can help
History of recurrent abdominal pain (type of pain or discomfort, site, radiation, severity, relationship with food, relieving and aggravating causes) and associated symptoms such as nausea and vomiting. Loss of body weight, heartburn. Past investigations for heartburn, e.g. endoscopy, barium meal. History of treatment for peptic ulcer disease	The aim is to assess if there is a history suggestive of peptic ulcer or gastritis. NSAIDs, aspirin and corticosteroids are associated with a high incidence of peptic ulcer and complications such as bleeding and perforation. Patients with a history of peptic ulcer or gastritis should not take these drugs
Past history of haematemesis or melaena	Indicating past history of bleeding peptic ulcer
	The main causes of haematemesis are: oesophageal varices; peptic ulcer; oesophagitis/gastritis; and Mallory–Weiss tears (oesophageal tear). Your aim should be to find out the cause for her haematemesis. Bleeding from oesophageal varices occurs in patients with liver cirrhosis and portal hypertension. Thus, you need to assess for alcohol-associated problems such as alcoholic liver cirrhosis. Patients with liver cirrhosis could develop portal hypertension and oesophageal varices

Drinking alcohol: amount, duration, frequency Treatment for alcoholism Any history of liver trouble	The effect of alcohol on the gastric mucosa is not actually known. Alcohol may stimulate gastrin release and acid secretion in some species but there is no evidence for a similar action in humans
Risk factors for hepatitis, e.g. tattooing, blood transfusion, travel overseas, sexual preference	Once again you need to assess for any history of chronic hepatitis and cirrhosis
Medications and allergies	Particularly medications that may cause liver injury, peptic ulcer and gastritis

NSAIDs, non-steroidal anti-inflammatory drugs.

 Q3: What investigations would be most helpful to you and why?

A3

Further investigations

- Full blood examination

- Blood group and cross-matching

- Blood urea, creatinine, sodium and potassium

- Gastroscopy.

 CASE 3.2 – It was not my appendix.

 Q1: What are the possible causes for the presenting problem?

A1

The following are possible causes (hypotheses) for Nicole's presentation:

- Acute Crohn's disease: this is the most likely hypothesis because of her presentation, the presence of inflammation of the terminal ileum and normal appendix, erythema nodosum, loss of body weight and changes in her bowel motions.

- Yersinia ileitis (acute inflammation of the ileum by organism *Yersinia pseudotuberculosis*): this presents with right iliac fossa pain which is clinically identical to acute appendicitis. Usually it is diagnosed at surgery, where the terminal ileum is thickened, red in colour and inflamed. The appearance of the terminal ileum may be very similar to Crohn's disease.

- Mesenteric adenitis (particularly important in children): a recent history of a sore throat or viral-type infection is usually present in mesenteric adenitis.

- Ulcerative colitis (less likely): patients may present with loose blood-stained stools and severe diarrhoea, often preceded by cramping abdominal pain. Anaemia, inflammation of the uveal tract of the eye and joint involvement may be present. The disease always involves the rectum but often extends proximally to involve the whole colon. Involvement of the terminal ileum may occur in 15–20 per cent of patients and is the result of secondary involvement. It is described as backwash ileitis.

- Ileocaecal tuberculosis: relatively rare in western countries but still seen in developing countries.

- Carcinoma of the caecum: less likely to occur in the patient's age group.

- Colitis, e.g. infectious colitis: colitis caused by *Shigella* or *Campylobacter* spp., invasive *Escherichia coli*, salmonellae or *Entamoeba histolytica* (less likely).

- Acute appendicitis (usually resulting from obstruction of the lumen of the appendix by faeces or faecolith): the mucosa is usually inflamed first. The inflammatory process may progress to involve the submucosa, muscular layer and serosa. It is obviously less likely.

Q2: What further questions would you like to ask to help you differentiate between your hypotheses?

A2

Table 3.9 Further history questions for Case 3.2

History questions	In what way answers can help
Could you indicate with your finger the site of the pain? How would you describe your abdominal pain? Could you rank the severity of your pain using numbers 1–10 (10 meaning very severe pain)? Are you aware of anything that triggers your pain? Have you tried anything to relieve your pain? Did it help you? Do you feel that you might have a fever?	Acute appendicitis usually runs a short course of a few hours to about 3 days. The patient with appendicitis usually presents with central abdominal pain and tenderness in the right iliac fossa. There may be fever between 37.3 and 38.5°C. Vomiting may occur one to three times
How long have you had loose bowel motions? Have you ever had similar bouts in the past? How many times per day do you normally pass stool? How many times did you pass one today? Any blood or mucus in your stool? Any changes in your appetite? Any changes in your body weight? Any history of joint pain, eye problems, back pain or skin changes	Patients with Crohn's disease may present with general ill health, anaemia, colicky abdominal pain and diarrhoea. Loss of appetite, weight loss, fever, joint pain, painful nodules/plaques about 2–5 cm on shins, thighs or arms (known as erythema nodosum), malaise, lassitude, uveitis and iritis are usually present when the disease is active. Erythema nodosum may occur in other conditions including: sarcoidosis; tuberculosis; leprosy; chlamydial infection; as a side effect of drugs such as sulphonamides, oral contraceptive pill, penicillin; histoplasmosis and coccidioidomycosis infections; and streptococcal infection
Have you ever had abdominal surgery? What surgery and when?	Previous abdominal surgery may be complicated, with adhesions resulting in intestinal obstruction and abdominal pain
Medications and allergies	Drugs such as sulphonamides, oral contraceptive pill, penicillin may produce erythema nodosum
Family history of inflammatory bowel disease	Approximately 15–20 per cent of patients with inflammatory bowel disease have positive family history and a first-degree relative affected by Crohn's disease or ulcerative colitis

Q3: What investigations would be most helpful to you and why?

A3

Further investigations

- Full blood examination
- Erythrocyte sedimentation rate
- Stool analysis
- Blood film
- Blood urea, creatinine, sodium and potassium
- Colonoscopy.

CASE 3.3 – I always feel tired and fatigued.

Q1: What are the possible causes for the presenting problem?

A1

The following are possible causes (hypotheses) for John's presentation:

- Colorectal cancer: tiredness, fatigue, alteration of bowel habit, increased constipation, spurious or false diarrhoea (caused by faecal impaction above the tumour mass and bacterial fermentation), diarrhoea alternating with constipation, colicky abdominal pain, anaemia, loss of body weight, abdominal distension/discomfort and bleeding per rectum are suggestive of carcinoma of the left half of the colon.
- Irritable bowel syndrome.
- Diverticular disease of the colon.
- Anaemia, possibly as a result of loss of blood from the gastrointestinal tract.
- Depression.

Q2: What further questions would you like to ask to help you differentiate between your hypotheses?

A2

Table 3.10 Further history questions for Case 3.3

History questions	In what way answers can help
Loss of appetite, loss of body weight, indigestion, bleeding per rectum, abdominal discomfort	Carcinoma of the right half of the colon usually presents with anaemia, weight loss and generalized fatigue, and may be a mass in the right iliac fossa. On the other hand, carcinoma of the left side of the colon usually presents with alteration of bowel habit, increased constipation, spurious or false diarrhoea (caused by faecal impaction above the tumour mass and bacterial fermentation), diarrhoea alternating with constipation, colicky abdominal pain, anaemia, loss of body weight, abdominal distension/discomfort and bleeding per rectum
Symptoms suggestive of intestinal obstruction, e.g. central abdominal pain, vomiting, abdominal distension, constipation	Acute intestinal obstruction most often occurs in later stages of the disease. It is likely to occur when tumours are close to the ileocaecal valve. Tenderness in the right iliac fossa in the presence of large bowel obstruction and anaemia is an indicator of cancer
Risk factors for the development of colorectal cancer, e.g. removal of benign polyps, ulcerative colitis, family history of polyposis coli	Patients with ulcerative colitis are at a higher risk of developing colon cancer in the 10 years after diagnosis
Past history of investigations, e.g. colonoscopy, barium meal and follow-through, barium enema	The results of these investigations will help as a baseline in assessment of the patient's condition

Q3: What investigations would be most helpful to you and why?

A3

Further investigations

- Full blood examination
- Erythrocyte sedimentation rate
- Blood urea, creatinine, sodium and potassium
- Colonoscopy
- Stool analysis
- Iron studies.

Further progress

CASE 3.1 – I've taken aspirin tablets because of my shoulder pain.

The A&E registrar arranges for some tests for Linda. The results of her tests are shown in Table 3.11.

Table 3.11 Test results for Case 3.1

Test	Linda's results	Normal range
Haemoglobin (Hb) (g/L)	88	115–160
Packed cell volume (PCV)	48	0.37–0.47
White blood cell count (WCC) ($\times 10^9$/L)	8.4	4.0–11.0
Platelet count ($\times 10^9$/L)	250	150–400
Serum sodium (mmol/L)	140	135–145
Serum potassium (mmol/L)	3.5	3.5–5.0
Blood urea (mmol/L)	18.8	2.5–8.3
Serum creatinine (mmol/L)	0.17	0.05–0.11

Gastroscopy report: no oesophageal tear or oesophageal varices, moderate amount of fresh blood in the stomach, active bleeding from a gastric ulcer, about 1 cm in diameter. The ulcer looks benign. The results of a rapid urease test performed on two antral biopsies are positive for *Helicobacter pylori*. The duodenum is normal. No other lesions found.

CASE 3.2 – It was not my appendix.

Further investigations confirmed that Nicole has Crohn's disease mainly involving about 60 cm of her terminal ileum. Three years later, she has two major episodes of recurrence of her symptoms, mainly diarrhoea, lower abdominal pain, arthritis, mild fever and generalized fatigue. As these symptoms are not controlled by medication, she undergoes resection of a major part of her ileum, and part of the ascending colon with ileocolic anastomosis. After the operation she has no fever or joint pains. Six months after the operation, Nicole travels with her husband to visit his home town in India. She has loose bowel motions on several occasions during her stay in India and stool analysis shows *Entamoeba histolytica*, for which she was treated with metronidazole tablets 800 mg three times a day for 7 days. Despite her treatment for amoebiasis as proved by negative several stool microscopy studies, she continues to have loose bowel motions. There is no blood or mucus in her stool but her stool is bulky and offensive in odour. She also complains of generalized fatigue.

The results of her current tests are shown in Table 3.12.

Table 3.12 Test results for Case 3.2

Test	Nicole's results	Normal range
Hb (g/L)	105	115–160
PCV	0.40	0.37–0.47
Mean corpuscular volume (MCV) (fL)	105	80–96

WCC ($\times 10^9$/L)	4.8	4.0–11.0
Platelet count ($\times 10^9$/L)	190	150–400
Erythrocyte sedimentation rate (ESR) (mm/h)	7	< 20
Stool collected over 72 h:		
Weight (g/day)	500	< 200
Fat content (g/day)	22	< 6 g/L
Stool microscopy (on three occasions)	No *Entamoeba histolytica*, or any other parasites or ova	
	Fat globules ++++	
	Undigested fibres ++	
	No red or white blood cells –	

● CASE 3.3 – I always feel tired and fatigued.

Dr Goodman arranges some tests for John. The results are shown in Table 3.13.

Table 3.13 Test results for Case 3.3

Test	John's results	Normal range
Hb (g/L)	95	115–160
WCC ($\times 10^9$/L)	8.9	4.0–11.0
Platelet count ($\times 10^9$/L)	321	150–400
Random distribution width (per cent)	21.3	11–15
ESR (mm/h)	97	< 20
Serum iron (μmol/L)	5	9–30
Serum transferrin (g/L)	5	2.0–4.0
Iron transferrin saturation (%)	< 10	15–50
Serum ferritin (μg/L)	5	10–120
Red blood cell folate (nmol/L packed cell)	880	317–1422
Serum vitamin B$_{12}$ (pmol/L)	312	148–616

Blood urea, creatinine, sodium and potassium: all within normal range.

Colonoscopy report: an annular tumour mass encircling the wall of the sigmoid colon is seen. The centre of the tumour mass shows two small ulcers; a separate mucosal polyp is seen near one of the ulcers.

Further questions

CASE 3.1 – I've taken aspirin tablets because of my shoulder pain.

Q4: In the light of the clinical presentation, how would you interpret the laboratory test results?

A4

Table 3.14 Interpretation of lab test results for Case 3.1

Test	Result	Interpretation
Hb	Low	The fact that only Hb is low whereas WCC and platelet counts are normal excludes bone marrow pathology as a cause of low Hb. The raised PCV indicates fluid loss and hypovolaemia
PCV	Raised	
WCC	Normal	
Platelet count	Normal	
Blood urea	Raised	The raised blood urea and creatinine are most probably a result of renal hypoperfusion (decreased glomerular filtration rate) caused by volume loss
Serum creatinine	Raised	

Table 3.15 Gastroscopy results for Case 3.1

Test	Result	Interpretation
Gastroscopy	No oesophageal tear or oesophageal varices, moderate amount of fresh blood in the stomach, active bleeding from a gastric ulcer, about 1 cm in diameter. The ulcer looks benign. The results of a rapid urease test performed on two antral biopsies are positive for *Helicobacter pylori*. The duodenum is normal. No other lesions found	The cause for her bleeding is an acute gastric ulcer caused by aspirin intake. It appears that Linda has an infection with *H. pylori* causing her abdominal discomfort and peptic ulcer before this presentation. Aspirin might have precipitated bleeding from a gastric ulcer; as a result of the intake of NSAIDs or aspirin such bleeding may occur in old people without prior infection with *H. pylori* *H. pylori* can be detected at endoscopy by histology, culture or urease test. Infection with *H. pylori* is usually patchy, so biopsy-based methods for detecting *H. pylori* are liable to sample error and may be negative despite the presence of infection

Q5: What is your final hypothesis?

A5

Acute upper gastrointestinal bleeding (haematemesis) caused by aspirin-induced gastric ulcer. The patient has *H. pylori* infection and the management plan should include treatment of this infection.

Q6: What issues in the given history, examination and laboratory tests support your final hypothesis?

A6

Supportive evidence

History

- Patient presented with vomiting blood and pallor

- Gives a history of recurrent pain in her right shoulder for which she takes aspirin tables

- Has used antacids containing magnesium and aluminium hydroxide for heartburn for some time

- Recently experienced abdominal pain and indigestion

- Has been drinking and feels depressed after the death of her husband.

Examination

- Looks pale

- No evidence of chronic liver disease (not jaundiced, no spider naevi or palmar erythema)

- Low blood pressure 100/60 (lying flat)

- Increased pulse rate and respiratory rate

- Afebrile

- Mild tenderness in the epigastrium

- Liver and spleen not palpable

- Cardiovascular and respiratory examinations normal.

Investigations

- Low Hb

- Raised blood urea and creatinine (hypovolaemia and decreased renal perfusion)

- Gastroscopy: no oesophageal tear or oesophageal varices, moderate amount of fresh blood in the stomach, active bleeding from a gastric ulcer, about 1 cm in diameter. The ulcer looks benign. The results of a rapid urease test performed on two antral biopsies are positive for Helicobacter pylori. The duodenum is normal. No other lesions found.

CASE 3.2 – **It was not my appendix.**

Q4: In the light of the clinical presentation, how would you interpret the laboratory test results?

A4

Table 3.16 Interpretation of lab test results for Case 3.2

Test	Result	Interpretation
Hb	Low	Anaemia may occur in patients with Crohn's disease as a result of: (1) malabsorption, (2) loss of appetite and lack of nutritional intake, (3) haemolysis and (4) blood loss from the gastrointestinal tract
MCV	Increased	Increased MCV may suggest macrocytic anaemia as a result of lack of vitamin B_{12} (normally vitamin B_{12} is absorbed in the terminal ileum). Further investigations are required for confirmation including serum vitamin B_{12} level, red blood folate and iron studies
ESR	Not raised	This might help in supporting the hypothesis that her loose bowel motions and generalized fatigue are not the result of recurrence of Crohn's disease. With regard to her generalized fatigue, we will need to assess her blood urea, creatinine, and serum sodium and potassium; this is because her loose bowel motions could have disturbed her fluid and electrolyte balance
Stool collection over 72 h	Increased fat content	Excessive fat loss in stool (steatorrhoea) is mainly caused by excessive loss of bile salts and interruption of the enterohepatic circulation of bile salts. Resection of the terminal ileum → failure of bile salts to be absorbed → excessive loss of bile salts in the large intestine → (1) irritation of the large bowel mucosa by bile salts → loose bowel motions + (2) interruption of the enterohepatic circulation of bile salts → decreased bile salt pool and poor digestion of fat (fat digestion requires bile salts and normal exocrine function of the pancreas) → loose bowel motions (steatorrhoea)
		The other possibility for her loose bowel is colitis caused by *E. histolytica* infection; however, patients with amoebiasis present with abdominal pain, dysentery, tenesmus, and some blood and mucus in stool
Stool microscopy	No *E. histolytica*, or any other parasites or ova	No evidence of infection as a cause of her loose bowel motions
		The increase in fat globules is consistent with the increased fat in stool (collected over 72 h)
	Fat globules ++++ Undigested fibres ++	
	No red or white blood cells	
Stool cultures for bacterial pathogens and serological tests for amoebiasis	Negative	

Q5: What is your final hypothesis?

A5

Crohn's disease of the terminal ileum presenting as acute appendicitis. The patient develops amoebiasis during her visit to India and is treated with metronidazole. Her loose bowel motions continue despite her treatment and are most probably the result of the interruption of the enterohepatic circulation of bile salts and malabsorption of fat (steatorrhoea). Other factors that might contribute to her loose bowel motions are (1) rapid transit time because of the resection of her small intestine, (2) irritation of the mucosa of the large intestine by bile salts lost in her stool and (3) stimulation of the sympathetic nervous system, possibly because of her anxiety. There is no evidence of *E. histolytica* infection or recurrence of her Crohn's disease activity.

Q6: What issues in the given history, examination and laboratory tests support your final hypothesis?

A6

Supportive evidence

History

- Presented with general ill health and abdominal pain – 1 month's duration
- Her pains are intermittent and mainly located in the right iliac fossa
- Skin: erythema nodosum
- Loose bowel motions, no rectal bleeding
- Diagnosed with Crohn's disease during a laparotomy (mainly involving about 60 cm of her terminal ileum)
- During her recent travel to India she had loose bowel motions caused by *E. histolytica* infection (treated with metronidazole)
- Her loose bowel motions continued.

Examination

- Looks ill
- Tenderness and guarding in the right iliac fossa
- Temperature 37.8°C
- Pulse rate 95/min.

Investigations

- Low Hb, increased MCV
- Normal WCC and platelets

- Normal ESR
- Increased faecal fat collected over 72 h
- Stool microscopy: increased fat globules +++, no red or white blood cells
- Stool culture and serology tests for amoebiasis are negative.

CASE 3.3 – I always feel tired and fatigued.

Q4: In the light of the clinical presentation, how would you interpret the laboratory test results?

A4

Table 3.17 Interpretation of lab test results for Case 3.3

Test	Result	Interpretation
Hb	Low	Anaemia may be the result of: blood loss from the tumour mass; decreased appetite and decreased nutrition intake; or bone marrow suppression
Random distribution width	Increased	The presence of red blood cells of different diameters indicates that the body is compensating by producing more blood cells. Increased random distribution width may be present in iron deficiency anaemia
ESR	Increased	Although the ESR is a very sensitive test, it is not specific. It indicates the presence of inflammation in the body but cannot help in indicating the site or nature of the inflammatory changes
Iron studies	Low serum iron, increased transferrin, low iron saturation, low ferritin	The findings indicate the presence of iron deficiency anaemia
Serum vitamin B_{12} and red blood cell folate	Normal	Anaemia is less likely to be megaloblastic or macrocytic. The findings are consistent with the clinical picture
Colonoscopy report	An annular tumour mass encircling the wall of the sigmoid colon is seen. The centre of the tumour mass shows two small ulcers; a separate mucosal polyp is seen near one of the ulcers	The site of the tumour may explain why the patient presented with changes in bowel habits

Q5: What is your final hypothesis?

A5

The clinical picture and the investigations support the diagnosis of colon cancer (sigmoid colon) causing alteration in the patient's bowel motions and iron deficiency anaemia.

Q6: What issues in the given history, examination and laboratory tests support your final hypothesis?

A6

Supportive evidence

History

- Progressive tiredness and fatigue for over 8 months

- Shortness of breath on little exercise

- No history of a cough, chest pain or palpitation

- Lost 4 kg in body weight over 6 months

- Changes in bowel movements

- Long history of dyspepsia and diagnosed with irritable colon

- Depressed as a result of a recent bereavement

- Colonoscopy, about 8 years ago, was normal.

Examination

- Looks pale

- Afebrile

- Abdominal examination: no tenderness or rigidity, no organomegaly or palpable masses

- Per rectum examination showed no melaena or rectal bleeding

- No finger clubbing

- Cardiovascular and respiratory examinations are normal.

Investigations

- Anaemia (low Hb)

- Normal WCC and platelets

- Raised random distribution width

- Raised ESR

- Iron studies: indicate the presence of iron deficiency anaemia

- Normal serum vitamin B_{12} and red blood folate

- Colonoscopy: an annular tumour mass encircling the wall of the sigmoid colon is seen. The centre of the tumour mass shows two small ulcers; a separate mucosal polyp is seen near one of the ulcers.

ÀÀ Integrated medical sciences questions

● CASE 3.1 – Discuss the role of parietal cells in the secretion of HCl and the different mechanisms by which pharmacological agents may control HCl secreted by parietal cells.

The main functions of the parietal cells are: the secretion of (1) HCl and (2) the gastric IF that facilitates the absorption of vitamin B_{12} in the ileum.

The process of secretion of HCl from the parietal cells can be summarized as follows:

1. At the intracellular level: CO_2 is produced by aerobic metabolism → CO_2 combines with H_2O → formation of H_2CO_3 → carbonic anhydrase acts on H_2CO_3 → H^+ and HCO_3^-.

2. At the membrane facing the stomach lumen (the apical membrane): the H^+/K^+ ATPase facilitates H^+ secretion into the gastric lumen.

3. At the membrane facing the blood supply (the basolateral membrane): the Cl^-/HCO_3^- exchanger facilitates the movement of HCO_3^- from the cell into the bloodstream and the movement of Cl^- to the parietal cells. The H^+ and Cl^- form the HCl in the stomach.

Table 3.18 summarizes the physiological factors stimulating HCl secretion from the parietal cells and the pharmacological agent used in the treatment of peptic ulcer.

Table 3.18 Physiological factors stimulating HCl secretion

Receptors/ transporters on the parietal cell	Chemical mediator	Mechanism of HCl control	Pharmacological agent used to treat peptic ulcer	Outcomes
Muscarinic receptors	ACh	ACh acts by (1) stimulating gastrin release and (2) direct stimulation of parietal cells	Atropine and related drugs	Atropine decreases the response of parietal cells to gastrin, histamine and ACh
H_2-receptors	Histamine (found in the ECl cells within the lamina propria of the gastric glands)	Histamine is a potent stimulator of parietal cell secretion. In the stomach, histamine release potentiates the effects of gastrin and ACh on the parietal cell	Cimetidine and all H_2-rceptor-blocking agents (ranitidine, afamotidine and nizatidine)	Cimetidine blocks the potentiated effects of histamine on parietal cells

Compared with atropine, cimetidine is a more effective inhibitor of acid secretion and has fewer side effects |
| Gastrin receptors | Gastrin: released from G-cells. The stimuli for its release are (1) GRP or bombesin and (2) protein digestion products (e.g. peptides, amino acids and amines may act directly on the G-cell to stimulate gastrin release) | Gastrin stimulates histamine release and synthesis and the growth of the ECl cells | Possibly as part of the action of atropine | Decreased HCl secretion |

	Note that somatostatin acts on the G-cell to inhibit gastrin release			
H⁺/K⁺ ATPase (H⁺ pump)	Allows the movement of H⁺ into the gastric lumen	An ATPase-dependent pump that allows H⁺ movement into the gastric lumen against concentration (uphill)	Proton-pump inhibitor blocks all acid secretion. Also has direct antibacterial activity against *H. pylori* but does not cure the infection when used alone	Omeprazole (a proton-pump inhibitor)

ACh, acetylcholine; ECl, enterochromaffin-like; GRP, gastrin-releasing peptide.

⬤ CASE 3.2 – **What are the long-term consequences of the surgical removal of the terminal ileum? Discuss the role of the terminal ileum in absorption.**

● Malabsorption of bile salts → interference with the enterohepatic circulation of bile salts → decreased bile salt in portal circulation → malabsorption of fat → steatorrhoea. It is also possible that the excessive loss of bile salts into the large bowel and stool causes irritation of the colorectal region and contributes to the pathogenesis of loose bowel motions.

● Increased bile salt synthesis to compensate for the loss of bile salts in stool.

● Increased oxalate absorption because of the presence of bile salts in the colon → renal oxalate stone.

● Decreased vitamin B_{12} absorption → failure of maturation of red blood cells → macrocytosis.

● Decreased bile concentration in bile → decreased micellar formation and relative increase in cholesterol concentration → increased lithogenic properties of bile → formation of gallbladder stones.

⬤ CASE 3.3 – **Discuss the risk factors for the development of colon cancer. Include in your answer the role of genetics in the pathogenesis of colorectal cancer.**

● Approximately 98 per cent of all cancers in the large intestine are adenocarcinomas.

● Most colorectal carcinomas occur sporadically.

● Populations that have a higher prevalence of adenomas are at a higher risk of developing colorectal cancer.

● The dietary factors that may contribute to the development of colorectal cancer are:

 – excess dietary caloric and fat intake

 – intake of food high in cholesterol

 – low content of fibres

 – high intake of red meat

 – decreased intake of micronutrients.

However, there is no strong evidence to support the notion that these dietary risk factors play a significant role in the development of colorectal cancer.

- Several studies have demonstrated that intake of aspirin or NSAIDs protects against the development of colorectal cancer.

- At the molecular level, the pathogenesis of colorectal cancer may include the following changes/mutations:

  - loss of the adenomatous polyposis coli (*APC*) gene: the first event in the formation of adenomas; about 80 per cent of colorectal carcinomas have an inactivated *APC* gene

  - mutation of K-*RAS* gene

  - loss of the *p53* gene: found in about 80 per cent of colorectal cancers

  - activation of telomerase: most colorectal carcinomas have increased telomerase activity.

- The most common sites for colon cancer are: the rectosigmoid region (40 per cent), caecum (35 per cent), descending colon (15 per cent) and transverse colon (10 per cent).

Further reading

Bell GM, Schnitzer TJ. Cox-2 inhibitors and other nonsteroidal anti-inflammatory drugs in the treatment of pain in the elderly. *Clinics in Geriatric Medicine* 2001;**17**:489–502.

Blanchard TG, Drakes ML, Czinn SJ. *Helicobacter* infection: pathogenesis. *Current Opinion in Gastroenterology* 2004;**20**:10–15.

Hawkey CJ. Non-steroidal anti-inflammatory drugs: who should receive prophylaxis? *Alimentary Pharmacology and Therapeutics* 2004;**20**(suppl 2):59–64.

Johnson LR. *Gastrointestinal Physiology. The Mosby physiology monograph series*, 6th edn. St Louis, MO: Mosby, 2001.

Jones J, Boorman J, Cann P *et al.* British society of gastroenterology guidelines for the management of the irritable bowel syndrome. *Gut* 2000;**47**(suppl 2):1–19.

Laine L. Proton pump inhibitor co-therapy with nonsteroidal anti-inflammatory drugs – nice or necessary? *Reviews in Gastroenterological Disorders* 2004;**4**(suppl 4):S33–S41.

Miller M, Windosor A. Ulcerative colitis. *Hospital Medicine* 2000;**61**:698–702.

Monteleone I, Vavassori P, Biancone L, Monteleone G, Pallone F. Immunoregulation in the gut: success and failure in human disease. *Gut* 2002;**50**(suppl III):60–64.

Nelson MR, Toukin AM, Cicultin FM, McNeil JJ. Cox-2 inhibitors: exemplars of drug-safety conundrum. *Medical Journal of Australia* 2005;**182**:262–263.

Okabe N. The pathogenesis of Crohn's disease. *Digestion* 2001;**63**(suppl 1):52–59.

Orlando RC. Mechanisms of epithelial injury and inflammation in gastrointestinal diseases. *Reviews in Gastroenterological Disorders* 2002;**2**(suppl 2):S2–S8.

Panchal PC, Forman JS, Blumberg DR, Wilson KT. *Helicobacter pylori* infection: Pathogenesis. *Current Opinion in Gastroenterology* 2003;**19**:4–10.

Schnitzer TJ. Cyclooxygenase-2-specific inhibitors: are they safe? *American Journal of Medicine* 2001;**110**(suppl 1):46 S–49S.

Talley NJ. Dyspepsia. *Gastroenterology* 2003;**125**:1219–1226.

Tarnawski AS, Caves TC. Aspirin in the XXI Century: Its major clinical impact, novel mechanisms of action, and new safer formulations. *Gastroenterology* 2004;**127**:341–343.

US Food and Drug Administration, Center for Drug Evaluation and Research. FDA alert practitioners on Celebrex (celecoxib). FDA Alert 12/17/04. Available at: www.fda.gov/cder/drug/infopage/celebrex-hcp.htm (accessed March 2005).

Windsor A. Ileal Crohn's disease is best treated by surgery. *Gut* 2002;**51**:11–12.

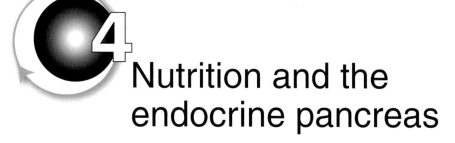

Nutrition and the endocrine pancreas

Q1: What are the possible causes for the presenting problem?
Q2: What further questions would you like to ask to help you differentiate between your hypotheses?
Q3: What investigations would be most helpful to you and why?
Q4: In the light of the clinical presentation, how would you interpret the laboratory test results?
Q5: What is your final hypothesis?
Q6: What issues in the given history, examination and laboratory tests support your final hypothesis?

Clinical cases

● CASE 4.1 – I do not know what is wrong with my child.

Nagi Mourice came with his mother, Mary, to see the local doctor. His mother is worried because Nagi is two and a half years old but is still unable to stand and walk. Further history reveals that Nagi has had six to seven attacks of loose bowel motions over the last 10 months and was admitted to hospital overseas on several occasions to treat his diarrhoea. The family migrated to Australia from southern Sudan as refugees a few months ago. Nagi has had no recent attacks of diarrhoea. On examination, there is an obvious delay in Nagi's growth and development. Only one tooth has erupted. There are no signs of dehydration and vital signs are normal.

● Abdomen is protruded but no tenderness.

● Both legs are bowed.

● Neurological examination is normal.

● Cardiovascular and respiratory systems are normal.

● CASE 4.2 – I was asked to see you by the insurance company.

Raj Succina, a 51-year-old train driver, comes in to see Dr Maureen Fisher for a routine check-up for life insurance. Raj migrated with his family to Australia 7 years ago. He has no complaints although he has noticed recently that he gets a little short of breath when walking. He also has gained 23 kg in body weight over the last 3 years. He has not seen a doctor for over 2 years. He has no family history of diabetes or high blood lipids. He does not drink alcohol. On examination, there is no pallor or yellowish discoloration of the sclera, and no spider naevi or palmar erythema. Examination of the cardiovascular and respiratory systems is normal. His body mass index (BMI) is 34 and his vital signs are shown in Table 4.1.

Table 4.1 Vital signs for Case 4.2

Vital signs	Raj's results	Normal range
Blood pressure (mmHg)	190/105	100/60–135/85
Pulse rate (/min)	95	60–100
Respiratory rate (/min)	18	12–16
Temperature (°C)	37	36.6–37.2

- His liver is palpable 3 cm below the costal margin. There are no signs of chronic liver disease.

- Spleen is not palpable; no shifting dullness on abdominal percussion.

- No palpable abdominal masses; no shifting dullness on percussion of the abdomen.

- No oedema of lower limbs.

CASE 4.3 – Sam was really sick when he arrived at the accident and emergency department.

Sam Michael, a primary school student in year 2, is brought by ambulance to the accident and emergency (A&E) department of a local hospital because of sudden severe shortness of breath and nausea; he vomited twice while on the way to the hospital. Sam's mother, Noreen, who came with him says: 'Sam had mild abdominal discomfort a few hours ago and then suddenly became short of breath. He drinks a lot of water and about eight to ten cans of Coca-Cola every day. He goes to the toilet a lot to pass water. I try to stop him from drinking soft drinks but he always feels thirsty and passes a lot of water.' Despite an increase in his appetite, he has recently lost about 2 kg in body weight.

On examination, Sam looks tired, pale and anxious. His tongue is dry. His vital signs are normal except for an increased respiratory rate (22/min). His breath smells sweet. Examination of the cardiovascular and respiratory systems is normal. Abdominal examination shows no rigidity or tenderness.

👥 Integrated medical sciences questions

⚫ CASE 4.1 – Briefly discuss the bone cells and their functions. Discuss the hormonal control of bone mineral metabolism. You may use diagrams to illustrate your answer.

⚫ CASE 4.2 – Discuss the mechanisms underlying Raj's raised blood glucose.

⚫ CASE 4.3 – Discuss the pathophysiological and pathological changes responsible for Sam's shortness of breath, vomiting and polyuria.

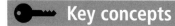 **Key concepts**

To work through the core clinical cases in this chapter, you will need to understand the following key concepts.

The vitamins

- Vitamins are organic compounds that occur in small concentrations in food.

- There are about 13 known vitamins and each one has specific physiological functions in the cells of our bodies.

- The lack or deficiency of one vitamin may interfere with the function of our body systems, producing diseases; in addition excessive intake of vitamins is not desirable and may produce undesirable toxic effects (e.g. vitamin A or vitamin B_6 toxicity).

The fat-soluble vitamins and diseases that may cause a deficiency of fat-soluble vitamins

- Vitamin A (retinol): its major sources are cod liver oil, lambs' liver and vitamin A precursors (carotenes).

- Vitamin D: several forms of vitamin D occur in nature – vitamin D_2 (ergocalciferol) and vitamin D_3 (cholecalciferol). Both these vitamins are formed by the ultraviolet irradiation of two provitamins: provitamin D_2 (ergosterol), found in yeasts, and provitamin D_3 (7-dehydrocholesterol), found in the skin. Other sources are butter, eggs and margarine.

- Vitamin E: exists in several forms. The main dietary sources of vitamin E are vegetable oils, polyunsaturated fatty acids and nuts.

- Vitamin K: two forms of vitamin K occur naturally, vitamin K_1 (phylloquinone) and vitamin K_2 (menoquinone), which is synthesized by the intestinal bacteria. The only synthetic form of vitamin K is known as vitamin K_3 (menadione). It has been estimated that about 50 per cent of our body requirement of vitamin K is obtained from the bacteria inhibiting the gut, while the other 50 per cent is obtained from the diet. The main nutritional sources of vitamin K are: green leafy vegetables, fruits and most animal products.

Diseases associated with malabsorption of fat and disturbance of the enterohepatic circulation of bile salts are associated with deficiency of fat-soluble vitamins and supplements of these vitamin may be provided by intramuscular injection.

The endocrine cells of the pancreas and their functions

Approximately 1 million islets of Langerhans are distributed throughout the human pancreas. These islets constitute the endocrine pancreas. The cells in Table 4.2 compose the parenchyma of the islet of Langerhans.

Table 4.2 Cells of the islets of Langerhans

Cells	Hormone produced by the cell	Function
α	Glucagon	Raises blood glucose level
β	Insulin	Lowers blood glucose level
δ	Somatostatin	Inhibits hormone release and reduces contractions of the gallbladder
PP	Pancreatic polypeptide	Inhibits exocrine secretion of the pancreas
G	Gastrin	Stimulates the production of hydrochloric acid by parietal cells of the stomach

The functions of insulin

Insulin is an anabolic hormone. It produces the following metabolic changes:

- Promotes the uptake of glucose by body cells (e.g. muscle and adipose tissue)
- Promotes glycogen synthesis
- Inhibits glycogenolysis and gluconeogenesis
- Promotes amino acid uptake and protein synthesis
- Promotes fatty acid, triglyceride (TG) and VLDL synthesis
- Inhibits pathways of fatty acid oxidation
- Inhibits pathways of fatty acid oxidation and the hormone-sensitive lipase in adipose tissue
- Stimulates lipoprotein lipase (located in the cell surface of vascular endothelium), causing release of free fatty acids from lipoprotein particles and therefore promotes storage of fat in the periphery (e.g. adipose tissue).

Does all body tissue require insulin receptors to facilitate the uptake of glucose?

Insulin promotes the uptake of glucose in muscle and adipose tissue. However, some cells lack receptors for insulin yet the insulin-independent cells are able to use glucose as a source of energy. These cells are:

- brain cells
- renal tubular cells
- red blood cells.

The metabolic consequences of a lack of insulin

- Activation of the glycogenolysis and gluconeogenesis pathways in the liver
- Inhibition of fatty acid and lipoprotein synthesis within the liver and activation of fatty acid oxidation and ketone formation
- Activation of hormone-sensitive lipase (in the periphery) causing breakdown of TGs to generate free fatty acids and glycerol. Both used by the liver in the gluconeogenesis pathway
- Breakdown of muscle protein resulting in the release of amino acids into the bloodstream; amino acids are used by the liver in the gluconeogenesis pathway.

Answers

 CASE 4.1 – I do not know what is wrong with my child.

Q1: What are the possible causes for the presenting problem?

A1

The following are possible causes (hypotheses) for Nagi's bowing legs and delayed teething:

- Malabsorption of fats and fat-soluble vitamins (e.g. vitamin D)

- Inadequate sunlight exposure (important in vitamin D metabolism)

- Kidney problem (impaired renal 1α-hydroxylation of 25-hydroxyvitamin D)

- Liver disease (impaired hepatic 25-hydroxylation of vitamin D)

- Nutritional deficiency (lack of intake of proteins, vitamin D and calcium-rich food)

- Problems with digestion, absorption and metabolism (decreased bioavailability of vitamin D)

- Impaired renal reabsorption of phosphorous (an X-linked disorder)

- Failure to thrive (repeated attacks of diarrhoea, lack of support, education, resources, health services, preventive measures, proper antenatal care and early management).

 ## Q2: What further questions would you like to ask to help you differentiate between your hypotheses?

A2

Further history questions: you may ask Nagi's mother about the questions in Table 4.3.

Table 4.3 Further history questions for Case 4.1

History questions	In what way answers can help
Nagi's nutritional intake (type and quantity of food including calcium-, protein- and vitamin D-rich food)	Assess nutritional intake and whether nutrition is responsible for his problem
Details of immunization, any illnesses since his birth, causes of hospital admission and any previous investigations	Recurrent illnesses such as vomiting, diarrhoea and fever could have contributed to his problem and possibly caused chronic changes in the absorptive surface of his small intestine. Vitamin D is activated in the liver and kidney, and diseases that may affect these organs should be excluded
Details of antenatal care and any illnesses during the mother's pregnancy	To assess for illnesses that may have occurred during pregnancy and affected his postnatal health and development

Exposure to sun rays, symptoms suggestive of kidney
troubles or malabsorption

Type of support available to the family, stresses in the family and possibly the need for a social worker to visit the family and help them	Failure to thrive may be related to lack of family support and financial troubles
Family history	To assess for familial and genetic diseases, and infectious diseases in the family
Any history of allergies?	
Medications	

 Q3: What investigations would be most helpful to you and why?

A3

Further investigations

- Full blood examination

- Blood urea and creatinine

- Blood calcium, phosphate and albumin levels

- Radiographs of both legs.

 CASE 4.2 – I was asked to see you by the insurance company.

Q1: What are the possible causes for the presenting problem?

A1

The following are possible causes (hypotheses) for Raj's presentation:

- Metabolic syndrome X

- Diabetes mellitus (type 2)

- Fatty infiltration of the liver (because of uncontrolled diabetes and possibly raised blood lipids)

- Alcohol-associated liver diseases (e.g. fatty liver).

The following are less likely causes:

- Anaemia causing shortness of breath (no pallor)

- Enlargement of the liver and shortness of breath of breath as a result of congestive heart failure (examination of cardiovascular system is normal and no oedema of lower limbs)

- Enlargement of liver as a result of chronic liver problem (no splenomegaly, no ascites, no stigmata of chronic liver disease, no jaundice); however, it will be necessary to do a few laboratory tests to exclude other conditions that might cause enlargement of the liver

- Chronic renal failure (however, it will be necessary to assess his kidney function because he is hypertensive).

 Q2: What further questions would you like to ask to help you differentiate between your hypotheses?

A2

Table 4.4 Further history questions for Case 4.2

History questions	In what way answers can help
Changes in calorie intake, eating habits, exercise, lifestyle and alcohol intake	Excessive eating of fats and proteins after immigration and shifting to western style of life. Excessive alcohol intake may cause steatohepatitis and fatty liver disease
Any recent symptoms, laboratory investigations or medications	Might help in diagnosis and duration of the problem (e.g. raised blood glucose, abnormal liver function tests, raised blood urea or creatinine, raised blood cholesterol or triglycerides [TGs])
Past history of blood transfusion, tattooing, intravenous drug use or viral infection	Useful in the assessment of his enlarged liver
Family history of diabetes mellitus, dyslipidaemia, metabolic disorders, obesity, high blood pressure	Type 2 diabetes mellitus is likely to occur in obese people particularly those with a family history of the disease

 Q3: What investigations would be most helpful to you and why?

A3

Further investigations

- Full blood examination
- Fasting blood glucose and blood lipids
- Liver function tests
- Blood urea, creatinine and electrolytes
- Ultrasound or magnetic resonance imaging (MRI) of the upper abdomen
- Liver biopsy
- Urinalysis.

⬤ **CASE 4.3 – Sam was really sick when he arrived at the A&E department.**

 Q1: What are the possible causes for the presenting problem?

A1

The following are possible causes (hypotheses) for Sam's presentation:

● Diabetic ketoacidosis and uncontrolled type 1 diabetes mellitus (may explain his acute illness as well as his polyuria, polyphagia, weight loss and sweet breath)

● Uncontrolled type 1 diabetes mellitus (may explain his polyuria, polyphagia and weight loss)

● Diabetes insipidus (lack of antidiuretic hormone [ADH] or failure of ADH to act on renal tubules, although diabetes insipidus cannot explain his acute illness, polyphagia and weight loss)

● Chronic renal failure

● Food poisoning, acute gastroenteritis (may explain his acute illness but not his polyuria, polyphagia and weight loss).

The following are less likely causes:

● Acute abdominal conditions such as acute appendicitis (no fever, no abdominal rigidity or tenderness)

● Pneumonia or other conditions affecting the respiratory system

● Acute viral hepatitis or biliary condition

● Renal colic

● Bowel obstruction

● Disturbance of the thirst regulatory system (caused by central nervous system problem).

Q2: What further questions would you like to ask to help you differentiate between your hypotheses?

A2

Table 4.5 Further history questions for Case 4.3

History questions	In what way answers can help
Constitutional symptoms (fatigue, tiredness, blurred vision, thirst, urine colour)	These symptoms might occur as a result of lack of insulin and the use of glucose as an energy source. The urine is extremely diluted in uncontrolled diabetes and in diabetes mellitus. Blurring of vision may occur in uncontrolled diabetes mellitus as a result of increased osmolality of the liquid in the eyeball
Any history of diarrhoea and past medical history	Food poisoning is usually associated with vomiting and loose bowel motions
Diet history and medications	To assess possible causes for his diarrhoea. Some medications may precipitate the appearance of diabetes, e.g. corticosteroids

Q3: What investigations would be most helpful to you and why?

A3

Further investigations

- Urinalysis (for glucose and ketone bodies)
- Fasting blood glucose
- Blood urea, creatinine and electrolytes
- Arterial blood gases
- Full blood examination.

Further progress

 CASE 4.1 – I do not know what is wrong with my child.

The doctor arranges some tests for Nagi. The results are shown in Table 4.6.

Table 4.6 Test results for Case 4.1

Test	Nagi's results	Normal range
Serum phosphate (mmol/L)	0.6	0.8–1.4
Serum calcium (mmol/L)	1.9	2.2–2.6
Serum alkaline phosphatase (ALP) (U/L)	270	30–150
Radiograph of lower limbs	Bowed femurs are evident bilaterally. At the distal ends of the femurs, the growth plates are wide and flared and display an irregular hazy appearance at the diaphyseal line	–

Full blood examination: normal

Blood urea, creatinine, sodium and potassium levels: normal

Serum bilirubin, albumin, aspartate transaminase (AST) and alanine transaminase (ALT) levels: normal.

CASE 4.2 – I was asked to see you by the insurance company.

Dr Fisher arranges for some tests for Raj. The results are shown in Table 4.7.

Table 4.7 Test results for Case 4.2

Test	Raj's results	Normal range
Urine glucose	++	Negative
Urine ketone bodies	Negative	Negative
Fasting blood glucose (mmol/L)	7.9	3.6–5.3
Blood cholesterol (mmol/L)	6.8	2.0–5.5
Blood TGs (mmol/L)	3.6	0.5–2.0
HDL-cholesterol (mmol/L)	0.65	0.9–2.2

Full blood examination: normal,

Blood urea, creatinine, sodium and potassium levels: normal,

Serum bilirubin, albumin, AST and alkaline phosphatase (ALP) levels: normal.

Ultrasound of the upper abdomen: normal shape and size of both kidneys. Pancreas is normal. Liver changes suggestive of hepatic steatosis.

CASE 4.3 – Sam was really sick when he arrived in the A&E department.

The A&E registrar arranges for some tests for Sam. The results are shown in Tables 4.8 and 4.9.

Table 4.8 Test results for Case 4.3

Test	Sam's results	Normal range
Urine glucose	++++	Negative
Urine ketone bodies	++++	Negative
Blood glucose (mmol/L)	47.8	3.6–5.3
Serum sodium (mmol/L)	133	135–145
Serum potassium (mmol/L)	5.4	3.5–5.0
Blood urea (mmol/L)	8.1	2.5–8.3
Serum creatinine (mmol/L)	0.11	0.05–0.11

Table 4.9 Arterial blood gases for Case 4.3

Test	Sam's results	Normal range
pH	7.13	7.38–7.44
P_{O_2} (mmHg)[a]	100 (13.3)	80–100 (10.6–13.3)
P_{CO_2} (mmHg)[a]	13 (1.7)	35–45 (4.5–6)
Bicarbonate (mmol/L)	9	21–28

[a]Values in parentheses are in kilopascals.

Full blood examination: normal.

Further questions

 CASE 4.1 – I do not know what is wrong with my child.

Q4: In the light of the clinical presentation, how would you interpret the laboratory test results?

A4

Table 4.10 Interpretation of lab test results for Case 4.1

Test	Change	Interpretation
Serum phosphate	Low	Low serum phosphate and serum calcium may be present in rickets
Serum calcium	Low	
Serum ALP	Raised	Serum ALP is raised in rickets and osteomalacia
Blood urea, creatinine and electrolytes	Normal	The bone problem (leg bowing) is not caused by chronic renal failure
Serum bilirubin, albumin, AST, ALT	Normal	The problem is less likely to result from liver disorders. 25-Hydroxylation of vitamin D normally occurs in the liver
Full blood count	Normal	No anaemia and chronic renal failure is less likely
Radiograph of lower limbs	Changes suggestive of rickets	Lack of mineralization of bone and cartilage

 Q5: What is your final hypothesis?

A5

The clinical picture and laboratory results are suggestive of rickets.

 Q6: What issues in the given history, examination and laboratory tests support your final hypothesis?

A6

Supportive evidence

History

- The patient is two and a half years old but is still unable to stand and walk.

- He has had six to seven attacks of loose bowel motions over the last 10 months.

- He was admitted to hospital overseas on several occasions to treat his diarrhoea.

- The family migrated to Australia from southern Sudan as refugees a few months ago.

- Nagi has had no recent attacks of diarrhoea.

Examination

- There is an obvious delay in the patient's growth and development

- Only one tooth has erupted.

- No signs of dehydration.

- Vital signs are normal.

- Abdomen is protruded but no tenderness.

- Both legs are bowed.

- Neurological examination is normal.

- Cardiovascular and respiratory systems are normal.

Investigations

- Serum calcium: low

- Serum phosphate: low

- Serum ALP: raised

- Blood urea, creatinine and electrolytes: normal

- Serum bilirubin, albumin, AST and ALT: normal

- Full blood examination: normal

- Radiograph of lower limbs: changes suggestive of rickets.

CASE 4.2 – I was asked to see you by the insurance company.

Q4: In the light of the clinical presentation, how would you interpret the laboratory test results?

A4

Table 4.11 Interpretation of test results for Case 4.2

Test	Changes	Interpretation
Urine glucose and ketone	Glucose ++	Suggestive of raised blood glucose above the renal threshold
	Ketone negative	Absence of ketone bodies suggests that insulin is not lacking and there is no excessive β oxidation of fatty acids
Fasting blood glucose	Raised	1. Insulin resistance secondary to obesity and possibly fewer insulin receptors in skeletal muscle, liver and adipose tissue
		2. Resistance may also be caused by abnormalities of the signalling pathways responsible for activation of cellular elements following receptor stimulation
		3. The β cells of the pancreas gradually become exhausted from secreting large amounts of insulin
		The effects of these three mechanisms are failure of effective utilization of glucose by body cells and increased blood glucose levels
Blood cholesterol and TGs	Raised	Mainly as a result of impaired VLDL clearance and downregulation of the LDL receptors
Ultrasound examination of the liver	Changes suggestive of hepatic steatosis	Fatty infiltration of the liver

LDL, low-density lipoprotein; VLDL, very-low-density lipoprotein.

Q5: What is your final hypothesis?

A5

The clinical picture and laboratory results are suggestive of metabolic syndrome X (obesity, uncontrolled type 2 diabetes mellitus, dyslipidaemia) and hepatic steatosis.

Q6: What issues in the given history, examination and laboratory tests support your final hypothesis?

A6

Supportive evidence

History

- The patient presents with shortness of breath, obesity, high blood pressure.
- There is no pallor or yellowish discoloration of the sclera.

Examination

- The cardiovascular and respiratory systems are normal.
- The liver is palpable 3 cm below the right costal margin.
- There is no splenomegaly, oedema of lower limbs or ascites.
- There are no stigmata of chronic liver disease (palmar erythema or spider naevi).

Investigations

- Fasting blood sugar: raised
- Blood cholesterol: raised
- Blood TGs: raised
- Urine glucose: ++, ketone bodies: negative
- Ultrasound examination of the liver: changes suggestive of hepatic steatosis.

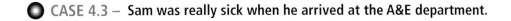 **CASE 4.3 – Sam was really sick when he arrived at the A&E department.**

 Q4: In the light of the clinical presentation, how would you interpret the laboratory test results?

A4

Table 4.12 Interpretation of lab test results for Case 4.3

Test	Changes	Interpretation
Urine glucose	++++	Lack of insulin secretion causes: failure of body cells such as muscle and liver cells to utilize glucose and use it as a source of energy; and accumulation of glucose in circulation (hyperglycaemia) as a result of these metabolic changes

Urine ketone bodies	++++	Insulin lack also causes excessive amounts of acetoacetic acid (a ketone body) to be formed in the liver cells. The mechanism responsible for the formation of ketone bodies is: Lack of insulin → excessive use of fat by liver cells as a source of energy → transport of fatty acids into the mitochondria of liver cells → β oxidation of the fatty acids in mitochondria → production of excess amounts of acetyl-CoA → formation of acetoacetic acid → release into the circulation. Some of the acetoacetic acid is converted to β-hydroxybutyric acid and acetone (ketone bodies). Excess ketone bodies in blood → acidosis → stimulation of compensatory mechanisms to correct blood pH back to normal: (1) secretion of ketone bodies in urine; (2) secretion of ketone bodies into stomach; (3) irritation of the stomach by ketone bodies and vomiting; and stimulation of chemoreceptors → increased respiratory rate (to get rid of CO_2 and hence help in correction of blood pH)
Blood glucose	Raised	Lack of insulin secretion from β cells of islet of Langerhans causes (1) failure of muscle and liver cells to use glucose as a source of: energy; (2) hyperglycaemia; and fat breakdown and the use of fat as a source of energy (lipolysis of storage fat and release of free fatty acids)
Serum sodium	Low	Secondary to loss of fluids in vomiting and urine
Serum potassium	Increased	Secondary to acidosis (decreased uptake of potassium by cells)
Blood urea	Close to upper normal limit	Possibly as a result of decreased renal perfusion (secondary to excessive loss of fluids in vomiting and urine)
Serum creatinine	Close to upper limit of normal	Possibly because of decreased renal perfusion (secondary to excessive loss of fluids in vomiting and urine)
Arterial blood gases	A picture suggestive of metabolic acidosis (low blood pH, low P_{CO_2} and low serum bicarbonate)	Increased ketone bodies in circulation → acidosis → stimulation of chemoreceptors → hyperventilation → CO_2 wash-out → helping in correction of acidosis

A5

Q5: What is your final hypothesis?

The clinical picture and laboratory results are suggestive of uncontrolled type 1 diabetes mellitus complicated with diabetic ketoacidosis.

Q6: What issues in the given history, examination and laboratory tests support your final hypothesis?

A6

Supportive evidence

History

- The patient presents with sudden severe shortness of breath and nausea; he vomited twice while on the way to the hospital.
- He has mild abdominal discomfort and is short of breath.
- He drinks a lot of water and about eight to ten cans of Coca-Cola every day.
- He goes to the toilet a lot to pass water.
- He always feels thirsty.
- Despite an increase in his appetite, he has recently lost about 2 kg in body weight.

Examination

- He looks tired, pale and anxious.
- His tongue is dry.
- His vital signs are normal except for increased respiratory rate (22/min).
- His breath smells sweet.
- Examination of the cardiovascular and respiratory systems is normal.
- Abdominal examination shows no rigidity or tenderness.

Investigations

- Fasting blood glucose: raised
- Urine glucose: ++++
- Urine ketone bodies: ++++
- Serum sodium: low

- Serum potassium: raised
- Blood urea and creatinine: upper limit of normal
- Arterial blood gases: a picture suggestive of metabolic acidosis (low blood pH, low $P\text{co}_2$ and low serum bicarbonate).

⁞⁞ Integrated medical sciences questions

● **CASE 4.1 –** **Briefly discuss the bone cells and their functions. Discuss the hormonal control of bone mineral metabolism. You may use diagrams to illustrate your answer.**

The main types of cells found in bone are shown in Table 4.12.

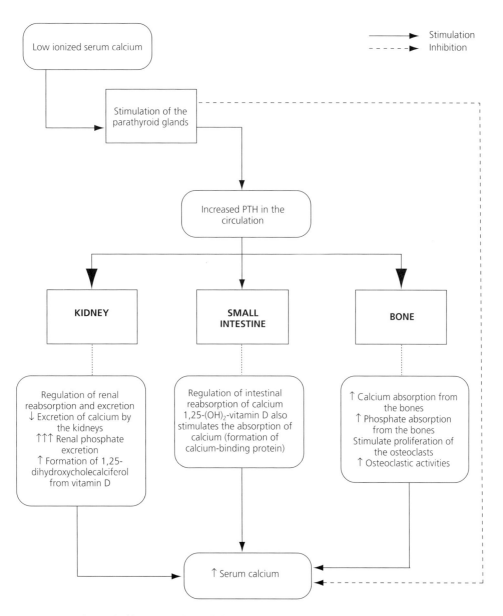

Figure 4.1 Hormonal control of bone mineral metabolism.

Table 4.12 Characteristics of main cells in bone

Bone cell	Characteristics	Function
Osteoclasts	Multinucleated giant cells	Specialized in reabsorption of bone
	Differentiated and non-dividing	Osteoclasts respond indirectly to parathyroid hormone (PTH) to mediate bone resorption
	Derived from granulocyte–macrophage stem cells in bone marrow	
Osteoblasts	Bone-forming cells	Responsible for secreting the matrix
	Arise from mesenchymal stem cells	
Osteocytes	When osteoblasts are surrounded by matrix, they become quiescent and become known as osteocytes	–

◉ CASE 4.2 – Discuss the mechanisms underlying Raj's raised blood glucose.

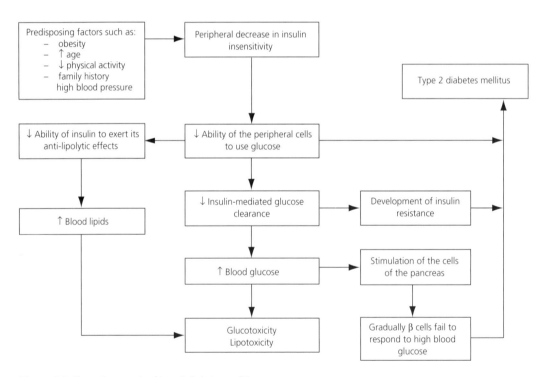

Figure 4.2 The pathogenesis of type 2 diabetes mellitus.

CASE 4.3 – Discuss the pathophysiological and pathological changes responsible for Sam's shortness of breath, vomiting and polyuria.

Predisposing factors

1. Genetic factors (e.g. HLA genes)

2. Environmental factors (e.g. viral infection, ingestion of toxins).

The genetic predisposing factors + environmental triggers (e.g. post-viral infection – Coxsackie virus, rubella or viral gastroenteritis) → development of autoantibodies to islet cells antigens + development of cell-mediated immunological reaction → insulinitis and destruction of the pancreatic β cells (mononuclear infiltration of the pancreatic islands) → decreased production of insulin by β cells of the pancreas ± increased glucagon hormone. The metabolic consequences of low blood insulin are:

- inhibition of protein synthesis

- increased protein breakdown and increased serum amino acids

- decreased uptake of glucose into muscles, liver and adipose tissue

- increased breakdown of fuel stores (glycogen and TG)

- inhibition of gluconeogenesis.

As a result of these metabolic changes → increased blood glucose + increased amino acids and free fatty acids in blood + loss of weight (caused by breakdown of proteins) → failure to use glucose by body cells to provide energy → the blood glucose concentration being higher than the normal renal threshold → appearance of large amounts of glucose in the urine → osmotic diuresis (*polyuria*).

The body starts to use free fatty acids to provide energy → fatty acids moving from blood to the liver → in the liver mitochondria, free fatty acids converted to coenzyme A thioesters → formation of ketone bodies (acetone, acetoacetic acid and β-hydroxybutyric acid) in the mitochondria → ketone bodies moving from the liver to the peripheral circulation (ketone bodies are acidic) → development of metabolic acidosis → stimulation of defence mechanisms to allow the blood pH return to normal range:

- Ketone bodies are excreted in the urine.

- Stimulation of the chemoreceptors → *reflex increase in the respiratory rate* (exhalation of ketone bodies in the lungs – characteristic odour of the patient's breath).

- Ketone bodies are used as a source of energy by the muscles and contribute to fuel homoeostasis.

- Ketone bodies are excreted into the stomach → irritation of the mucosal membrane lining the stomach → *nausea and vomiting*. Ketone bodies may also act centrally and stimulate the vomiting centre in the brain stem → *nausea and vomiting*.

Normally, the brain cells use glucose as the main source of energy. With the lack of insulin, the brain cells fail to find their fuel (glucose). Ketone bodies cannot be used by the brain cells because they lack an enzyme that enables the conversion of ketone bodies to acetyl-CoA. If the condition continues, as in starvation, within 4–5 days the enzyme is induced and ketone bodies are used by the brain cells as a source of energy.

Further reading

Fisher RM, Gertow K. Fatty acid transport and insulin resistance. *Current Opinion in Lipidology* 2005;**16**:173–178.

Freeland BS. Diabetes ketoacidosis. *Diabetes Educator* 2003;**29**:384 –392, 394–395.

Guthrie RA, Guthrie DW. Pathophysiology of diabetes mellitus. *Critical Care Nursing Quarterly* 2004;**27**:113–125.

Hensrud DD. Diet and obesity. *Current Opinion in Gastroenterology* 2004;**20**:119–124.

Kaufman FR. Type 1 diabetes mellitus. *Pediatrics in Review* 2003;**24**:291–300.

Ladhani S, Srinivasan L, Buchanan C, Allgrove J. Presentation of vitamin D deficiency. *Archives of Disease in Childhood* 2004;**89**:781–784.

Mastorakos G, Zapanti E. The hypothalamic–pituitary–adrenal axis in the neuroendocrine regulation of food intake and obesity: The role of corticotrophin releasing hormone. *Nutritional Neuroscience* 2004;**7**:271–280.

Pettifor JM. Nutritional rickets: deficiency of vitamin D, calcium or both? *American Journal of Clinical Nutrition* 2004;**80**(suppl 6):1725S–1729S.

Shaw NJ. Vitamin D deficiency rickets. *Endocrine Development* 2003;**6**:93–104.

Sjoholm A, Nystrom T. Endothelial inflammation in insulin resistance. *Journal of Nephrology* 2005;**12**:610–612.

Tsakiris D, Ioannon K. An underdiagnosed type of diabetes: The MODY syndrome. Pathophysiology, clinical presentation and renal disease progression. *American Journal of Nephrology* 2004;**17**:637–641.

Wharton B, Bishop N. Rickets. *Lancet* 2003;**362**:1389–1400.

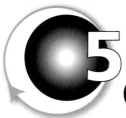

5 Cardiovascular system

? **Questions for each of the case scenarios given**

Q1: What are the possible causes for the presenting problem?
Q2: What further questions would you like to ask to help you differentiate between your hypotheses?
Q3: What investigations would be most helpful to you and why?
Q4: In the light of the clinical presentation, how would you interpret the laboratory test results?
Q5: What is your final hypothesis?
Q6: What issues in the given history, examination and laboratory tests support your final hypothesis?

Clinical cases

● CASE 5.1 – Suddenly I became short of breath.

Desmond Farrell, a 56-year-old manager, undergoes a right hip replacement for severe degenerative joint disease. On day 4 after surgery, he develops sudden shortness of breath and chest pain. He smoked 30 cigarettes per day for over 20 years but ceased smoking 3 years ago. He had a past history of bronchial asthma during primary school.

On examination, he looks anxious and breathless. His body mass index (BMI) is 30. His vital signs are shown in Table 5.1.

Table 5.1 Vital signs for Case 5.1

Vital signs	Desmond's results	Normal range
Blood pressure (mmHg)	100/70	100/60–135/85
Pulse rate (/min)	140, regular	60–100
Respiratory rate (/min)	28	12–16
Temperature (°C)	37	36.6–37.2

- Lung examination: normal.

- Cardiac examination: no abnormality apart from tachycardia.

- Lower limb examination: the surgical wound on the right leg is healing well. Calf muscles on the right side are tender, warm and swollen. The left leg is normal.

● CASE 5.2 – I was treated with warfarin for deep venous thrombosis.

Mr Brendan McCallum, a 77-year-old pensioner, is brought by ambulance to the accident and emergency (A&E) department because of low blood pressure, shortness of breath, fever and rigors. Brendan has a recent history of deep venous thrombosis and has been on warfarin tablets for the last 2 months. He also has a history of hypertension and diabetes for over 15 years. He was catheterized on two recent occasions because of urinary retention.

On examination, he is pale and breathless. His vital signs are shown in Table 5.2.

Table 5.2 Vital signs for Case 5.2

Vital signs	Brendan's results	Normal range
Blood pressure (mmHg)	70/60	100/60–135/85
Pulse rate (/min)	120	60–100
Respiratory rate (/min)	28	12–16
Temperature (°C)	38.8	36.6–37.2

Cardiovascular and respiratory examinations

- Inaudible heart sounds

- Bilateral crackles on both lung bases.

Abdominal examination

- Fullness and tenderness in both loins

- He was unable to pass urine for laboratory analysis.

● CASE 5.3 – My heart has never fluttered like this before.

Ozlem Maden, a 25 year old, is brought by ambulance to a local hospital because of a sudden onset of palpitations, severe shortness of breath and coughing. Ozlem arrived by aeroplane last night from Turkey and she intends to spend 4 weeks with her married sister who lives in Victoria. She gives a history of palpitations for over a year, lasting a few hours to a maximum of 2 days but she has never had shortness of breath. She coughs repeatedly and produces a small amount of whitish, frothy sputum with streaks of blood. Her last menstrual period was 10 days ago.

On examination, she has ruddy cheeks, cyanosed lips and her vital signs are shown in Table 5.3.

Table 5.3 Vital signs for Case 5.3

Vital signs	Ozlem's results	Normal range
Blood pressure (mmHg)	100/60	100/60–135/85
Pulse rate (/min)	120, irregularly irregular	60–100
Respiratory rate (/min)	24	12–16
Temperature (°C)	36.9	36.6–37.2

Cardiovascular and respiratory examination

- Jugular venous pressure (JVP) not raised

- Apex beat at the left fifth intercostal space midclavicular line

- Heart rate irregularly irregular

- Loud S1 (first hear sound) and low-pitched rumbling diastolic murmur at the apex
- Bilateral inspiratory crackles heard over both lungs.

Abdominal examination

- Normal

ii Integrated medical sciences questions

● CASE 5.1 – Discuss the mechanism underlying Desmond's shortness of breath.

● CASE 5.2 – Briefly list the changes that may occur in peripheral circulation in septic shock.

● CASE 5.3 – Briefly discuss the pathogenesis and the pathology underlying Ozlem's condition.

Key concepts

In order to work through the core clinical cases in this chapter, you will need to understand the following key concepts.

Heart failure

Heart failure is defined as cardiac dysfunction resulting in inadequate perfusion of tissue with oxygen and nutrients. Most causes of heart failure result from dysfunction of the left ventricle (left-sided heart failure). The right ventricle may also become dysfunctional (right-sided heart failure or congestive heart failure). Heart failure is usually a consequence of left ventricular failure. Right-sided heart failure may also occur as a consequence of pulmonary hypertension resulting from pulmonary parenchymal or pulmonary vascular disease (cor pulmonale or pulmonary heart disease). Some conditions cause inadequate perfusion despite normal or elevated cardiac out put (high output failure).

Left ventricular hypertrophy

Left ventricular hypertrophy may occur as a result of: (1) high blood pressure, (2) aortic valve stenosis and (3) cardiomyopathy. In patients with aortic stenosis or hypertension, the stimulus to ventricular hypertrophy is sustained load on the left ventricle, resulting in mechanical effects and release of growth factors. Hypertrophy renders the myocardium stiff and, as a result, ventricular compliance and stroke volume are both decreased.

Causes of cell injury

- Hypoxia
- Microbial agents (viruses, bacteria, fungi, rickettsiae and parasites)
- Immunological reactions
- Nutritional deficiencies
- Ageing
- Physical agents, e.g. trauma, extremes of temperature
- Chemical agents
- Genetic defects
- Necrosis.

A number of sequences of morphological changes follow cell death in living tissues (e.g. coagulative necrosis). The processes responsible for necrosis are (1) enzyme digestion of the cell or (2) denaturation of the cell proteins.

Myocardial infarction

This is the development of a definite area of myocardial necrosis caused by local cardiac ischaemia (a decreased blood and oxygen supply). Myocardial infarction usually results from coronary artery thrombosis.

Table 5.4 The differences between a blood clot and a thrombosis

Item	Blood clot	Thrombosis
Occurrence	In tissue when blood escapes out of vessels In blood vessels after death In a test tube	Within the heart or blood vessels of a living organism
Composition	A blood clot is composed of fibrin with entrapped platelets and red cells	A thrombus is composed of layers of aggregated platelets and fibrin
Formation	Blood stasis outside blood vessels	Requires the so-called Virchow's triad: (1) endothelial damage; (2) stasis; and (3) blood hypercoagulability

Table 5.5 The main histological differences of arteries, arterioles and large veins

Artery	Tunica intima	Tunica media	Tunica adventitia
Aorta (elastic arteries)	Endothelium Basal lamina Subendothelial layer Internal elastic lamina	Elastic membrane Smooth muscle cells Thin external elastic lamina	Thin Mainly fibroelastic connective tissue Vasa vasorum Lymphatics Nerve fibres
Arteriole	Endothelium Basal lamina Thin subendothelial layer Some elastic fibres (no internal elastic lamina)	One to two layers of smooth muscle cells	Loose connective tissues Nerve fibres
Large vein	Endothelium Basal lamina Valves Subendothelial connective tissue	Connective tissue Smooth muscle cells	Smooth muscle cells (longitudinal bundles) Collagen Few fibroblasts

The risk factors responsible for the development of atherosclerosis

Age: risk increases after the age of 40.

Sex: males are much more prone to atherosclerosis.

Familial/genetics: most probably polygenic.

Hyperlipidaemia: high levels of low-density lipoprotein (LDL)-cholesterol and low levels of high-density lipoprotein (HDL).

Hypertension: both high systolic and high diastolic blood pressure increase the risk.

Diabetes mellitus: increased risk of atherosclerosis, myocardial infarction and strokes.

Cigarette smoking: heavy smoking increases the risk of death from ischaemic heart disease.

Obesity: possibly because of the development of diabetes and hyperlipidaemia.

Multiple risk factors may be present and cause a multiplicative effect.

Table 5.6 The main differences between warfarin and heparin

Item	Warfarin	Heparin
What are they?	Oral anticoagulant Acts only in vivo	A family of sulphated glycosaminoglycans (mucopolysaccharides). Doses are specified in units of activity. Given by subcutaneous or intravenous routes (intramuscular injections cause haematomas) Acts in vivo and in vitro
Mechanisms of action	Warfarin interferes with the post-translational γ-carboxylation of glutamic acid residues in clotting factors II, VII, IX and X Warfarin prevents the reduction of vitamin K (warfarin is structurally similar to vitamin K)	Heparin activates anti-thrombin III and accelerates the rate of action of anti-thrombin III (heparin – anti-thrombin III complex) → inhibition of thrombin (IIa) and Xa Low-molecular-weight (LMW) heparins increase the action of anti-thrombin III on factor Xa but not its action on thrombin (IIa)
Effect	Warfarin's effect is not immediate (takes a few days) This will depend on the half-lives of these factors. Factor VII is the first to be affected (half-life = 6 hours)	Acts immediately after intravenous injections (follows saturation kinetics) Heparin: half-life 40–85 min LMW heparin: the half-life is longer and dosing is less frequent (once a day)
Factors that potentiate their actions	Liver diseases Agents that inhibit hepatic metabolism of drugs, e.g. cimetidine and amiodarone Drugs that inhibit reduction of vitamin K (e.g. cephalosporins) Drugs interfering with vitamin K availability and suppress the intestinal flora (e.g. broad-spectrum antibiotics)	Haemorrhage may occur in patients with bleeding tendencies and severe liver diseases

	Drugs that displace warfarin from binding sites on plasma albumin (e.g. non-steroidal anti-inflammatory drugs)	
	Drugs that inhibit platelet function (e.g. aspirin)	
Factors that decrease their actions	Hypothyroidism	Anti-thrombin III deficiency (is rare)
	Vitamin K	Platelets, plasma proteins and fibrin may interfere with the action of heparin
	Drugs that induce hepatic cytochrome P-450 enzymes (e.g. barbiturates, rifampicin)	
	Drugs interfering with absorption of vitamin K (e.g. cholestyramine)	
Side effects	Haemorrhage: brain, bowel	Heparin: thrombocytopenia and thrombosis, osteoporosis (long-term treatment) and possibly hypersensitivity
	Necrosis of tissues may occur	
		LMW heparin: less likely to cause thrombocytopenia and thrombosis

The main causes of pulmonary oedema

- Changes in permeability of blood capillaries, e.g. infections, acute inflammation, liquid aspiration, shock, radiation, inhaled gases

- Increased capillary hydrostatic pressure, e.g. massive myocardial infarction, severe mitral stenosis, volume overload, pulmonary vein obstruction

- Decreased oncotic pressure, e.g. liver disease, nephritic syndrome

- Other causes, e.g. high altitude.

The consequences of right-sided heart failure

- Systemic venous congestion (clinically: raised JVP)

- Liver congestion (clinically: liver is palpable and tender)

- Venous stasis, decreased venous return, increased capillary permeability (clinically: pitting oedema). Usually becomes apparent first in the dependent areas of the body (feet and lower limbs). With more severe conditions, oedema becomes generalized and pleural effusion and pericardial effusion may be present. Oedema of right-sided heart failure has low protein content.

The risk factors for pulmonary embolism

- Surgery, especially major surgery (e.g. lower limb orthopaedic surgery)

- Malignancy: pelvic, abdominal, metastatic

- History of previous venous thromboembolism
- Lower limb problems: fracture, varicose veins.

Other minor risk factors

- Congenital heart disease
- Use of oral contraceptives, hormone replacement therapy
- Obesity
- Occult malignancy.

Answers

 CASE 5.1 – Suddenly I became short of breath.

 Q1: What are the possible causes for the presenting problem?

A1

Possible causes (hypotheses) for his shortness of breath:

- Pulmonary embolism

- Acute myocardial infarction

- Postoperative pulmonary collapse/pleurisy

- Bronchial asthma (less likely).

 Q2: What further questions would you like to ask to help you differentiate between your hypotheses?

A2

Table 5.7 Further history questions to ask Case 5.1

History questions	In what way answers can help
Details about his chest pain including site, character, duration, severity and radiation of his pain, and what brings his pain on and what relieves it	This might help to differentiate between chest pain caused by myocardial infarction and pain caused by pulmonary embolism and pleurisy
Any associated symptoms such as fainting and excessive sweating	Patients with massive pulmonary embolism may present with fainting and sympathetic stimulation (excessive sweating)
Any history of sweating, cough and fever	To assess for the possibility of infection (e.g. pneumonia)
Any history of angina	Desmond has a number of risk factors for cardiovascular disease and atherosclerosis (obesity, male sex, age and long history of smoking); he might also have angina or have been investigated for chest pain
Medications and allergy	To assess his current medications and drugs that may interfere with the management of his pulmonary embolism/myocardial infarction

Q3: What investigations would be most helpful to you and why?

A3

Further investigations

- Chest radiograph
- Arterial blood gases
- Ventilation–perfusion scan
- ECG
- Venous duplex scanning, lower limbs
- Cardiac enzymes.

CASE 5.2 – I was treated with warfarin for deep venous thrombosis.

Q1: What are the possible causes for the presenting problem?

A1

Possible causes (hypotheses) for his shortness of breath:

- Septic shock (urinary tract infection causing septicaemia)
- Myocardial infarction
- Pulmonary embolism
- Pneumonia
- Hypovolaemia (peripheral vasodilatation)
- Pericardial tamponade (bleeding into the pericardium).

Q2: What further questions would you like to ask to help you differentiate between your hypotheses?

A2

Table 5.8 Further history questions for Case 5.2

History questions	In what way answers can help
Any changes in conscious state, confusion and disorientation	In septic shock, patients develop encephalopathy and become disoriented and confused
Details about warfarin therapy and whether he is taking proper dose and regular review with his doctor for the INR test. What was the result of his most recent INR test?	If he was not talking warfarin therapy, he would be at a higher risk of pulmonary embolism

Any history of nose bleeding or skin spots	If he is taking an overdose of warfarin, he will be at risk of bleeding (e.g. nose bleeding, easily bruising and possibly pericardial tamponade)
Any history of fever, rigors, sweating and loin pain or pain on passing urine	To assess him in regard to upper urinary tract infection (ascending infection)
If he is aware about the cause of his urine retention and investigation results	Most probably he has an enlarged prostate
Medications	A number of drugs can interfere with warfarin's action

INR, international normalized ratio.

 Q3: What investigations would be most helpful to you and why?

A3

Further investigations

- Full blood examination
- Urea, electrolytes and creatinine
- Liver function tests
- Blood glucose (fasting)
- Blood culture
- Urine culture
- Urinalysis
- ECG, chest radiograph, echocardiogram
- International normalized ratio (INR)
- Ultrasound of the kidneys and upper abdomen.

 CASE 5.3 – My heart has never fluttered like this before.

 Q1: What are the possible causes for the presenting problem?

A1

Possible causes (hypotheses) for Ozlem's presentation:

- Rheumatic heart, mitral stenosis, left ventricular failure, pulmonary oedema and atrial fibrillation
- Pneumonia (less likely because of the auscultatory signs and absence of fever)
- Congestive, right-sided heart failure (less likely because there is no increased JVP, enlarged tender liver or oedema of lower limbs).

Q2: What further questions would you like to ask to help you differentiate between your hypotheses?

A2

Table 5.9 Further history questions for Case 5.3

History questions	In what way answers can help
Any history of shortness of breath and cough precipitated by severe exertion	Patients with mitral stenosis (MS) usually presents with shortness of breath and cough, particularly precipitated by excitation, fever, anaemia, pregnancy, sexual intercourse and atrial fibrillation (AF)
Any history of shortness of breath at night when the patient is in the recumbent position	This is likely to occur in patients with MS. It is also known as orthopnoea and paroxysmal nocturnal dyspnoea. It is the result of redistribution of blood from the dependent portions of the body to the lungs, causing pulmonary congestion and increased interstitial fluids in the lungs
Past history of rheumatic fever when a child	MS is generally rheumatic in origin. It is very rarely congenital
Any history suggestive of systemic embolization	In MS, systemic embolization may be the presenting complaint particularly in the presence of AF. Usually thrombi are formed in the left atrium of MS patients. The contributing factors for thrombi formation in the left atrium are: dilatation of the left atrium; calcification and rigidity of the mitral valve; narrowing of the mitral orifice and stagnation of blood in left atrium; and AF
Any history of coughing up blood (haemoptysis)	Coughing up blood may result from rupture of the pulmonary–bronchial venous connections secondary to pulmonary venous hypertension
Any history of swelling of her lower limbs or a feeling of nausea and upper abdominal discomfort	Patients with MS may develop right-sided heart failure manifested by oedema of the lower limbs and congestion of the liver (patient may complain of nausea and upper abdominal discomfort because of liver congestion). On examination, the liver is enlarged and tender

 Q3: What investigations would be most helpful to you and why?

A3

Further investigations

- Chest radiograph
- Echocardiography
- ECG
- Full blood examination.

Further progress

 CASE 5.1 – **Suddenly I became short of breath.**

The treating doctor arranges some tests for Desmond. The results are shown in Tables 5.10 and 5.11.

Table 5.10 Full blood examination and cardiac enzymes for Case 5.1

Test	Desmond's results	Normal range
Haemoglobin (Hb) (g/L)	130	115–160
Packed cell volume (PCV)	0.42	0.37–0.47
White blood cell count (WCC) ($\times 10^9$)	9.0	4.0–11.0
Platelet count ($\times 10^9$)	480	150–400
Serum creatine kinase (CK) (IU/L)	25	30–200
Creatine kinase MB (CK-MB) (%)	1	< 5

Table 5.11 Other test results for Case 5.1

Test	Desmond's results
Chest radiograph	Hyperinflated chest, flat diaphragm, increased anteroposterior chest diameter and a widened retrosternal air space. No lung collapse
	No changes compared with a chest radiograph taken of the patient 2 months ago
ECG	Sinus tachycardia, heart rate is 150/min. No ischaemic changes
Echocardiogram	Normal
Ventilation–perfusion scan	Normal ventilation scan
	Large defect in perfusion involving the inferior aspect of the right lung
Venous duplex scanning, lower limbs	Evidence of deep venous thrombosis above the right knee

Arterial blood gases: hypoxaemia and hypocapnia.

 CASE 5.2 – **I was treated with warfarin for deep venous thrombosis.**

The treating doctor arranges some tests for Brendan. The results are shown in Tables 5.12–5.14.

Table 5.12 Full blood examination for Case 5.2

Test	Brendan's results	Normal range
Hb (g/L)	9	115–160
PCV	0.36	0.37–0.47
WCC ($\times 10^9$)	18	4.0–11.0
Platelet count ($\times 10^9$)	120	150–400

Table 5.13 Serum biochemistry for Case 5.2

Test	Brendan's results	Normal range
Serum CK (IU/L)	45	30–200
CK-MB (per cent)	3	< 5
Serum glucose (fasting) (mmol/L)	9	3.6–5.3
Serum bilirubin (mmol/L)	21	0–19
Serum aspartate aminotransferase (AST) (IU/L)	55	0–40
Serum alanine aminotransferase (ALT) (IU/L)	45	0–55
Blood urea (mmol/L)	15	2.5–8.3
Serum creatinine (mmol/L)	0.12	0.05–0.11
Serum sodium (mmol/L)	132	135–145
Serum potassium (mmol/L)	4.5	3.5–5.0
INR	1.5	Ratio of patient time to control time

Table 5.14 Other tests for Case 5.2

Test	Brendan's results
Chest radiograph	Diffuse bilateral infiltrates
ECG	Sinus tachycardia; non-specific S-T wave abnormalities
Echocardiogram	Normal
Blood culture	No growth detected
Urine culture	Gram-negative bacilli > 10^8/L (sensitive to norfloxacin and cefazoline; resistant to ampicillin and Augmentin (amoxicillin with potassium clavulanate)

Urinalysis: protein +++, blood +++, nitrates +++, white blood cells (WBCs) +++, glucose +++, ketone bodies ++, specific gravity elevated.

● CASE 5.3 – My heart has never fluttered like this before.

The treating doctor arranges some tests for Ozlem. The results are shown in Table 5.15.

Table 5.15 Test results for Case 5.3

Test	Ozlem's results
Chest radiographs (taken after treating the patient with intravenous furosemide [Lasix] in the A&E department)	Straightening of the left border of the cardiac silhouette, prominence of the main pulmonary arteries, dilatation of the upper lobe pulmonary veins, Kerley B lines (fine, opaque, horizontal lines, most prominent in the lower and mid-lung zones)
ECG	Evidence of AF
Echocardiogram	Evidence of dilatation of left atrium, mitral valve area 0.9 cm² (normally 4–6 cm²), normal left ventricular function, no significant regurgitation from mitral valves, other heart chambers normal

Full blood examination: normal.

Further questions

 CASE 5.1 – Suddenly I became short of breath.

Q4: In the light of the clinical presentation, how would you interpret the laboratory test results?

A4

Table 5.16 Interpretation of test results for Case 5.1

Test	Change	Interpretation
Full blood examination	Normal except for the raised platelet count	His shortness of breath is less probably a result of anaemia, acute blood loss, coronary thrombosis or massive pulmonary embolism
		There is no evidence of anaemia
		Platelet count is usually raised after surgical operations
		The rise of the platelet count may have contributed to the development of deep venous thrombosis (DVT)
Serum CK and CK-MB	Normal	Myocardial infarction is less likely
Chest radiograph	Hyperinflated chest, flat diaphragm, increased anteroposterior chest diameter, and a widened retrosternal air space; no lung collapse	These changes are suggestive of emphysema
		The fact that there are no changes in his current chest radiograph compared with an old one is expected in pulmonary embolism
	No changes compared with a chest radiograph taken of the patient 2 months ago	
ECG	Sinus tachycardia, heart rate 150/min, no ischaemic changes	In patients with pulmonary embolism the most common finding on the ECG is sinus tachycardia
Ventilation–perfusion scan	Normal ventilation scan	Normally, the ventilation and perfusion of any lung segment are proportional; in pulmonary embolism, perfusion of the lung is decreased but ventilation remains normal, so the findings are consistent with pulmonary embolism
	Large defect in perfusion involving the inferior aspect of the right lung	

Arterial blood gases	Hypoxaemia and hypocapnia	These results are typical in pulmonary embolism: the extent of increase in the alveolar–arterial oxygen gradient correlates linearly with the severity of pulmonary embolism
		If the arterial blood gases are normal we cannot exclude the diagnosis because about 30 per cent of patients with pulmonary embolism have normal arterial blood gas results
Venous duplex scanning, lower limbs	Evidence of DVT above the right knee	Pulmonary embolism originates from lower limbs. The finding of DVT could help in confirming the clinical findings

 Q5: What is your final hypothesis?

A5

Deep venous thrombosis of the right leg complicated by a pulmonary embolism.

 Q6: What issues in the given history, examination and laboratory tests support your final hypothesis?

A6

Supportive evidence

History

- The patient (aged 56) undergoes a right hip replacement and develops sudden shortness of breath and chest pain on day 4 after surgery.
- A man who smoked 30 cigarettes per day for over 20 years.
- A man with a past history of bronchial asthma during primary school.

Examination

- BMI = 30
- Pulse rate = 150/min, low blood pressure and increased respiratory rate
- Afebrile
- Chest is clear on auscultation
- The surgical wound is healing well
- Right calf muscles are tender: ++
- Left leg is normal.

Investigations

- Chest radiograph: changes consistent with emphysema. No changes compared with a previous chest radiograph.

- ECG and cardiac enzymes: no evidence of myocardial infarction

- Ventilation–perfusion scan: normal ventilation scan. Large defect in perfusion involving the inferior aspect of the right lung.

- Venous duplex scanning, lower limbs: evidence of DVT above the right knee.

CASE 5.2 – I was treated with warfarin for deep venous thrombosis.

 Q4: In the light of the clinical presentation, how would you interpret the laboratory test results?

A4

Table 5.17 Interpretation of the test results for Case 5.2

Test	Change	Interpretation
Full blood examination	Low Hb, increased WCC, decreased platelet count	Low Hb may be the result of haemolysis (caused by septicaemia)
		Increased WCC is typical in sepsis but leukopenia may occur in overwhelming sepsis particularly in people with alcohol problems and elderly people
		Low platelet count is consistent with coagulopathy, commonly present in Gram-negative septicaemia
Serum CK and CK-MB	Normal range	Myocardial infarction is less likely; however, patients with sepsis are at higher risk of developing myocardial infarction
Fasting blood sugar	Raised	In sepsis, the blood glucose homoeostasis is usually impaired in people with diabetes and hyperglycaemia may occur. Hypoglycaemia is rare
Liver function tests (serum bilirubin, AST and ALT)	Mild rise of serum bilirubin and transaminases	Mild impairment of liver function tests may be present in sepsis
		The rise in serum bilirubin in patients with septicaemia may be the result of: increased haemolysis; decreased uptake of bilirubin by liver cells; impaired conjugation of bilirubin; or cholestasis
Blood urea and creatinine	Raised	In patients with septicaemia, raised blood urea may be: the result of acute tubular necrosis; secondary to hypotension and decreased renal perfusion; or caused by tubulointerstitial disease

Chest radiograph	Diffuse bilateral infiltrates	Pulmonary complications of sepsis syndrome include adult respiratory distress syndrome with hypoxaemia and diffuse alveolar infiltrates; this is mainly because of increased capillary permeability and accumulation of fluids in the interalveolar spaces and diffuse alveolar infiltrates. The underlying mechanism is the inflammatory cytokines released as a result of sepsis
		Arterial blood gases are important in the assessment of the patient, who may have respiratory alkalosis in the beginning but, when he develops respiratory muscle fatigue, his blood gases show metabolic acidosis (because of accumulation of lactic acid in his respiratory muscles) and increased anion gap
ECG and echocardiogram	Sinus tachycardia, no evidence of ischaemia	No evidence of acute myocardial infarction
Urinalysis	Increased red blood cells, WBCs, nitrates, ketone bodies and glucose	Evidence of urinary tract infection
Urine culture	Gram-negative bacilli > 10^8/L	Gram-negative septicaemia is more likely to occur in: diabetes mellitus; invasive procedures; indwelling urinary catheter; diverticulitis; burns; and liver cirrhosis

 Q5: What is your final hypothesis?

A5

- Gram-negative septic shock as a consequence of upper urinary tract infection
- On warfarin for 2 months before admission because of DVT
- No evidence of acute myocardial infarction or pulmonary embolism.

 Q6: What issues in the given history, examination and laboratory tests support your final hypothesis?

A6

Supportive evidence

History

- The patient presents with low blood pressure, shortness of breath, fever and rigors.
- He has been treated recently for DVT (on warfarin, for 2 months).
- He has a history of hypertension and diabetes of 15 years.
- He has been catheterized on two occasions because of urinary retention.

Examination

- Low blood pressure, increased pulse rate and respiratory rate
- Febrile: 38.8°C
- Inaudible heart sounds
- Bilateral crackles on both lung bases
- Fullness and tenderness in both loins
- Unable to pass urine for laboratory analysis.

Investigations

- Low Hb and increased WCC
- Low platelet count
- Mild rise in serum bilirubin and transaminases
- ECG, echocardiogram and cardiac enzymes: no evidence of myocardial infarction or cardiac tamponade
- Urine culture: evidence of infection with Gram-negative bacteria.

● CASE 5.3 – My heart has never fluttered like this before.

Q4: In the light of the clinical presentation, how would you interpret the laboratory test results?

A4

Table 5.18 Interpretation of the lab test results for Case 5.3

Test	Change	Interpretation
Chest radiograph	Straightening of the left border of the cardiac silhouette, prominence of the main pulmonary arteries, dilatation of the upper lobe pulmonary veins, Kerley B lines (fine, opaque, horizontal lines most prominent in the lower and mid-lung zones)	The following findings suggest mitral stenosis, pulmonary congestion and back pressure on the pulmonary artery: left atrial enlargement; and prominence of the main pulmonary arteries and dilatation of the upper lobe of pulmonary veins The Kerley B lines are the result of interalveolar filtration of fluid
ECG	Evidence of AF	AF is usually associated with MS Embolization is more frequently seen in MS patients with AF

| Echocardiogram | Evidence of dilatation of left atrium, mitral valve area 0.9 cm² (normally 4–6 cm²), normal left ventricular function, no significant regurgitation from mitral valves, other heart chambers normal | Echocardiography is the most sensitive and useful non-invasive tool in diagnosis of MS; it can provide information about: mitral orifice size; severity of MS; whether there is mitral regurgitation accompanying MS; the degree of restriction of movement of valve leaflets; and the size of other cardiac chambers |

 Q5: What is your final hypothesis?

A5

Rheumatic fever, severe MS complicated with left ventricular failure (pulmonary oedema) and AF. No evidence of right-sided heart failure.

 Q6: What issues in the given history, examination and laboratory tests support your final hypothesis?

A6

Supportive evidence

History

- A 25-year-old woman from Turkey

- Presents with a sudden onset of palpitations, severe shortness of breath and coughing

- History of a recent travel from Turkey

- Has had palpitations for over a year

- Cough produces small amount of whitish, frothy sputum with streaks of blood

- She is not pregnant; her last menstrual period was 10 days ago.

Examination

- Ruddy cheeks, cyanosed lips

- Blood pressure 100/60 mmHg

- Pulse irregularly irregular

- Respiratory rate 24/min, afebrile

- No evidence of right-sided heart failure: no rise of her JVP, liver not enlarged or tender, no oedema of her lower limbs

- Apex beat at the left fifth intercostal space, midclavicular line

- Loud first heart sound (S1) and low-pitched rumbling diastolic murmur at the apex
- Evidence of acute left heart failure: bilateral inspiratory crackles heard over both lungs.

Investigation

- Chest radiograph: evidence of pulmonary oedema, and changes suggestive of MS and enlargement of left atrium
- ECG: evidence of AF
- Echocardiogram: evidence of severe MS.

👥 Integrated medical sciences questions

⬤ CASE 5.1 – Discuss the mechanism underlying Desmond's shortness of breath.

Predisposing factors

- Lower limb orthopaedic surgery (right hip replacement)

- Obesity (BMI 30)

- Heavy smoking.

The presence of stasis, hypercoagulability and intimal injury (Virchow's triad) has contributed to the development of DVT as follows: damage of the intimae of the blood vessels of lower limbs + blood stasis + changes in the blood coagulability because of surgery (a rise in coagulation factors and platelets) → the veins of the lower abdomen, pelvis and legs most frequently affected → thrombi formation in the deep veins (deep venous thrombosis) → small fragments of thrombi moving in the venous system as emboli → pelvic veins → inferior vena cava → right atrium → tricuspid valve → right ventricle → pulmonary valve → pulmonary artery → the right and left branches of the pulmonary artery → interference with the flow of venous blood in the lungs → interference with the oxygenation of blood in the alveoli (decreased perfusion) → decreased oxygenated blood returning to the left atrium via pulmonary veins → decreased oxygenated blood entering the left ventricle → decreased cardiac output → low blood pressure + decreased blood in the carotids and vertebral arteries supplying the brain (syncope may occur).

Decreased cardiac output → decrease of arterial blood pressure → less pressure on the stretch receptors located in the carotid body and aortic arch → less firing of activated receptors → fewer signals to the vasomotor centres of the central nervous system → more stimulation via the sympathetic nerve → peripheral vasoconstriction (increased vasoconstriction) + increased heart rate + increased respiratory rate

In addition, the chemoreceptors (located in the carotid and aortic bodies) are stimulated by O_2 lack, CO_2 excess and increased H^+ concentration. Stimulation of the chemoreceptors → sympathetic impulses → increased rate and depth of respiration + peripheral vasoconstriction.

Both chemoreceptor and baroreceptor systems aim at blood pressure correction back to normal. However, the baroreceptor and chemoreceptor systems are not able to maintain the blood pressure control long term via the above mechanisms.

⬤ CASE 5.2 – Briefly list the changes that may occur in peripheral circulation in septic shock.

- Presence of endotoxin (the lipopolysaccharide moiety in the outer membrane of the Gram-negative bacteria and the O side chain) → activation of the complement system and contact coagulation system → endothelial damage.

- Endothelial damage causes the release of a number of inflammatory mediators including platelet activation factor, thromboxane A_2, prostaglandins, interferon-γ and leukotrienes

- Release of interleukins IL-1, IL-2, IL-6, IL-8, IL-12, interferon-γ, platelet-activating factor → stimulation of nitric oxide synthesis → vasodilatation despite low blood pressure.

- Low systolic vascular resistance.

- Leakage of plasma into the extravascular space contributes to hypovolaemia.

- Plasma vasopressin levels are not increased in septic shock. Vasopressin levels are usually raised in all other types of shocks to augment vasoconstriction.

● CASE 5.3 – Briefly discuss the pathogenesis and the pathology underlying Ozlem's condition.

During childhood, upper respiratory tract infection with group A β-haemolytic streptococci → immunopathological changes of the disease (not fully understood) → antibody reaction to the streptococci → antibodies cross-reacting with unidentified antigen present in connective tissues of the heart, joints and subcutaneous tissues → changes in connective tissues including the following:

● Oedema of the ground substance

● Fragmentation of collagen fibres

● Cellular infiltration

● Fibrinoid degeneration

● Focal perivascular inflammation (Aschoff's nodules, which are pathognomonic of rheumatic fever).

These changes → the changes in rheumatic fever which may involve the following structures of the heart: (1) the pericardium, (2) myocardium, (3) the endocardium and (4) the cardiac valves, e.g. mitral and aortic valves.

The changes in the valve (e.g. the mitral valve) are: (1) thickened valve, (2) deformed valve, (3) shortened chordae tendinea, (4) fused commissures and (5) narrowed or stenosed valve (aperture < 0.9 cm² as is the case here)

Mitral stenosis → increased obstruction of left ventricle filling → increased left atrial pressure + a persistent gradient between the left atrium and left ventricle → decreased left ventricle filling → decreased cardiac output + stagnation of blood in the left atrium → left atrial dilatation + congestion of pulmonary veins → congestion of pulmonary vessels → increased pressure in pulmonary capillaries → passage of fluids across pulmonary capillary walls into the alveoli and interstitial spaces → fluids filling alveoli and interstitial spaces (development of pulmonary oedema) → interference with oxygenation of blood in alveoli and gas exchange → decreased oxygenated blood returning to the heart (cyanosis) → decreased cardiac output → reflex decreased pressure on the specialized receptors (baroreceptors) located in the carotid body and aortic arch → reflex sympathetic stimulation → increased heart rate + increased respiratory rate.

A stretch of the left atrium and hypoxaemia may contribute to the development of AF → AF also responsible for the low cardiac output.

Portion of the mechanism that may occur later as the condition deteriorates

If pulmonary hypoxaemia continues → arteriolar vasoconstriction → increased pulmonary pressure (development of pulmonary hypertension) → increased resistance to the flow of blood from the right ventricle into the pulmonary artery. As the process continues → left ventricular hypertrophy and then failure → accumulation of blood in right ventricle and atrium → increased JVP and liver congestion (nausea, right upper abdominal discomfort) + venous stagnation in lower limbs → increased venous hydrostatic pressure → increased tendency of fluids to transudate into interstitial spaces → development of oedema of lower limbs.

Further reading

Al-Saady NM, Obel OA, Camm AJ. Left atrial appendage: structure, function and role in thromboembolism. *Heart* 1999;**82**:547–555.

Farber HW, Loscalzo J. Mechanisms of disease: Pulmonary arterial hypertension. *New England Journal of Medicine* 2004;**351**:1655–1665.

Goldhaber SZ. Medical progress: Pulmonary embolism. *New England Journal of Medicine* 1998;**339**:93–104.

Humbert M, Sitbon O, Simonneau G. Drug therapy: Treatment of pulmonary arterial hypertension. *New England Journal of Medicine* 2004;**351**:1425–1436.

Jessup M, Brozena S. Medical progress: Heart failure. *New England Journal of Medicine* 2003;**348**:2007–2018.

Laughlin MH. Cardiovascular response to exercise. *Advances Physiology Education* 1999;**22**:S244–S259.

Ross R. Mechanisms of disease: atherosclerosis-an inflammatory disease. *New England Journal of Medicine* 1999;**340**:115–126.

Schrier RW, Wang W. Mechanisms of disease: Acute renal failure and sepsis. *New England Journal of Medicine* 2004;**351**:159–169.

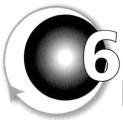

Respiratory system

Clinical cases

● CASE 6.1 – Jasmine was diagnosed with asthma at the age of 6.

Jasmine Barton is a 14-year-old primary school pupil who is brought by her mother, Noreen, to see a local doctor, Dr Linda Kriegsman. This is the first time that they had seen Dr Kriegsman because the Barton family moved to Melbourne from Queensland 5 months ago. Noreen is concerned that Jasmine's blue puffer is not working any more. Jasmine was diagnosed with asthma at the age of 6 and since that time has been using a blue puffer on a regular basis. Over the last 15 months she has had recurrent upper and lower respiratory tract infections and has been treated with antibiotics on four occasions. Further questioning reveals that Jasmine has been coughing up thick, greenish sputum and sometimes has trouble bringing it up. Yesterday, her mother also noticed that she was a little bit feverish and flushed. Jasmine quietly mentions that, on some mornings, the sputum contains streaks of blood.

On examination, Jasmine looks flushed and ill, and her lips are not cyanosed. Her vital signs are shown in Table 6.1.

Table 6.1 Vital signs for Case 6.1

Vital signs	Jasmine's results	Normal range
Blood pressure (mmHg)	110/70	100/60–135/85
Pulse rate (/min)	90	60–100
Respiratory rate (/min	19	12–16
Temperature (°C)	38.5	36.6–37.2

Respiratory examination

- Crackles on both sides of the lungs
- Dullness on percussion at both bases
- Clubbing of fingers.

Cardiovascular and abdominal examination: normal.

● CASE 6.2 – For over 20 years, I've had passion for breeding birds.

Changlong Phong, an unemployed 54 year old who worked as a mechanical assistant for over 30 years, comes in to see Dr James Watson. Changlong has noticed progressive shortness of breath, particularly after walking for about 10–15 minutes.

He smoked 10 cigarettes per day for over 20 years but stopped smoking 5 years ago. He has had a cough for a number of years, particularly early in the morning. He has not coughed up any blood and has never been in hospital. He emigrated with his family from Vietnam about 15 years ago. For over 20 years, he has had a passion for breeding birds in his own backyard. Although it is a life-long hobby, he also sells the animals for extra income.

On examination, he is short of breath and cyanosed. His vital signs are summarized in Table 6.2.

Table 6.2 Vital signs for Case 6.2

Vital signs	Changlong's results	Normal range
Blood pressure (mmHg)	120/70	100/60–135/85
Pulse rate (/min)	95	60–100
Respiratory rate (/min)	23	12–16
Temperature (°C)	37.5	36.6–37.2

The patient has finger clubbing and auscultation of his chest reveals bilateral coarse end-inspiratory crackles and wheezes throughout the chest.

The cardiovascular examination is normal.

⬤ CASE 6.3 – I have to stop to catch my breath after walking 10–12 steps.

Mr Philip Turner, a 57-year-old retired factory worker, comes in to see his GP, Dr Norm Gregor, because of progressive shortness of breath on exertion and ankle swelling over the last 4 months. Philip says: 'My shortness of breath has increased over the last month and I have to stop to catch my breath after walking 10–12 steps.' He also has a long history of a morning cough with some white sputum, which he believes is related to his smoking. Further history questions reveal that his ankle swelling has increased over the past 3–4 months. It is painless and usually swells more towards the end of the day. He denies any history of fever, chills, worsening cough, haemoptysis, nausea and jaundice.

Philip smoked 30 cigarettes per day for over 35 years but ceased smoking 2 years ago after three hospital admissions for treatment of chest infections.

On examination, his lips are cyanosed. His vital signs are shown in Table 6.3.

Table 6.3 Vital signs for Case 6.3

Vital signs	Philip's results	Normal range
Blood pressure (mmHg)	140/90	100/60–135/85
Pulse rate (/min)	95	60–100
Respiratory rate (/min)	19	12–16
Temperature (°C)	36.7	36.6–37.2

Respiratory examination: increased anteroposterior diameter of the chest. Widespread crackles on both sides.

Cardiovascular examination: loud second heart sound.

Lower limbs: pitting oedema of both lower limbs.

👥 Integrated medical sciences questions

● CASE 6.1 – Discuss the pathophysiological mechanisms underlying Jasmine's presentation.

● CASE 6.2 – Discuss the pathophysiological mechanisms underlying Changlong's presentation.

● CASE 6.3 – Discuss the pathophysiological mechanisms underlying the development of ankle swelling in a patient with a long history of heavy smoking.

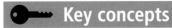

Key concepts

To work through the core clinical cases in this chapter, you will need to understand the following key concepts.

The cells forming the walls of alveoli

Table 6.4 The functions of each cell and their clinical significance

Cell	Main features	Function	Clinical significance
Type I alveolar cells (also known as type I pneumocytes)	Make up 93–96 per cent of the lining cells Thin cytoplasm Nucleus is relatively large Cell's organelles: a small number of mitochondria, a small amount of rough endoplasmic reticulum (RER) and a less-developed Golgi apparatus	They form occluding junctions with each other and this structure prevents any tissue fluid entering the alveolar lumen They form the stem cells from which type II pneumocytes are formed	Not known
Type II alveolar cells (also known as type II pneumocytes, septal cells)	Much less numerous than type I cells Found at the junctions of alveolar septa (hence also known as septal cells) Cuboidal cells Have a centrally placed nucleus, an abundance of RER and a well-developed Golgi apparatus and mitochondria Also have lamellar bodies that contain pulmonary surfactant	Produce pulmonary surfactant, which decreases surface tension, preventing the collapse of the alveolus Phagocytose excess surfactant Undergo mitosis to regenerate themselves	Immature newborns (those born before 28 weeks' gestation) usually have inadequate production of surfactant in their lungs and are at a high risk of developing respiratory distress syndrome Glucocorticoids stimulate type II pneumocytes to produce pulmonary surfactant
Alveolar macrophages (also known as dust cells)	Monocytes that become alveolar macrophages after their access to the pulmonary interstitial tissue	Phagocytose particles, e.g. dust and bacteria. Help type II pneumocytes in the uptake of surfactant	In patients with pulmonary congestion and heart failure, alveolar macrophages play a role in phagocytosing red blood cells that are extravasated because of pulmonary congestion

What is the blood–gas barrier?

The thinnest region of the interalveolar septum where exchange of gases, O_2 (in the alveolar lumen) and CO_2 (in the blood capillaries), takes place is known as the blood–gas barrier. It comprises:

- Type I pneumocytes and surfactant
- Fused basal laminae of type I pneumocytes and endothelial cells of blood capillaries
- Endothelial cells of blood capillaries.

The factors affecting the O_2 dissociation curve

The O_2 dissociation curve (also known as the oxyhaemoglobin dissociation curve) is obtained by exposing blood to a number of partial pressures of O_2 and measuring how much of its total O_2-carrying capacity is occupied. The curve also allows us to study a number of changes (conditions) that can shift the dissociation curve and change the loading (at the lungs) and the unloading (at the tissue) of oxygen. The factors affecting the O_2 dissociation curve are summarized as follows:

- Hydrogen ion concentration ($[H^+]$): increased $[H^+]$, which also means decreased pH and increased acidity of blood, displaces the curve to the right (more O_2 available to the body tissues). This is because H^+ ions act on the haemoglobin (Hb) molecule and decrease its affinity for O_2 (Bohr shift). This is important clinically, particularly in patients with acidity (e.g. low blood pressure and shock state) because, for a decrease of 0.2 pH unit, there is an increase of O_2 release by 25 per cent at low P_{O_2}.

- Carbon dioxide: CO_2 reacts with Hb to form carbamino-Hb, moving the curve to the right. If increased P_{CO_2} continues for several hours with chronic acidosis, red blood cell 2,3-diphosphoglycerate (DPG) is decreased, shifting the curve to the left.

- Temperature: a decrease in body temperature shifts the curve to the left. On the other hand, a rise in body temperature, as in fevers, causes a shift of the curve to the right.

- DPG in red blood cells reacts with HbO_2, causing a release of oxygen by shifting the oxygen dissociation curve to the right. Examples of the clinical significance of DPG are:

  - residence in high altitude which causes an increase in DPG in red blood cells, resulting in a shift to the right

  - prolonged exercise which causes an increase in DPG in red blood cells, resulting in a shift to the right

  - blood stored in blood banks, in which red blood cells contain less DPG, is not efficient in O_2 delivery to tissues compared with a fresh blood transfusion.

- Fetal Hb (two γ-polypeptide chains in place of the β chains of adult Hb): this Hb is hungry for O_2 causing a shift of the O_2 dissociation curve to the left. The physiological reason for the presence of fetal Hb rather than adult Hb in the human fetus is the fact that the latter is dependent on its mother for O_2 and is always threatened by the possibility of hypoxia in the mother. Fetal Hb is able to alleviate this risk by its high affinity for O_2 and facilitating the release of O_2 from mother to fetus even if the mother's P_{O_2} is low.

The pathophysiological changes in patients with acute asthma

- Recurrent 'reversible' obstruction of airways is characterized by bronchial hyperresponsiveness together with inflammatory changes in the airways. This airway hyperresponsiveness is usually initiated by non-specific irritants such as cold air, allergen, smoke and exercise. Between attacks the patient has no symptoms.

● The pathological changes in the lungs during an acute attack are:

  – spasm of bronchial smooth muscles

  – swelling of the mucous gland lining

  – increased secretion of mucus

  – activation of parasympathetic postganglionic fibres to release acetylcholine, which stimulates muscarinic receptors on the smooth muscle fibres, causing them to contract

  – mast cell degranulation: allergens interact with IgE antibodies on their surface, causing them to degranulate releasing a number of inflammatory mediators including serotonin, heparin, histamine, lysosomal enzymes and chemotactic factors

  – degranulation of eosinophils and release of neutrophil chemotactic factors (play a significant role in asthma).

Table 6.5 The pharmacological differences between salbutamol and beclomethasone in bronchial asthma

Characteristic	Salbutamol (blue puffer)	Beclomethasone (brown puffer)
Active substance	β_2-Adrenoceptor agonist	Glucocorticoids
Primary effect	Bronchodilator	Anti-inflammatory agent
	Effective in reversing the bronchospasm of immediate phase	Inhibits and prevents the inflammatory components of both phases (airway inflammation + release of mediators + epithelial damage)
		Glucocorticoids are *not* effective in the treatment of immediate response/changes in asthma
Mechanisms	Dilates bronchi by a direct action on β_2-adrenoceptors on smooth muscles	Decreases the formation of cytokines (T-helper 2 or Th2 cytokines that recruit and activate esinophils and are responsible for the production and expression of IgE receptors)
	Increases mucus clearance by action on cilia	Inhibits the generation of vasodilators
		Inhibits the production of spasmogens, leukotrienes LTC_4 and LTD_4
		Reduces recruitment and activation of inflammatory cells
Benefits of long-term use	Not proved	Mainly reduces the synthesis of IL-3 and the early phase response to allergens, and prevents exercise-induced asthma
Unwanted side effects	Tremors	Oropharyngeal candidiasis
	Tolerance	Dysphonia (voice change)
		Adrenal suppression (as a result of long-term use)

The pathological changes in chronic obstructive pulmonary disease

Predisposing factors are:

- Smoking: cigarette smoking is the most common cause. The mechanisms by which smoking can cause chronic obstructive pulmonary disease (COPD) are: smoking impairs ciliary movement; smoking inhibits the function of alveolar macrophages; smoking causes hyperplasia of the mucus-secreting glands; smoking damages the alveolar walls (causes local inflammation and stimulates polymorphonucleocytes to secrete proteolytic enzymes resulting in damage of alveolar walls); and smoking increases airway resistance

- Air pollution

- Occupational exposure to chemicals

- Recurrent chest infections

- Familial and genetic causes, e.g. α_1-antitrypsin deficiency.

The pathological changes associated with chronic bronchitis may include:

- Hypertrophy and hyperplasia of the mucus-secreting glands in the submucosa of airways

- A high Reid index (the mean ratio of the thickness of the submucosal glands to that of the bronchial wall is 0.55 ± 0.09)

- Goblet cell hyperplasia

- Local increase of mucosal and submucosal inflammatory cells

- Oedema of the mucus lining and peribronchial fibrosis

- Intraluminal mucus plugs

- Increased smooth muscle in small airways

- Decreased FEV_1/FVC (forced expiratory volume in 1 s:forced vital capacity) ratio.

In emphysema the changes may be:

- Centriacinar (centrilobular) emphysema: involves airspaces in the centre of lobules. It is commonly seen in association with cigarette smoking and coal-workers' pneumoconiosis.

- Panacinar (panlobular) emphysema: involves the whole acinus and is present in the central and peripheral portions of the acinus. Thus, it is associated with a reduction in the alveolar–capillary gas exchange surface and a loss of the elastic recoil properties. It usually involves the bases of the lungs and is seen in patients with α_1-antitrypsin deficiency.

Answers

CASE 6.1 – Jasmine was diagnosed with asthma at the age of 6.

 Q1: What are the possible causes for the presenting problem?

A1

The following are possible causes (hypotheses) for Jasmine's presentation:

- Bronchiectasis (may explain her symptoms including fever and coughing up greenish sputum with streaks of blood, as well as the clinical findings including bilateral basal crackles, dullness on percussion at both bases and clubbing of fingers), most probably caused by cystic fibrosis (CF)

- Lung abscess.

Less probable causes are:

- Bronchitis

- Pneumonia

- Acute asthma

- COPD

- Pulmonary tuberculosis (TB).

 Q2: What further questions would you like to ask to help you differentiate between your hypotheses?

A2

Table 6.6 Further history questions for Case 6.1

History questions	In what way the answers can help
History of recurrent cough, upper respiratory tract infections, recurrent sinusitis, decreased appetite, and weight loss	Patients with cystic fibrosis (CF) may present during childhood with failure to thrive, decreased appetite, weight loss, chronic cough and recurrent respiratory infections
	Episodes of cough tend to persist longer than expected for an acute respiratory illness and despite treatment with antibiotics
	Failure of the exocrine function of the pancreas, mainly because of obstruction of the pancreatic duct, occurs in about 85 per cent of patients
	It is particularly present in homozygous patients with the $\Delta F508$ mutation
	This obstruction may result in the following pathological changes: loss of acinar cells; pancreatic enzyme deficiency; malabsorption of protein, fat and fat-soluble vitamins; and foul-smelling stools caused by excessive loss of fat in stool (steatorrhoea) and loss of bodyweight

Any history of hospital admission because of chest infections and investigations, e.g. chest radiographs, sputum microbiology, respiratory function tests, etc.	This may help in assessing the patient and progression in the disease Patients with CF are at a high risk of developing recurrent chest infections for the following reasons: thick mucus secreted in CF causes damage to the respiratory lining and impaired mucociliary clearance; increased binding of bacteria to airway epithelia; development of chronic inflammatory state and loss of cilia of the airways;colonization of the lungs and airways with micro-organisms; and micro-organisms colonized in the patient's airways may develop altered characteristics and resistance to antibiotics
Antenatal care, any problems during neonatal period, growth and development, and immunization	Patients with CF may present as newborns with meconium ileus or children with poor appetite and failure to thrive
Family history of CF and chronic respiratory illness	CF is an autosomal recessive genetic disease The defect in CF is in the gene encoding the CF transmembrane conductance regulator (CFTR)
Medication and allergy	Patients with CF usually present with recurrent respiratory infections and will require antibiotic therapy. It is important to know if they have a history of allergy to any medication.

 Q3: What investigations would be most helpful to you and why?

A3

Further investigations

- Chest radiograph
- High-resolution chest computed tomography (CT)
- Full blood examination
- Sputum microbiological studies
- Blood culture
- Arterial blood gases.
- Lung function tests.
- Sweat Cl⁻ measurement
- DNA testing (using buccal swab specimens).

CASE 6.2 – For over 20 years, I've had a passion for breeding birds.

 Q1: What are the possible causes for the presenting problem?

A1

The following are possible causes (hypotheses) for Changlong's presentation:

- Bird fanciers' lung (extrinsic allergic alveolitis)
- Cryptogenic lung fibrosis (idiopathic lung fibrosis)
- COPD (heavy smoking)
- Other occupational diseases such as asbestosis and silicosis
- Pulmonary TB.

Less likely causes:

- Lung fibrosis associated with rheumatoid arthritis or systemic lupus erythematosus (SLE)
- Pneumoconiosis.

Q2: What further questions would you like to ask to help you differentiate between your hypotheses?

A2

Table 6.7 Further history questions for Case 6.2

History questions	In what way answers can help
More details regarding his cough and expectoration, amount and colour of his sputum, and any increase in the amount of his sputum	Chronic bronchitis is defined as coughing for at least 3 months of the year for at least 2 consecutive years in the absence of any other disease
	We need to assess whether he has chronic bronchitis because of his long history of smoking; quitting smoking does alter the subsequent loss of lung function to the same rate as in non-smokers but, if there has been lung damage because of smoking, cessation might not be that effective
Duration of his shortness of breath	Helps in clinical assessment of the severity of his lung problem
What types of activities might bring on his shortness of breath?	

Details regarding his job and any exposure to chemicals, asbestos or silica at work	Exposure to chemicals, silica (silicon dioxide) and asbestos may cause pulmonary fibrosis and result in diseases such as silicosis and asbestosis
Details regarding his hobby (e.g. types of birds that he breeds in his backyard)	His hobby could also be the source of his illness; the antigens are usually proteins present on the feathers and in the excreta
Are there systemic symptoms such as arthritis, joint deformity, morning stiffness, skin rash, muscle pain, muscle weakness, mucous membrane ulcers or generalized fatigue?	The association of systemic rheumatic diseases and pulmonary fibrosis is well established It is important to assess if his condition is related to a systemic disorder such as SLE, systemic sclerosis, polymyositis and rheumatoid arthritis
Past history of hospital admission, investigations (e.g. chest radiographs) and treatment for his cough/shortness of breath (e.g. treatment for TB)	Chest radiograph may be very useful in assessing the cause of his chest problem, e.g. in patients with asbestosis, the chest radiograph may be normal or show pleural thickening, unilateral pleural effusion or diffuse bilateral streaky shadows; in patients with silicosis, the chest radiograph may show thin streaks of calcification around the hilar lymph nodes (eggshell calcification); and in patients with progressive massive fibrosis, the chest radiograph may show round masses of several centimetres in diameter with necrosis in the centre, usually present in the upper lobe
Medications and allergy	Drugs may produce a wide range of respiratory disorders; the mechanism by which drugs may cause pulmonary disorders may be: direct toxicity ,e.g. bleomycin; immune complex formation, e.g. hydralazine; diffuse lung fibrosis, e.g. amiodarone; opportunistic infection, e.g. corticosteroids, azathioprine; and respiratory depression, e.g. sedatives

 Q3: What investigations would be most helpful to you and why?

A3

Further investigations

- Chest radiograph

- Full blood examination

- Lung function tests

- Arterial blood gases

- Avian precipitins, antinuclear factor, rheumatoid factor

- Sputum: Gram stain and Ziehl–Neelsen (ZN) stain

- Chest CT.

CASE 6.3 – I have to stop to catch my breath after walking 10–12 steps.

A1

The following is the possible cause (hypotheses) for Philip's presentation:

- COPD (e.g. chronic bronchitis/emphysema) complicated by increased pulmonary pressure and the development of cor pulmonale (cyanosis, loud second heart sound and pitting oedema)

Unlikely causes are:

- Congestive heart failure
- Hypertensive heart disease
- Left-sided heart failure.

Q2: What further questions would you like to ask to help you differentiate between your hypotheses?

A2

Table 6.8 Further history questions for Case 5.3

History questions	In what way answers can help
More details about his cough and expectoration: amount and colour of his sputum, any increase in the amount of his sputum	Chronic bronchitis is defined as coughing for at least 3 months of the year for at least 2 consecutive years in the absence of any other disease
	We need to assess whether he has chronic bronchitis because of his long history of smoking.
Exposure to chemicals or air pollution	The causes of COPD are: smoking; air pollution; occupational exposure to chemicals; recurrent chest infections; and familial and genetic causes
Past history of hospital admission, investigations (e.g. chest radiographs) and treatment	Helps in assessment of the progression of his illness
Family history of COPD at an early age	Patients with diseases such as α_1-antitrypsin deficiency may present with emphysema and COPD-like illness at an early age

Q3: What investigations would be most helpful to you and why?

A3

Further investigations

- Chest radiograph
- Full blood examination
- Lung function tests
- Arterial blood gases
- Chest CT
- ECG.

Further progress

CASE 6.1 – Jasmine was diagnosed with asthma at the age of 6.

Dr Kriegsman arranges some tests for Jasmine. The results are shown in Tables 6.9–6.11.

Table 6.9 Full blood examination for Case 6.1

Test	Jasmine's tests	Normal range
Haemoglobin (Hb) (g/L)	130	115–160
Packed cell volume (PCV)	0.42	0.37–0.47
White cell count (WCC) ($\times 10^9$/L)	12.0	4.0–11.0
Platelet count ($\times 10^9$/L)	290	150–400

Table 6.10 Arterial blood gases (on oxygen, 2 L/min) for Case 6.1

Test	Jasmine's tests	Normal range
pH	7.40	7.38–7.44
P_{CO_2} (mmHg)[a]	33 (4.4)	35–45 (4.7–6.0)
P_{O_2} (mmHg)[a]	57 (7.6)	80–100 (10.6–13.3)
Bicarbonate (mmol/L)	20	21–28

[a]Values in parentheses are in kilopascals.

Table 6.11 Lung function tests for Case 6.1

Test	Jasmine's tests	Normal range
FEV$_1$ (L)	1.23 (33)[a]	3.70
FVC (L)	1.83 (41)[a]	4.48
FEV$_1$/FVC (per cent)	67.2	> 70 (age dependent)
CO diffusion	Normal	

[a]Values in parentheses are percentages.
FVC, forced vital capacity; FEV$_1$, forced expiratory volume in 1 s.

Chest radiograph: hyperinflation, peribronchial cuffing; no evidence of pneumothorax.

High-resolution chest CT: widespread bronchiectasis; no hilar lymphadenopathy; no changes suggestive of pulmonary hypertension.

Sputum Gram stain: Gram-negative bacilli and inflammatory cells seen.

Sputum culture: *Pseudomonas aeruginosa* isolated and the organisms are sensitive to aminoglycosides.

Blood culture: no growth.

Sweat test: the sweat is high in Cl$^-$ and sodium.

DNA testing (using buccal swab specimens): a $\Delta F508$ mutation is found (a loss of the codon for phenylalanine at the 508 position of the protein).

● CASE 6.2 – For over 20 years, I've had a passion for breeding birds.

The treating doctor arranges some tests for Changlong. The results are shown in Tables 6.12–6.15.

Table 6.12 Full blood examination for Case 6.2

Test	Changlong's results	Normal range
Hb (g/L)	130	115–160
PCV	0.42	0.37–0.47
WCC ($\times 10^9$/L)	10.0 (relative rise in eosinophils)	4.0–11.0
Platelet count ($\times 10^9$/L)	290	150–400

Table 6.13 Arterial blood gases for Case 6.2

Test	Changlongs's results	Normal range
pH	7.30	7.38–7.44
Pco$_2$ (mmHg)[a]	41 (5.5)	35–45 (4.7–6.0)
Po$_2$ (mmHg)[a]	72 (9.6)	80–100 (10.6–13.3)
Bicarbonate (mmol/L)	19	21–28

[a]Values in parentheses are in kilopascals.

Table 6.14 Lung function tests for Case 6.2

Test	Changlongs's results	Normal range
FEV$_1$ (L)	1.9	3.70
FVC (L)	2.5	4.48
FEV$_1$/FVC (per cent)	76	> 70 (age dependent)
CO diffusion	Reduced	

Table 6.15 Other tests for Case 6.2

Test	Changlongs's results
Avian precipitins	IgG antibodies against pigeon protein
Antinuclear factor	Negative
Rheumatoid factor	Negative

Chest radiograph: bilateral basal fine reticular shadowing.

High-resolution CT: peripheral reticular and ground glass opacification.

Sputum (Gram stain): negative

Sputum (ZN stain): no acid-fast bacilli found on three occasions.

CASE 6.3 – I have to stop to catch my breath after walking 10–12 steps.

Dr Gregor arranges some tests for Philip. The results are shown in Tables 6.16–6.18.

Table 6.16 Full blood examination for Case 6.3

Test	Philip's results	Normal range
Hb (g/L)	195	115–160
PCV	0.51	0.37–0.47
WCC ($\times 10^9$/L)	5.9	4.0–11.0
Platelet count ($\times 10^9$/L)	310	150–400

Table 6.17 Arterial blood gases for Case 6.3

Test	Philip's results	Normal range
pH	7.37	7.38–7.44
Pco$_2$ (mmHg)[a]	53 (7.1)	35–45 (4.7–6.0)
Po$_2$ (mmHg)[a]	59 (7.8)	80–100 (10.6–13.3)
Bicarbonate (mmol/L)	31	21–28

[a]Values in parentheses are in kilopascals.

Table 6.18 Lung function tests for Case 6.3

Test	Philip's results	Normal range
FEV$_1$ (L)	1.6 (FEV$_1$ does not attain normal values after salbutamol inhalation)	3.70
FVC (L)	3.2	4.48
FEV$_1$/FVC (per cent)	50	> 70 (age dependent)
Alveolar volume (per cent)	4.9	90
CO diffusion	Decreased	

Chest radiograph: increased anteroposterior diameter, hyperinflation of lungs and flat diaphragm.

High-resolution axial CT: multiple dark holes in the lung surrounded by normal parenchymal appearance. Both sides are affected but the right side is more severely affected.

ECG: evidence of right ventricular hypertrophy.

Further questions

 CASE 6.1 – Jasmine was diagnosed with asthma at the age of 6.

Q4: In the light of the clinical presentation, how would you interpret the laboratory test results?

A4

Table 6.19 Interpretation of lab test results for Case 6.1

Test	Change	Interpretation
Full blood examination	Normal Hb, increased WCC	There is no evidence of anaemia or polycythaemia; the increase in WCC supports the hypothesis of infection
Arterial blood gases	Hypoxaemia	Hypoxaemia can be the result of:
		1. Gas exchange abnormalities, e.g. ventilation–perfusion mismatch as in CF, asthma and pulmonary embolism; right-to-left shunts and pulmonary A-V shunts; loss of A/C membrane as in emphysema and thick A/C membrane as in pulmonary fibrosis; the CO diffusion is normal in the ventilation–perfusion mismatch and A-V shunts; it is usually decreased in conditions associated with thick A/C membrane or loss of the A/C membrane as in emphysema
		2. Hypoventilation which is mostly associated with raised P_{CO_2}; this is less likely here because Jasmin's P_{CO_2} is low rather than high, so the most likely cause for her hypoxaemia is ventilation–perfusion mismatch
Lung function tests	Low FEV_1, FVC and FEV_1/FVC	Evidence of obstruction of airways
Chest radiograph	Hyperinflation, peribronchial cuffing, no evidence of pneumothorax	The radiological findings are suggestive of bronchiectasis; its development in patients with CF is related to: mucus plugging of small airways; persistence of inflammation and infection; postobstructive cystic dilatations and parenchymal destruction; interference with mucocilliary clearance mechanisms; and bronchial wall destruction by inflammation, infection and mucus plugging
		Pneumothorax may be present in 10 per cent of patients with CF
High-resolution chest CT	Widespread bronchiectasis, no hilar lymphadenopathy, no changes suggestive of pulmonary hypertension	The CT changes may reveal early changes of bronchiectasis before conventional radiographs show any changes

Sputum Gram stain	Gram-negative bacilli and inflammatory cells seen	Initially the lower respiratory tract of patients with CF is colonized with *Staphylococcus aureus* and *Haemophilus influenzae* and, ultimately, *Pseudomonas aeruginosa* (a Gram-negative bacillus)
Sputum culture	*Pseudomonas aeruginosa* isolated and the organisms are sensitive to aminoglycosides	The abnormal thick and viscous secretions cause luminal obstruction and destruction of the alveoli and terminal respiratory bronchioles → destructive changes in the elastic and muscular layers of bronchial walls
		Pseudomonas aeruginosa is usually found in the sputum of patients with CF
Blood culture	No growth	In about 20–30 per cent of patients with CF, the blood culture is expected to be negative even in the presence of chest infection
Sweat test (Cl⁻ in sweat)	Increased	In CF, the sweat is high in Cl⁻ and Na⁺ concentrations. A sweat Cl⁻, concentration > 60 mmol/L together with the clinical manifestation is usually sufficient to make the diagnosis
DNA test	A ΔF508 mutation is found (see text)	The mutation in CF occurs in a single gene encoding the CFTR, which regulates the chloride channel normally present in the apical surface of epithelial cells
		Failure to produce this transporter results in defective Cl⁻ transport in epithelial cells and an increase in Na⁺ reabsorption in pancreatic duct, airways and other ductal epithelia → thick and viscous secretions in the pancreatic duct and the respiratory, hepatobiliary, gastrointestinal and reproductive tracts

A/C, alveo-capillary; A-V, atrioventricular; CF, cystic fibrosis; CFTR, cystic fibrosis transmembrane conductance regulator.

 Q5: What is your final hypothesis?

A5

The clinical picture and laboratory results are suggestive of CF.

Q6: What issues in the given history, examination and laboratory tests support your final hypothesis?

A6

Supportive evidence

History

- The patient was diagnosed with asthma at the age of 6.
- The blue puffer is not working any more.
- Treated for recurrent upper and lower respiratory infections over last 15 months.
- Coughing up thick greenish sputum.
- Feverish and flushed.
- Her sputum contains streaks of blood.

Examination

- Not cyanosed.
- Temperature 38.5°C
- Increased respiratory and pulse rate
- Crackles on both sides
- Dullness on percussion at both bases
- Clubbing of fingers.

Investigations

- Chest radiograph: hyperinflation, peribronchial cuffing; no evidence of pneumothorax
- High-resolution chest CT: widespread bronchiectasis, no hilar lymphadenopathy, no changes suggestive of pulmonary hypertension.
- Sputum (Gram stain): Gram-negative bacilli and inflammatory cells
- Sputum culture: *Pseudomonas aeruginosa* isolated and the organisms sensitive to aminoglycosides
- Blood culture: no growth
- Sweat test: sweat is high in Cl^- and Na^+ concentrations
- DNA test: a $\Delta F508$ mutation is found (a loss of the codon for phenylalanine at position 508 of the protein).

CASE 6.2 – For over 20 years, I've had a passion for breeding birds.

Q4: In the light of the clinical presentation, how would you interpret the laboratory test results?

A4

Table 6.20 Interpretation of lab test results for Case 6.2

Test	Change	Interpretation
Full blood examination	Relative increase in eosinophils	Eosinophils are raised in extrinsic allergic alveolitis, such as bird fanciers' lung
Arterial blood gases	Hypoxaemia	CO_2 retention is rare, even late in the disease Hypoxaemia is usually the result of abnormal ventilation–perfusion or diffusion abnormalities
Lung function tests	FEV$_1$/FVC raised CO diffusion decreased	In interstitial lung diseases, the CO diffusion is decreased and FEV$_1$/FVC is raised, suggesting a restrictive lung disease
Avin precipitins, ANAs and rheumatoid factor	Only positive for avin precipitins	The presence of avin precipitins supports the diagnosis of bird fanciers' lung disease ANAs and rheumatoid may be raised in other interstitial lung diseases
Chest radiograph	Bilateral basal fine reticular shadowing	In most cases of interstitial lung disease, the chest radiograph shows infiltrates in the lower lung zones A diffuse ground-glass pattern is seen early in the disease A reticulonodular infiltrate may be also seen in interstitial lung disease
HRCT	Peripheral reticular and ground glass opacification	In interstitial lung disease, HRCT abnormalities may be present before pulmonary function tests are abnormal, although a normal HRCT does not exclude interstitial lung disease
Sputum Gram stain	Negative	The possibility of infection is less likely
Sputum ZN stain.	No acid-fast bacilli	The possibility of pulmonary TB is not likely, which is also consistent with the chest radiograph findings.

ANA, antinuclear antibody; HRCT, high-resolution CT; ZN, Ziehl–Neelsen.

Q5: What is your final hypothesis?

A5

The clinical picture and laboratory results are suggestive of an interstitial lung disease (a restrictive lung disease), most probably bird fanciers' lung.

Q6: What issues in the given history, examination and laboratory tests support your final hypothesis?

A6

Supportive evidence

History

- Worked as a mechanical assistant for over 30 years
- Progressive shortness of breath, particularly after walking for about 10–15 min
- Smoked 10 cigarettes per day for over 20 years; stopped smoking 5 years ago
- Has had a cough for a number of years
- Never coughed blood or been treated in hospital
- Emigrated from Vietnam about 15 years ago
- Breeds birds in his own backyard.

Examination

- He is cyanosed
- Temperature 37.5°C
- Increased pulse and respiratory rates
- Finger clubbing
- Bilateral coarse end-inspiratory crackles and wheezes throughout the chest
- Cardiovascular examination normal.

Investigations

- Relative increase in eosinophils.
- FEV_1/FVC is raised (consistent with a restrictive lung disease)
- Avin precipitins: positive
- Chest radiograph: bilateral basal fine reticular shadowing

- High-resolution CT: peripheral reticular and ground-glass opacification

- Arterial blood gases: hypoxaemia

- Sputum (Gram stain): negative

- Sputum (ZN stain): no acid-fast bacilli found on three occasions.

● CASE 6.3 – I have to stop to catch my breath after walking 10-12 steps.

 Q4: In the light of the clinical presentation, how would you interpret the laboratory test results?

A4

Table 6.21 Interpretation of lab test results for Case 6.3

Test	Change	Interpretation
Full blood examination	Increased Hb	Chronic hypoxaemia stimulates the release of erythropoietin (Epo) → excessive production of red blood cells by bone marrow (secondary polycythaemia, also known as secondary erythrocytosis)
Arterial blood gases	Low P_{O_2} and high P_{CO_2}	These changes suggest the development of respiratory failure
Lung function tests	FEV_1 does not attain normal values after salbutamol inhalation	In COPD, FEV_1 does not attain normal values after salbutamol inhalation, whereas it can return to normal in patients with asthma
	FEV_1/FVC is low (< 70%)	Airway obstruction (FEV_1/FVC < 70) in a person with a long history of smoking, at least 20 cigarettes per day, is always suggestive of COPD
	Decreased CO diffusion	
Chest radiograph	Increased antero-posterior diameter, hyperinflation of lungs and flat diaphragm	This is typical of COPD; other findings include: increased retrosternal space; small vertical heart; and signs of pulmonary hypertension may be present (mainly prominent pulmonary artery)
HRCT	Multiple dark holes in the lung surrounded by normal parenchymal appearance	Helpful in assessment of distribution and extent of emphysema
	Both sides are affected but the right side more severely	
ECG	Evidence of right ventricular hypertrophy	This may indicate the development of pulmonary arteriolar vasoconstriction and pulmonary hypertension, and the presence of a resistance to the blood flow in the pulmonary artery

Q5: What is your final hypothesis?

A5

The clinical picture and laboratory results are suggestive of COPD complicated by right-sided heart failure (cor pulmonale).

Q6: What issues in the given history, examination and laboratory tests support your final hypothesis?

A6

Supportive evidence

History

- Progressive shortness of breath on exertion
- Has to stop to catch his breath after walking 10–12 steps
- Long history of a morning cough with some white sputum
- Ankle swelling over the last 4 months; ankles usually swell more towards the end of the day
- He denies any history of fever, chills, worsening cough, haemoptysis, nausea and jaundice
- He has smoked 30 cigarettes per day for over 35 years but ceased smoking 2 years ago.

Examination

- His lips are cyanosed.
- His blood pressure is 140/90 mmHg, his pulse rate and respiratory rates are increased.
- He is afebrile.
- Respiratory examination shows increased anteroposterior diameter of the chest, widespread crackles on both sides.
- Cardiovascular examination shows a loud second heart sound.
- Lower limbs: pitting oedema of both lower limbs.

Investigations

- Full blood examination: increased Hb (secondary polycythaemia)
- Lung function tests: FEV_1 does not attain normal values after salbutamol inhalation; FEV_1/FVC low (< 70 per cent)
- Arterial blood gases: evidence of respiratory failure (hypoxaemia and CO_2 retention)
- Decreased CO diffusion: picture consistent with obstructive lung disease
- Chest radiograph: increased anteroposterior diameter, hyperinflation of lungs and flat diaphragm
- High-resolution CT: multiple dark holes in the lung surrounded by normal parenchymal appearance; both sides affected but the right side more severely
- ECG: evidence of right ventricular hypertrophy.

👥 Integrated medical sciences questions

⬤ CASE 6.1 – Discuss the pathophysiological mechanisms underlying Jasmine's presentation.

A $\Delta F508$ mutation in the gene encoding the CFTR (a loss of the codon for phenylalanine at the 508 position of the protein) → absence of the transporter responsible for Cl^- transport in the apical surface of epithelial cells → defective transport of Cl^- in the epithelial cells in airways → production of thick and viscous secretions → mucus plugging of small airways → (1) mucus plugging small airways, (2) interference with the mucociliary clearance mechanisms and (3) increased susceptibility for chest infection → inflammation + gradual destruction in the wall of bronchial walls → persistence of inflammation and infection → progression of airway damage and recurrence of infection and inflammation → cough and expectoration.

The organisms responsible for the infection are *Staphylococcus aureus* and *Haemophilus influenzae* and, ultimately, *Pseudomonas aeruginosa*.

Infection usually persists and the recurrence of inflammation, infection and airway damage results in the development of bronchiectasis, changes in the lung function tests (decreased FEV_1, FVC FEV_1/FVC) and hypoxaemia → shortness of breath.

CASE 6.2 – Discuss the pathophysiological mechanisms underlying Changlongs's presentation.

Breeding birds → chronic exposure to animals and their excreta → inhalation of proteins (antigens) present on feathers and in excreta → development of immune reaction → immune attack to epithelial and endothelial cells → recruitment of inflammatory response and immune effector cells → development of alveolitis (accumulation of inflammatory and immune effector cells within the alveolar walls) → the accumulation of white cells which causes the following changes: (1) distortion of normal alveolar cells, (2) release of mediators and injury of parenchymal cells and (3) stimulation of fibrosis → alveoli being replaced by cystic spaces separated by thick fibrous bands and inflammatory cells. The alveolar macrophages also increase in number and play a role in fibrosis → restrictive lung disease → decreased FEV_1, FVC, increased FEV_1/FVC and decreased CO diffusion + hypoxaemia → stimulation of shortness of breath.

CASE 6.3 – Discuss the pathophysiological mechanisms underlying the development of ankle swelling in a patient with a long history of heavy smoking.

● The mechanism by which smoking produces lung damage may include the following:

    – direct injury by oxidant gases

    – increased elastase activity

    – decreased antiprotease activity.

● Chronic history of smoking → a number of pathological changes including: loss of cilia, mucous gland hyperplasia, increased number of goblet cells in the central airways, mucus plugging of small airways and destruction of alveoli.

● These changes result in damage of the alveoli and the gradual development of emphysema and chronic bronchitis → interference with ventilation–perfusion and gas diffusion → hypoxaemia and CO_2 retention.

● Chronic hypoxaemia → pulmonary arteriolar vasoconstriction → pulmonary hypertension → increased resistance to flow of blood from right ventricle via pulmonary artery to pulmonary vessels → development of right ventricular hypertrophy, which gradually results in right-sided ventricular failure → right-sided venous congestion → stagnation of blood in leg veins (effect of gravity) and increased pressure → increased flow of blood from blood capillaries to interstitial fluids → development of lower limb oedema.

- The development of right-sided heart failure (increased JVP, congested tender liver and oedema of lower limbs) as a consequence of a lung disease is known as cor pulmonale.

Further reading

Barnes PJ. Chronic obstructive pulmonary disease. *New England Journal of Medicine* 2000;**343**:269–280.

Beckett WS. Occupational respiratory disorders. *New England Journal of Medicine* 2000;**342**:406–413.

Busse WW, Lemnske RF Jr. Asthma. *New England Journal of Medicine* 2001;**344**:350–362.

Doherty DE. The pathophysiology of airway dysfunction. *American Journal of Medicine* 2004;**20**:117; **12A**(suppl):11S–23S.

Gross TJ, Hunninghake GW. Idiopathic pulmonary fibrosis. *New England Journal of Medicine* 2001;**345**:517–525.

Kay AB. Advances in immunology: allergic disease-first of two parts. *New England Journal of Medicine* 2001;**344**:30–37.

Ratjen F, Doring G. Cystic fibrosis. *Lancet* 2003;**361**:681–689.

Stoller JK. Acute exacerbation of chronic obstructive pulmonary disease. *New England Journal of Medicine* 2002;**346**:988–994.

Wagner GR. Asbestosis and silicosis. *Lancet* 1997;**349**:1311–1315.

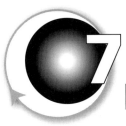

Renal system

Q1: What are the possible causes for the presenting problem?
Q2: What further questions would you like to ask to help you differentiate between your hypotheses?
Q3: What investigations would be most helpful to you and why?
Q4: In the light of the clinical presentation, how would you interpret the laboratory test results?
Q5: What is your final hypothesis?
Q6: What issues in the given history, examination and laboratory tests support your final hypothesis?

Clinical cases

CASE 7.1 – Was it because of the motor-car accident?

Linda Michael, a 66-year-old retired physical education teacher is brought by ambulance to the accident and emergency (A&E) department of a local hospital. Linda has fractured her left femur, tibia and fibula in a motor-car accident. She also has a number of lacerations on her body and has lost over 2 litres of blood. Linda has a past history of high blood pressure for which she takes Lasix (furosemide; a loop diuretic) and enalapril (an angiotensin-converting enzyme or ACE inhibitor). Her blood pressure is always in the range 140/90–150/95 mmHg. She has chronic shoulder pain for which she takes naproxen (a non-steroidal anti-inflammatory drug or NSAID). On arrival at the hospital she is conscious but in severe pain. Her vital signs on arrival are shown in Table 7.1.

Table 7.1 Vital siqns for Case 7.1

Vital signs	Linda's results	Normal range
Blood pressure (mmHg)	90/60	100/60–135/85
Pulse rate (/min)	120	60–100
Respiratory rate (/min)	23	12–16
Temperature (°C)	36.5	36.6–37.2

Cardiovascular and respiratory examinations are normal.

Her abdomen is soft and there is no tenderness or rigidity. There is no evidence of intra-abdominal bleeding. Neurological examination is normal.

No other fractures found.

The A&E registrar starts an intravenous infusion of a plasma substitute to expand her plasma volume and takes blood for laboratory tests, blood grouping and cross-matching. Over the next few hours, Linda's blood pressure responds to the intravenous fluid infusion but her urine output, collected via a bladder catheter, remains very low (5–10 mL/h).

Urinalysis: blood +++, protein +++.

● CASE 7.2 – I always feel tired and lack energy.

Sam Griggs, a 56-year-old scientist, comes in to see a local GP, Dr Michael Loscalloz, because of generalized fatigue, muscle aches and headaches over the last 6 months. He also gives a recent history of nausea, loss of appetite, changes in his taste and tingling and numbness of both lower limbs. Sam has been undergoing treatment for type 2 diabetes mellitus and high blood pressure for over 18 years. On examination, his conjunctivae are pale, his mouth is dry and itching marks are noted on his body. His skin is pale with yellow complexion. His vital signs are shown in Table 7.2.

Table 7.2 Vital signs for Case 7.2

Vital signs	Sam's results	Normal range
Blood pressure (mmHg)	180/110	100/60–135/85
Pulse rate (/min)	90	60–100
Respiratory rate (/min)	19	12–16
Temperature (°C)	36.5	36.6–37.2

Cardiovascular and respiratory examination:

- Jugular venous pressure (JVP) raised
- Auscultation of the heart: both first and second heart sounds are heard; no murmurs
- Mild pitting oedema of both lower limbs.

Abdominal examination: soft and not tender.

Upper and lower limbs: glove and stocking hypothesia.

● CASE 7.3 – I have swollen legs and I can't get my shoes on.

Farah Al Aion Anwar is a 22-year-old international university student who comes in to see the GP, Dr Candice Morri, at her clinic at the student union building. Farah noticed swelling of her feet the morning after celebrating her best friend's birthday. This was about 3 weeks ago. Since then she has noticed that the swelling is increasing and she is unable to get her shoes on. She has also noticed that her fingers have become swollen and she is unable to get any of her rings off her fingers. Two mornings ago, one of her friends who lives with her at college noticed that Farah Al Aion's eyelids were more swollen than usual. Farah gives a history of type 1 diabetes and has been on insulin since the age of 6. On examination, Farah has a swollen face and oedema of the eyelids, fingers and lower limbs. Her vital signs are shown in Table 7.3.

Table 7.3 Vital signs for Case 7.3

Vital signs	Farah Al Aion's results	Normal range
Blood pressure (mmHg)	180/110	100/60–135/85
Pulse rate (/min)	88	60–100
Respiratory rate (/min)	18	12–16
Temperature (°C)	37.1	36.6–37.2

Cardiovascular and respiratory systems: normal.

Pitting oedema of both lower limbs and hands.

Slight puffiness of her eyelids.

Urinalysis: protein +++.

👥 Integrated medical sciences questions

● CASE 7.1 – Discuss the mechanisms underlying the pathogenesis of Linda's presenting problems. You can use flow diagrams to outline your answers.

● CASE 7.2 – Discuss the mechanisms underlying the pathogenesis of Sam's presenting problems. You can use flow diagrams to outline your answers.

● CASE 7.3 – Discuss the mechanisms underlying the pathogenesis of Farah Al Aion's presenting problems. You can use flow diagrams to outline your answers.

🔑 Key concepts

In order to work through the core clinical cases in this chapter, you will need to understand the following key concepts.

The functions of the kidney

- Filtrate blood and remove toxic by-products of metabolism from the blood, e.g. urea and creatinine

- Conserve salts, glucose, proteins and water

- Monitor and respond to changes in blood pressure (e.g. via the production of renin)

- Contribute to acid–base balance of the body (remember that the heart, lung and liver are very important in acid–base balance; the kidney is important in long-term acid–base homoeostasis)

- Produce a hormone called erythropoietin, which is the key regulator of red blood cell production

- Produce renin, erythropoietin and prostaglandins and convert precursors of vitamin D to active vitamin D (1,25-dihydroxyvitamin D); thus the kidney plays an important role in calcium and phosphate homoeostasis

- Contribute to detoxification and excretion of many drugs and their metabolites.

The main characteristics of the cells forming the different parts of a uriniferous tubule and the functions of each of these cells

Table 7.4 Cells making up the uriniferous tubules

Region of a tubule	Cell type	Main characteristics/transporters	Function
Renal capsule	Simple squamous epithelium	Fused basal laminae and podocyte formation	Filtration
Proximal tubule	Simple cuboidal epithelium	Basolateral membrane transporters: Na^+/K^+ ATPase GLUT2 (early proximal tubule cells) Apical (luminal) transporters: Na^+/glucose co-transporter Na^+/inorganic phosphate co-transporter Na^+/amino acid co-transporter Na^+/H^+ exchanger Cl^-/base exchanger	Reabsorption of 70–80 per cent of water, sodium and chloride. Reabsorption of 100 per cent of amino acids, inorganic phosphate, proteins, glucose and bicarbonate Hydrogen extrusion
Descending thin limb of the loop of Henle	Simple squamous epithelium	Cells have numerous, long, radiating processes that interdigitate with those of neighbouring cells. Cells bulge into the lumen of the tubule. Their nuclei stain less densely	Completely permeable to water and salts

Ascending thin limb of the loop of Henle	Simple squamous epithelium	Cells have numerous, long, radiating processes that interdigitate with those of neighbouring cells	Impermeable to water; permeable to sodium and chloride
Ascending thick limb of the loop of Henle	Simple cuboidal epithelium	Basolateral membrane transporters: Na⁺/K⁺ ATPase Cl⁻ channels K⁺ channels Cl⁻/K⁺ co-transporters Apical (luminal) transporters: Na⁺/2Cl⁻/K⁺ co-transporter Na⁺/H⁺ exchanger K⁺ channels	Impermeable to water Sodium and chloride leave renal tubule to enter renal interstitium
Distal convoluted tubule	Simple cuboidal epithelium	Basolateral membrane transporters: Na⁺/K⁺ ATPase Cl⁻ channels Apical (luminal) transporters: Na⁺/Cl⁻ co-transporter Na⁺/H⁺ exchanger	Pumps sodium to the interstitial fluid Antidiuretic hormone (ADH) acts on the distal convoluted tubules allowing water and urea to leave the lumen and enter the renal interstitium
Collecting tubules	Simple cuboidal epithelium	Basolateral membrane transporters: Na⁺/K⁺ ATPase Apical (luminal) transporters: Na⁺ channel K⁺ channels	Pumps sodium to the interstitial fluid ADH acts on the collecting tubules. allowing water and urea to leave the lumen and enter the renal interstitium

The structure and function of the juxtaglomerular apparatus

The juxtaglomerular (JG) apparatus consists of the following:

- The macula densa of the distal tubule (tall, narrow cells with centrally placed nuclei)
- The JG cells of the adjacent afferent glomerular arteriole (modified smooth muscle cells located in the tunica media of afferent glomerular arterioles)
- The extraglomerular mesangial cells, which contain granules and occupy the space bounded by the afferent arteriole, macula densa, efferent arteriole and vascular arteriolar pole of the renal capsule).

The JG apparatus plays an important role in blood pressure regulation.

The possible mechanisms by which the kidney contributes to blood pressure control

- A fall in systemic blood pressure → decreased renal afferent arteriole perfusion pressure → decreased glomerular capillary hydrostatic pressure → decreased glomerular filtration rate (GFR) → decreased sodium and water delivered in the renal tubule → less salt in renal tubules → the macula densa cells sensing a decreased concentration of sodium → triggering of the following:

  - dilatation of the afferent arteriole

  - release of renin from the juxtaglomerular cells → increased production of angiotensin I and angiotensin II → vasoconstriction of the efferent arteriole and stimulation of aldosterone secretion. Aldosterone acts on the distal tubules and collecting ducts resulting in increased sodium, chloride and water reabsorption and increased potassium secretion.

- A fall of blood pressure → stimulates sympathetic innervation to the kidney → resulting in these changes:

  - vasoconstriction of the afferent and efferent arterioles

  - increased sodium reabsorption in the proximal tubule and thick ascending limb of the loop of Henle

  - increased renin secretion and hence angiotensin II formation.

  This mechanism is stimulated in severe hypotension.

- A fall in blood pressure → decreased cardiac output and haemoconcentration → increased osmolality of blood → stimulation of antidiuretic hormone (ADH) secretion from the posterior pituitary → ADH acting on the distal convoluted tubules and collecting ducts → water channels being inserted into the apical plasma membrane → uptake of water from the tubular fluid → maximal amount of water being reabsorbed from the tubular fluid → concentrated urine secreted.

The possible causes for anaemia in chronic renal failure

- Increased haemolysis (shortened red cell survival)
- Failure to synthesize erythropoietin (the sensor for O_2-carrying capacity is in the medulla, allowing the kidney to send impulses when there is a need for the production of additional red blood cells; erythropoietin secreted by the kidney travels via the bloodstream to the bone marrow where it stimulates erythropoiesis)
- Decreased bone marrow activity
- Decreased appetite and dietary deficiency (e.g. folate)
- Increased blood loss (from the gut, in urine and during repeated haemodialysis).

What is renal failure?

Renal failure means failure of the renal excretory functions as a result of decreased GFR. Chronic renal failure may be associated with failure of erythropoietin production (anaemia), lack of vitamin D hydroxylation (bone changes, bone pain, renal osteodystrophy), disturbed acid–base regulation (acidosis), abnormal regulation of salt and water balance (fluid retention, heart failure, polyuria and oedema), abnormal platelet function (bruising, epistaxis), skin changes (pigmentation, pruritus) and loss of blood pressure control (high blood pressure). The presence of these changes may help in differentiating chronic from acute renal failure.

The causes of acute renal failure?

The main causes of acute renal failure may be summarized as follows:

- Prerenal disorders (also known as prerenal azotaemia): this may be caused by total volume loss, e.g. blood loss, excessive vomiting and diarrhoea, pancreatitis, burns and congestive heart failure

- Intrarenal disease (also known intrinsic renal azotaemia): this may be caused by: glomerular disease, e.g. acute glomerulonephritis, vascular disease, e.g. vasculitis, and tubulointerstitial disease, e.g. acute tubular necrosis, drug-induced interstitial nephritis, damage of the renal tissue by immunoglobulin light chains, etc.

- Postrenal disease (also known as postrenal azotaemia): this may be caused by prostatic enlargement in males, pelvic or retroperitoneal malignancy causing occlusion of the two ureters, and urethral obstruction caused by stones.

The main differences between prerenal azotaemia and intrinsic renal azotaemia (Table 7.5)

Table 7.5 Main differences between prerenal and intrinsic renal axotaemia

Characteristic	Prerenal azotaemia	Intrinsic renal azotaemia
Urinary sediment	No casts	Granular and hyaline casts
	No red blood cells	Red blood cells +++
Urinary Na+ concentration (mmol/L)	< 20	> 40
Urinary specific gravity	> 1.020	< 1.010
Urine osmolality (mosmol/L)	> 500	< 300

The main causes of chronic renal failure

- Hypertensive nephropathy
- Primary glomerular disease
- Secondary glomerular disease, e.g. diabetes mellitus, systemic lupus erythematosus (SLE)
- Reflux nephropathy
- Vasculitis
- Polycystic kidney disease
- Renal tuberculosis
- Nephrocalcinosis
- Drug-induced interstitial nephritis.

Answers

 CASE 7.1 – Was it because of the motor-car accident?

Q1: What are the possible causes for the presenting problem?

A1

The following are possible causes (hypotheses) for Linda's presentation:

- Acute renal failure secondary to hypovolaemia (blood loss), hypotension and decreased renal perfusion
- Acute tubular necrosis (precipitated by blood loss, intake of naproxen which inhibits local prostaglandin production, intake of enalapril, an ACE inhibitor, and Lasix (furosemide), a loop diuretic): these three drugs have interfered with the renal autoregulatory mechanisms and precipitate acute tubular damage
- Acute-on-chronic renal failure: we need to assess whether or not Linda has had renal failure before the accident
- Damage to her kidneys, ureters, bladder and urethra because of the accident.

 Q2: What further questions would you like to ask to help you differentiate between your hypotheses?

A2

Table 7.6 Further history questions for Case 7.1

History questions	In what way answers can help
Any past history of renal impairment, past investigations or treatment for renal failure	Renal function is monitored by measurement of serum creatinine, blood urea nitrogen and urinalysis, and by several quantification tests of urinary protein excretion. It is important to consider in our assessment Linda's renal function before the accident. Pre-existing renal failure will aggravate the degree of her renal impairment
The patient's blood pressure readings before the accident	We need to know the degree of her blood pressure drop as a result of the blood loss. We might also measure her blood pressure on sitting and lying in bed. A significant difference, > 30 mmHg systolic and > 15 mmHg diastolic, indicates significant volume loss and postural drop of blood pressure
How long has the patient been on naproxen and enalapril? Is she on any other medications?	Naproxen is a non-steroidal anti-inflammatory drug (NSAID). It acts by inhibiting the enzyme cyclo-oxygenase (COX). Prostaglandins have vasodilator effects on the kidney. This is particularly important in the presence of renal impairment, e.g. in patients with renal impairment, glomerular filtration is decreased. The body corrects this impairment by afferent arteriolar vasodilatation, mediated by prostaglandins, and by efferent arteriolar vasoconstriction, mediated by angiotensin II. Thus, intake of naproxen and enalapril will interfere with these two compensatory mechanisms, resulting in renal impairment, decreased urine output and raised blood creatinine

	Naproxen also interferes with renal function by a number of mechanisms including: NSAIDs cause salt and water retention → hypertension and oedema; inhibition of renin release → hypoaldosteronism → impaired potassium excretion → hyperkalaemia; and NSAIDs may cause interstitial nephritis
Any increases in the patient's urine output per hour after treating her volume loss?	If there is an improvement in her urine output after treating volume loss, her renal impairment is most likely caused by decreased renal perfusion (acute renal failure caused by decreased renal perfusion)

 Q3: What investigations would be most helpful to you and why?

A3

Further investigations

- Full blood examination
- Serum sodium, potassium, urea and creatinine
- Urine sodium, urine osmolality
- Arterial blood gases
- Urine microscopy
- Urinalysis including urine specific gravity and osmolality
- Ultrasound of the abdomen
- Radiograph of fractured bones.

 CASE 7.2 – I always feel tired and lack energy.

 Q1: What are the possible causes for the presenting problem?

A1

The following are possible causes (hypotheses) for Sam's presentation:

- Chronic renal failure secondary to diabetic glomerulosclerosis
- Chronic renal failure secondary to hypertensive nephropathy
- Chronic renal failure caused by primary glomerulonephritis.

Q2: What further questions would you like to ask to help you differentiate between your hypotheses?

A2

Table 7.7 Further history questions for Case 7.2

History questions	In what way answers can help
Any history of breathlessness	Shortness of breath in patients with chronic renal failure are the result of: fluid and sodium retention; development of heart failure because of fluid and sodium overload and high blood pressure; and anaemia. Anaemia is common in patients with chronic renal failure, and the possible causes are: deficiency of erythropoietin; decreased erythropoiesis; reduced red cell survival; increased blood loss because of capillary fragility; and decreased dietary intake and possibly malabsorption
Any history of bone pain	Renal osteodystrophy (metabolic bone disease) may occur in chronic renal failure. This is usually in the form of osteomalacia, hyperparathyroid bone disease, osteoporosis and osteosclerosis:
	Osteomalacia: results from diminished activity of α_1-hydroxylase enzyme and failure of formation of active vitamin D (1,25-dihydroxycholecalciferol)
	Osteitis fibrosa: results from secondary hyperparathyroidism
	Osteoporosis: may be related to malnutrition
	Osteosclerosis: cause is unknown
Any history of muscle cramps, particularly at night	In chronic renal failure, patients may complain of muscle cramps and 'restless leg syndrome' at night. This may be the result of poor nutrition, hyperparathyroidism, electrolyte imbalance, vitamin D deficiency or motor neuropathy
Loss of libido and sexual functions	In patients with chronic renal failure, loss of libido and sexual function is caused by: disturbance of the pituitary gonadal axis or hyperprolactinaemia
Any changes in the patient's urine	Patients with chronic renal failure may notice these changes: nocturia, which is usually an early symptom of chronic renal failure and results from renal loss of concentrating ability and increased osmotic load per nephron; or urine, usually frothy, indicating excessive loss of protein in urine
Any bleeding or increased tendency to ecchymoses and mucosal bleeding	Patients with chronic renal failure may notice increased bleeding tendency, caused by platelet malfunction, prolonged bleeding time or capillary fragility
Medications and allergies	The half-life of a large number of drugs is affected by the renal function, e.g. the half-life of insulin is prolonged in chronic renal failure as a result of reduced metabolism of insulin in renal tubules. Thus, insulin requirements may be reduced. However, a post-receptor defect in insulin action may be present leading to a relative resistance to insulin action

Q3: What investigations would be most helpful to you and why?

A3

Further investigations

- Full blood examination
- Serum sodium, potassium, calcium, phosphorus and albumin
- Blood urea and creatinine
- Fasting blood glucose level
- Urinalysis and urine microscopy
- Renal ultrasound
- Renal computed tomography (CT)
- ECG.

 CASE 7.3 – I have swollen legs and I can't get my shoes on.

 Q1: What are the possible causes for the presenting problem?

A1

A possible cause (hypothesis) for Farah Al Aion's presentation is development of nephrotic syndrome. The causes of her nephrotic syndrome may be:

- Diabetic nephropathy
- Focal and segmental glomerulonephritis
- Minimal change nephropathy
- Membranous nephropathy
- Other causes: systemic lupus erythematosus (SLE) and amyloidosis.

Less likely causes for her lower limb oedema:

- Congestive heart failure
- Liver failure.

Q2: What further questions would you like to ask to help you differentiate between your hypotheses?

A2

Table 7.8 Further history questions for Case 7.3

History questions	In what way answers can help
Any past history of renal trouble during childhood	Minimal change nephropathy may occur during childhood
Past investigations and treatment	
Recent changes in bodyweight	The increase in bodyweight is likely to be the result of fluid retention and oedema. The mechanisms responsible for oedema formation in these patients are: lowered oncotic pressure of blood because of low serum albumin; increased capillary fragility, leakage of protein in the interstitium and reduced oncotic pressure gradient; and increased hydrostatic pressure, fluid retention and intravascular volume expansion
Any history of recurrent infections or increased susceptibility to infections	Patients with nephrotic syndrome are at higher risk of infection, especially pneumococci, usually caused by hypogammaglobinaemia
Any history of thromboembolism, or arterial or venous occlusion	Patients with nephrotic syndrome may present with arterial or venous occlusion caused by increased blood coagulability or development of hypercholesterolaemia
Any changes in urine	The presence of excessive amounts of protein in urine may produce frothy urine

 Q3: What investigations would be most helpful to you and why?

A3

Further investigations

- Full blood examination
- Serum sodium, potassium, calcium and phosphorus
- Blood urea and creatinine
- Serum albumin
- Blood cholesterol
- Urine microscopy
- Urine protein/24 h
- Ultrasound of kidneys
- Renal biopsy.

Further progress

● CASE 7.1 – Was it because of the motor-car accident?

The registrar arranges some tests for Linda. The results are shown in Tables 7.9–7.11.

Table 7.9 Full blood examination: results for Case 7.1

Test	Linda's results	Normal range
Haemoglobin (Hb) (g/L)	95	115–160
Packed cell volume (PCV)	0.56	0.37–0.47
White cell count (WCC) ($\times 10^9$/L)	8.3	4.0–11.0
Platelet count ($\times 10^9$/L)	540	150–400

Table 7.10 Biochemical test results for Case 7.1

Test	Two months before the accident	On admission	Normal range
Serum sodium (mmol/L)	142	138	135–145
Serum potassium (mmol/L)	4.7	6.4	3.5–5.0
Serum chloride (mmol/L)	101	94	95–110
Blood urea (mmol/L)	5.5	46	2.5–8.3
Serum creatinine (mmol/L)	0.08	0.48	0.05–0.11

Table 7.11 Urine test on admission for Case 7.1

Test	Linda's results	Normal range
Volume (mL/h)	5	30–150
Colour	Dark	Pale amber
pH	5	5–7
Nitrates	Negative	Negative
Blood	+++	Negative
Protein	+++	Negative
Urine sodium (mmol/L)	43	20–200
Urine osmolality (mosmol/L)	300	80–800
Urine specific gravity	1.010	1.010–1.030

Urine microscopy: granular and hyaline casts are present.

Abdomen ultrasound examination: normal; no evidence of trauma to internal organs.

CASE 7.2 – I always feel tired and lack energy.

Dr Loscalloz arranges some tests for Sam. The results are shown in Tables 7.12–7.14.

Table 7.12 Full blood examination: results for Case 7.2

Test	Sam's results	Normal range
Hb (g/L)	93	115–160
PCV	0.39	0.37–0.47
WCC ($\times 10^9$/L)	4.1	4.0–11.0
Platelet count ($\times 10^9$/L)	290	150–400

Table 7.13 Biochemical test results for Case 7.2

Test	Sam's results	Normal range
Serum sodium (mmol/L)	139	135–145
Serum potassium (mmol/L)	4.9	3.5–5.0
Serum chloride (mmol/L)	104	95–110
Blood urea (mmol/L)	42	2.5–8.3
Serum creatinine (mmol/L)	0.78	0.05–0.11
Fasting blood glucose (mmol/L)	5.3	3.6–5.3
Blood calcium (mmol/L)	1.9	2.1–2.6
Blood phosphate (mmol/L)	2.9	0.9–1.35
Serum albumin (g/L)	18	35–50

Table 7.14 Urine test results for Case 7.2

Test	Sam's results	Normal range
Volume (mL/h)	20	30–150
Colour	Pale	Pale amber
pH	6	5–7
Nitrates	Negative	Negative
Blood	+++	Negative
Protein	+++	Negative
Urine specific gravity	1.010	1.010–1.030

Renal ultrasound examination: both kidneys are small and shrunken. No evidence of back-pressure or obstruction. No urinary calculi.

ECG: evidence of left ventricular hypertrophy. No ischaemic changes.

● CASE 7.3 – I have swollen legs and I can't get my shoes on.

Dr Morris arranges some tests for Farah Al Aion. The results are shown in Tables 7.15 and 7.16.

Table 7.15 Full blood examination: results for Case 7.3

Test	Farah Al Aion's results	Normal range
Hb (g/L)	120	115–160
PCV	0.35	0.37–0.47
WCC (× 10⁹/L)	8.7	4.0–11.0
Platelet count (× 10⁹/L)	190	150–400

Table 7.16 Biochemical test results for Case 7.3

Test	Farah Al Aion's results	Normal range
Serum sodium (mmol/L)	138	135–145
Serum potassium (mmol/L)	3.6	3.5–5.0
Serum chloride (mmol/L)	105	95–110
Blood urea (mmol/L)	16.2	2.5–8.3
Serum creatinine (mmol/L)	0.15	0.05–0.11
Fasting blood glucose (mmol/L)	8.5	3.6–5.3
Serum albumin (g/L)	17	35–50
Blood cholesterol (mmol/L)	9.6	0.0–5.5
Blood triglycerides (mmol/L)	2.0	0.5–2.0

Table 7.17 Urine test results for Case 7.3

Test	Farah Al Aion's results	Normal range
Casts	Mainly hyaline and few red cell casts	Negative
Urine protein excretion/24 h (g)	5.5 (consisted mainly of albumin)	< 3.5

Renal ultrasound examination: both kidneys are not shrunken. No evidence of renal stones or obstructive uropathy.

Renal biopsy: not performed.

Further questions

● CASE 7.1 – Was it because of the motor-car accident?

Q4: In the light of the clinical presentation, how would you interpret the laboratory test results?

A4

Table 7.18 Interpretation of lab test results for Case 7.1

Test	Change	Interpretation
Hb	Low	The patient lost over 2 L blood and this has caused volume depletion, decreased renal perfusion and acute renal failure. Prolonged renal hypoperfusion could also result in acute tubular necrosis
Platelet count	Raised	Platelet count may be raised when the body is exposed to severe acute stress/damage, e.g. after surgery, trauma
Serum potassium	Raised	In acute renal failure, the serum potassium level is raised (hyperkalaemia). The mechanism by which hyperkalaemia occurred in the patient's condition are: abrupt shift of potassium from the ICF to the ECF, which occurs in acidosis or circumstances resulting in cell destruction, e.g. trauma; hyperkalaemia may be the result of intake of NSAIDs and ACE inhibitors; and impaired secretion of potassium by renal tubules
		Metabolic acidosis in renal failure can be the result of decreased net acid excretion (mainly excretion of organic and inorganic anions such as phosphates and sulphates)
Blood urea	Raised	Blood urea is affected by several factors including: blood volume and renal perfusion (increase in hypovolaemia and hypotension); liver function (decrease in liver failure); cardiac function (increase in congestive heart failure); protein intake; and renal function (increase in impaired renal function)
		Raised blood urea in her condition could be caused by decreased renal perfusion (hypovolaemia and hypotension) or acute tubular damage and back leak of solutes such as urea and creatinine into the circulation
		Tubular damage may be caused by: renal ischaemia; lack of ATP required for normal tubular cell function; vasoconstriction; presence of 'free radicals'; damage of renal tubules by myoglobin released from damaged muscles; and presence of a 'second insult', e.g. intake of NSAIDs and ACE inhibitors resulting in failure of the autoregulatory mechanisms

Serum creatinine	Raised	Serum creatinine is derived from the high-energy phosphate compound, phosphocreatine, which maintains the level of ATP in muscle. Loss of phosphocreatine's phosphate → a waste product 'creatinine' being created and excreted by the kidney
		Creatinine is filtered and passed thought the nephron without any reabsorption. Only a small amount is added to urine by tubular secretion
		The serum creatinine levels are affected by two main factors: (1) rate of creatinine production and (2) rate of creatinine clearance (decreased GFR results in increased serum creatinine level), reflecting renal impairment
Urine sodium	> 40 mmol/L (raised)	In prerenal acute failure, urinary sodium is < 20 mmol/L and urinary osmolality > 500 mosmol/L, whereas in acute tubular necrosis urinary sodium is > 40 mmol/L (sodium lost in urine) and urinary osmolality < 300 mosmol/L
Urine osmolality and urine specific gravity	Low (expected to be raised because of the volume loss)	The failure of the kidney to preserve sodium and water (low urine osmolality) in the presence of low blood pressure and hypovolaemia indicate acute renal tubular damage
Urinalysis	Red blood cells +++, protein +++ Granular and hyaline casts are present	The presence of red blood cells (+++), protein (+++) and granular casts indicate renal tubular damage. In prerenal acute renal failure, the urinalysis usually shows negative red blood cells, negative protein and no granular casts

ACE, angiotensin-converting enzyme; ATP, adenosine triphosphate; ECF, extracellular fluid; GFR, glomerular filtration rate; ICF, intracellular fluid; NSAID, non-steroidal anti-inflammatory drug.

 Q5: What is your final hypothesis?

A5

The clinical picture and laboratory results are supportive of acute tubular necrosis.

 Q6: What issues in the given history, examination and laboratory tests support your final hypothesis?

A6

Supportive evidence

History

● Patient fractured her left femur, tibia and fibula in a motor-car accident

● A number of lacerations on her body

● Lost over 2 L blood

- Past history of chronic shoulder pain
- On naproxen (for shoulder pain), and enalapril and Lasix (furosemide; for high blood pressure).

Examination

- Low blood pressure
- Increased heart rate and respiratory rates
- Afebrile
- No evidence of internal bleeding
- No other fractures
- Very little urine despite volume replacement and correction of her blood pressure.

Investigations

- Evidence of acute renal failure: raised blood urea and creatinine after the accident, raised serum potassium. The patient has no renal trouble before the accident; the precipitating factor is blood loss (low Hb).
- Evidence of acute tubular necrosis: urine specific gravity is low despite hypovolaemia and low blood pressure (kidney lost its ability to concentrate urine). Increased sodium loss in urine (kidney is unable to retain sodium). Urine microscopy: Red blood cells +++, protein +++, granular and hyaline casts present (indicating tubular damage).

CASE 7.2 – I always feel tired and lack energy.

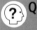 **Q4: In the light of the clinical presentation, how would you interpret the laboratory test results?**

A4

Table 7.19 Interpretation of lab test results for Case 7.2

Test	Change	Interpretation
Hb	Low	Anaemia in patients with chronic renal failure may be the result of: deficiency of erythropoietin; decreased erythropoiesis caused by toxic effects of anaemia on bone marrow precursor cells; increased blood loss resulting from capillary fragility and poor platelet function; decreased dietary intake; reduced red cell survival; and malabsorption
Serum potassium	Upper limit of normal range	In chronic renal failure, hyperkalaemia does not occur until the GFR has reached a low level of < 15 ml/L. Several factors may precipitate hyperkalaemia in patients with chronic failure including development of acidosis, impaired secretion of potassium by collecting duct segment and injudicious administration of intravenous fluids containing potassium

Blood urea	Raised	Raised blood urea and serum creatinine indicate the presence of chronic renal impairment (see comments on previous case). Urea itself is relatively non-toxic but its serum level is a good surrogate indicator of how the kidney could handle products of protein metabolism
Fasting blood glucose	Upper limit of normal	Patients with diabetes usually require less exogenous insulin as chronic renal failure progresses (because of decreased production of renal insulinase and decreased degradation of insulin in their bodies). The patient has type 2 diabetes and is most probably on oral hypoglycaemic agents. As a result of the prolonged half-life of oral hypoglycaemic agents in patients with chronic renal failure, great caution should be taken if there is a need to raise the dose. In most patients the dose needs to be decreased
Blood calcium	Low	The causes of low blood calcium in chronic renal failure are: phosphate retention; poor nutrition; malabsorption of calcium absorption; and lack of α_1-hydroxylase enzyme. Lack of α_1-hydroxylase $\rightarrow$ lack of 1,25-dihydroxyvitamin D $\rightarrow$ decreased absorption of calcium from the intestine
Blood phosphate	Raised	Decreased filtration of phosphate as GFR falls $\rightarrow$ phosphate retention $\rightarrow$ increased blood phosphate concentration $\rightarrow$ relative decrease of blood calcium concentration $\rightarrow$ augmentation of parathyroid hormone (PTH) synthesis and secretion $\rightarrow$ increased blood PTH concentration $\rightarrow$ increased activity of osteoclasts $\rightarrow$ acceleration of bone resorption
Serum albumin	Low	Increased loss of albumin in urine as a result of glomerular damage
Urine blood and Protein	+++	Glomerular damage causing loss of blood and protein in urine
Urine specific gravity	Low	This is mainly the result of loss of renal-concentrating ability and decreased osmotic load per nephron. Both factors result in excessive loss of water
Renal ultrasound	Both kidneys are small. No evidence of back pressure or obstruction. No urinary calculi	In chronic renal failure both kidneys are usually small in size
ECG	Left ventricular hypertrophy	Left ventricular hypertrophy is probably related to high blood pressure. Hypertension in chronic renal failure is usually the result of: sodium retention; hypersecretion of renin; increased secretion of angiotensin II and aldosterone; fluid retention; sympathetic stimulation via afferent renal reflexes; impaired renal endothelial function with decreased nitric oxide and increased endothelin production; and atherosclerosis and hyperlipidaemia

Q5: What is your final hypothesis?

A5

The clinical picture and laboratory results are suggestive of chronic renal failure.

Q6: What issues in the given history, examination and laboratory tests support your final hypothesis?

A6

Supportive evidence

History

- Generalized fatigue, muscle aches over the past 6 months
- Recent history of nausea, loss of appetite, changes in taste, tingling and numbness of both lower limbs
- Treated for type 2 diabetes and high blood pressure for over 18 years.

Examination

- Conjunctivae are pale
- Patient's mouth is dry
- Itching marks noted on his body
- His skin is pale and yellow in complexion
- Blood pressure 180/110 mmHg
- Raised pulse and respiratory rates
- JVP raised
- Mild pitting oedema of both lower limbs
- Glove-and-stocking hypothesia.

Investigations

- Hb low
- Serum potassium upper limit of normal
- Raised blood urea and creatinine
- Low serum calcium
- Raised serum phosphate
- Low serum albumin
- Urine specific gravity low (1.010)

- Urine: blood +++, protein +++, nitrates negative

- Renal ultrasound examination: both kidneys are small and shrunken; no evidence of back pressure or obstruction; no urinary calculi.

- ECG: evidence of left ventricular hypertrophy; no ischaemic changes.

● CASE 7.3 – I have swollen legs and I can't get my shoes on.

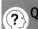 **Q4: In the light of the clinical presentation, how would you interpret the laboratory test results?**

A4

Table 7.20 Interpretation of lab test results for Case 7.3

Test	Change	Interpretation
Blood urea and serum creatinine	Mildly raised	Moderate azotaemia may be present in patients with nephrotic syndrome (usually related to hypoalbuminaemia and intravascular volume depletion)
Fasting blood glucose	Raised	Diabetes may be responsible for the development of nephrotic syndrome
Serum albumin	Low	Nephrotic syndrome is characterized by: heavy proteinuria; hypoalbuminaemia; severe oedema; and hypercholesterolaemia
		Hypoalbuminaemia is the result of excessive loss of albumin from damaged glomeruli
Blood cholesterol	Raised	Most patients with nephrotic syndrome have elevated total and LDL-cholesterol + low or normal HDL-cholesterol
		Serum triacylglycerols may be raised
		The mechanisms responsible for raised blood lipids in patients with nephrotic syndrome are: (1) overproduction and impaired catabolism of apolipoprotein β-containing lipoproteins, (2) decreased catabolism of chylomicrons and VLDLs, and (3) decreased plasma oncotic pressure which stimulates hepatic lipoprotein synthesis and hyperlipidaemia
Urine microscopy	Casts (mainly hyaline and red cell cast)	The presence of red cell casts indicates glomerular disease
Urine protein excretion/24 h	Raised (5.5 g/24 h)	Increased protein loss in urine > 3.5 g/24 h indicates nephrotic syndrome

HDL, high-density lipoprotein; LDL, low-density lioprotein; VLDL, very low-density lipoprotein.

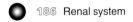

 Q5: What is your final hypothesis?

A5

The clinical picture and laboratory results are suggestive of nephrotic syndrome.

 Q6: What issues in the given history, examination and laboratory tests support your final hypothesis?

A6

Supportive evidence

History

- Noticed swelling of her feet – 3 weeks ago
- Swelling is increasing and she is unable to get her shoes on
- Her fingers have become swollen
- Her eyelids are swollen and look different from usual
- On insulin for type 1 diabetes mellitus since the age of 6.

Examination

- Blood pressure 180/110 mmHg
- Afebrile
- Cardiovascular and respiratory systems are normal
- Pitting oedema of both lower limbs and hands
- Slight puffiness of her eyelids
- Urinalysis: protein +++.

Investigations

- Normal Hb
- Mildly raised blood urea and creatinine
- Raised fasting blood sugar
- Low serum albumin
- Raised blood cholesterol
- Urinalysis: hyaline and few red cell casts
- Urine protein excretion high (5.5 g/24 h)
- Renal ultrasound examination: both kidneys are not shrunken; no evidence of renal stones or obstructive uropathy
- Renal biopsy: not performed.

⚇ Integrated medical sciences questions

⬤ CASE 7.1 – Discuss the mechanisms underlying the pathogenesis of Linda's presenting problems. You can use flow diagrams to outline your answers.

Acute haemorrhage (> 2 L) → intravascular volume depletion → fall in mean arterial pressure → decreased GFR → decreased urine output.

The decrease in mean arterial pressure resulting from blood loss → decreased venous return → decreased cardiac output → decreased renal perfusion → decreased GFR → decreased urine output.

The fall in mean arterial pressure caused by reflex → decrease of pressure on stretch receptors in carotid sinus and aortic arch → neurohormonal response → the following changes:

- Activation of the sympathetic nervous system.

- Activation of renin–angiotensin–aldosterone system.

- Release of vasopressin (ADH)

- Release of endothelin.

These biochemical changes → vasoconstriction of mucocutaneous and visceral blood vessels + salt and water retention → maintain cerebral perfusion and GFR.

The fall in mean arterial pressure → decreased stretch receptors in the afferent arteriole → decreased perfusion pressure + relaxation of the arteriolar smooth muscle cells (the release of prostacyclin, prostaglandin E_2 and nitric oxide) → vasodilatation of afferent arteriole.

Although angiotensin II causes preferential vasoconstriction to efferent arteriole, intraglomerular pressure is preserved + increased renal filtration by glomeruli → enhancement of renal filtration (autoregulation).

Autoregulation of the kidney depends on the following:

- Secretion of prostaglandin locally

- Secretion of nitrogen oxide

- Secretion of angiotensin II.

The patient is on an ACE inhibitor → inhibition of the production of angiotensin II → failure to cause vasoconstriction of the efferent arterioles. He is also on naproxen (an NSAID) → inhibition of prostaglandin secretion → failure to dilate the afferent arterioles → decreased glomerular filtration + decreased urine output.

Also the decreased mean arterial pressure → progressive renal ischaemia → decreased oxygenation of epithelial cells + decreased glomerular ultrafiltration pressure → necrosis of epithelial cells, particularly affecting these two areas:

1. The terminal straight portion of the proximal tubules.

2. The thick ascending limb of the loop of Henle.

These two structures are particularly present in the corticomedullary junction and outer medulla (these areas normally require less O_2 compared with the renal cortex) → the mechanisms responsible for the development of necrosis which are:

- Disturbance of ion transport

- Increased intracellular Ca^{2+}
- Altered phospholipids metabolism
- Formation of free radicals.

Necrosis of epithelial cells → back leak of solutes such as urea and creatinine → increased levels of urea and creatinine in blood.

Necrotic epithelial cells and tubular casts may block the renal tubules → obstruction of their lumen → no flow + intraluminal pressure → further resistance to glomerular filtration → further decrease in urine output.

In summary, the main pathological features of acute tubular necrosis are:

- Focal necrosis of tubular epithelium
- Occlusion of renal tubules by casts and cellular debris
- Epithelial swelling
- Detachment of epithelial cells from basement membrane
- Epithelial necrosis
- Presence of inflammatory reaction, oedema and WBC infiltration. (See Figure 7.1, p. 189.)

● **CASE 7.2 – Discuss the mechanisms underlying the pathogenesis of Sam's presenting problems. You can use flow diagrams to outline your answers.**

(See Figure 7.2 on p. 190.)

● **CASE 7.3 – Discuss the mechanisms underlying the pathogenesis of Farah Al Aion's presenting problems. You can use flow diagrams to outline your answers.**

Diabetes mellitus → development of diabetic glomerulonephritis → disturbance in size- and charge-selective barriers of glomerular capillary wall → excessive glomerular leakage → loss of proteins in urine (mainly albumin). Other proteins that may be lost in urine are:

- thyroxine-binding globulin → disturbance of thyroid function test results
- metal-binding proteins → disturbance of serum levels of zinc, copper, iron, etc.
- anti-thrombin III → increased tendency for thrombosis.

The loss of proteins in urine (>3.5 g/24 h indicates glomerular damage) → hypoalbuminaemia → decreased plasma oncotic pressure → disturbance of Starling's forces across capillaries → fluid travel across capillaries to interstitial tissues → generalized oedema (face, fingers and feet).

Excessive fluid loss → hypovolaemia → the following:

- Activation of the renin–angiotensin–aldosterone system → release of angiotensin II
- Stimulation of the sympathetic nervous system

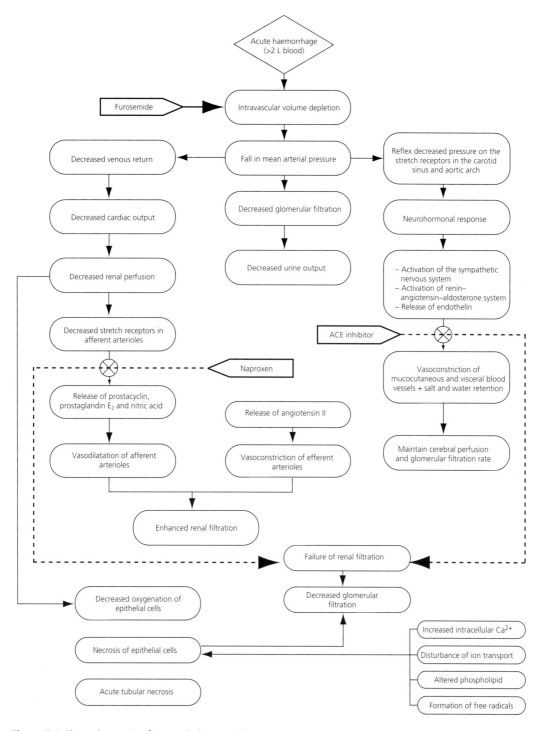

Figure 7.1 The pathogenesis of acute tubular necrosis.

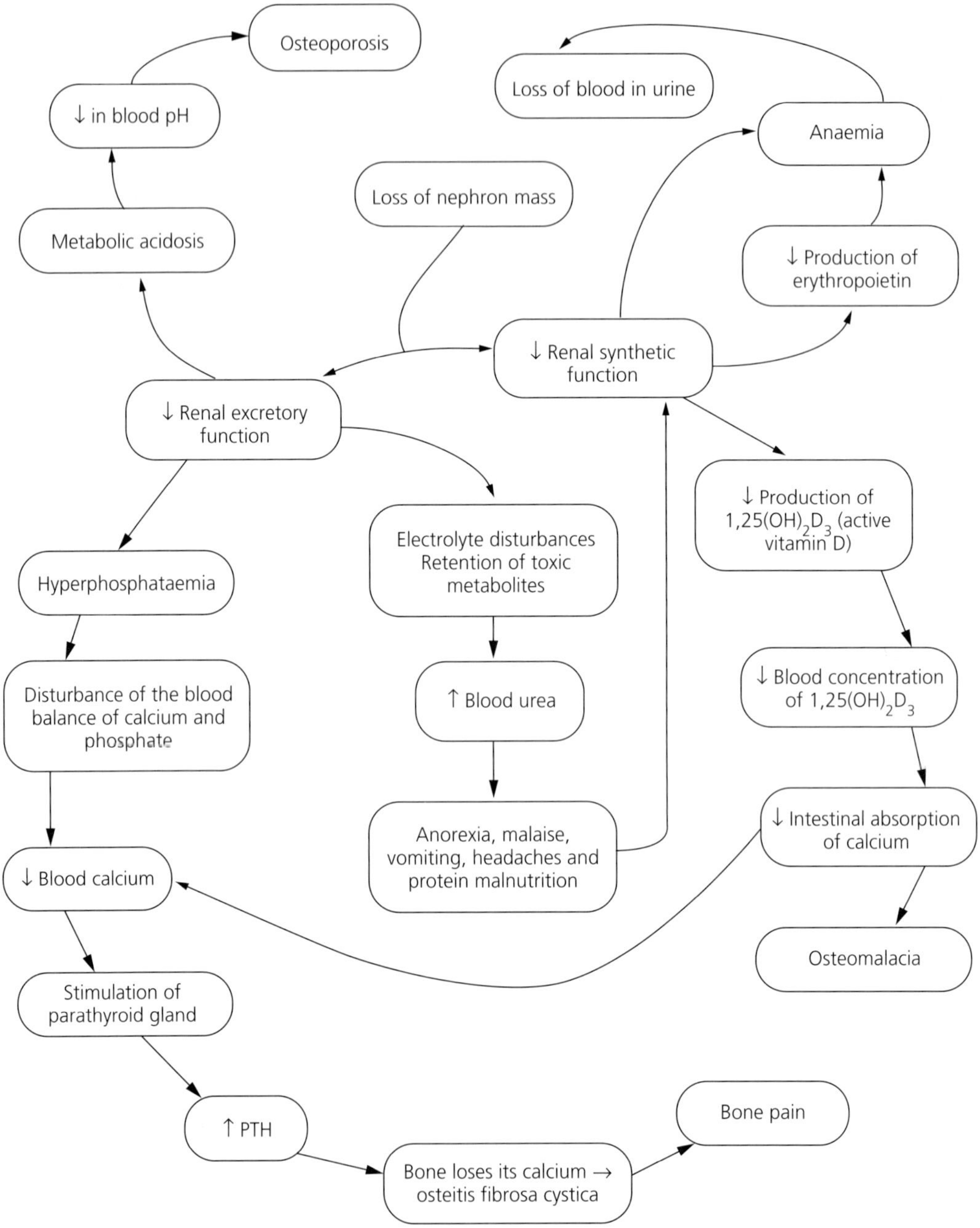

Figure 7.2 The pathogenesis of chronic renal failure.

- Decreased secretion of natriuretic hormone.

These changes result in sodium and water retention → more development of oedema and volume depletion.

However, the current evidence shows that there is no hypovolaemia in nephrotic syndrome. The evidence in support of hypervolaemia rather than hypovolaemia may be summarized as follows:

- There is an increase in blood pressure which is consistent with hypervolaemia.

- The level of circulating atrial natriuretic peptide is often elevated, causing overfilling rather than hypovolaemia.

- The pharmacological blockade of the renin–angiotensin–aldosterone system does not cause natriuresis.

In conclusion, the exact mechanism underlying nephrotic syndrome has not yet been completely understood and further research is needed to explain these differences in views.

Further reading

Akhtar M, Mana H. Molecular basis of proteinuria. *Advances in Anatomic Pathology* 2004;**11**:304–309.

Asanuma K, Mundel P. The role of podocytes in glomerular pathobiology. *Clinical and Experimental Nephrology* 2003;**7**:255–259.

Bock HA. Pathophysiology of acute renal failure in septic shock: from prerenal to renal failure. *Kidney International Supplement* 1998;**64**:S15–S18.

Brady HR, Singer GG. Acute renal failure. *Lancet* 1995;**346**:1533–1540.

Cho S, Atwood JE. Peripheral edema. *American Journal of Medicine* 2002;**113**:580–586.

Esson ML, Schrier RW. Diagnosis and treatment of acute tubular necrosis. *Annals of Internal Medicine* 2002;**137**:744–752.

Filler G. Acute renal failure in children: aetiology and management. *Paediatric Drugs* 2001;**3**:783–792.

Ichihara A, Kobori H, Nishiyama A, Navar LG. Renal renin–angiotensin system. *Contributions to Nephrology* 2004;**143**:117–130.

Komlosi P, Fintha A, Bell PD. Renal cell-to-cell communication via extracellular ATP. *Physiology* 2005;**20**:86–90.

Koomans HA. Pathophysiology of edema in idiopathic nephritic syndrome. *Nephrology, Dialysis, Transplantation* 2003;**6**(suppl):vi30–32.

Murray MD, Brater DC. Effects of NSAIDs on the kidney. *Progress in Drug Research* 1997;**49**:155–171.

Palapattu GS, Barbaric Z, Rajfer J. Acute bilateral renal cortical necrosis as a cause of postoperative renal failure. *Urology* 2001;**58**:281.

Persson PB. Renin: origin, secretion and synthesis. *Journal of Physiology* 2003;**552**(Pt 3):667–671.

Silva FG. Chemical-induced nephrology. A review of the renal tubulointerstitial lesions in humans. *Toxicologic Pathology* 2004;**32**(suppl 2):71–84.

Sladen RN, Landry D. Renal blood flow regulation, autoregulation and vasomotor nephrology. *Anesthesiology Clinics of North America* 2000;**18**:791–807.

Slapak M. Acute renal failure in general surgery. *Journal of the Royal Society of Medicine* 1996;89(suppl 29):13–15.

Stark J. Acute renal failure. Focus on advances in acute tubular necrosis. *Critical Care Nursing Clinics of North America* 1998;**10**:159–170.

Tsar V, Zima T, Kalousova M. Pathobiochemistry of nephrotic syndrome. *Advances in Clinical Chemistry* 2003;**37**:173–218.

Wan L, Bellomo R, Di Giantomasso D, Ronco C. The pathogenesis of septic acute renal failure. *Current Opinion in Critical Care* 2003;**9**:496–502.

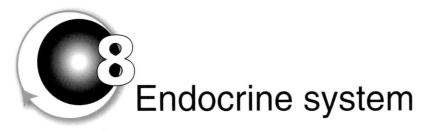

Endocrine system

? **Questions for each of the case scenarios given**

Q1: What are the possible causes for the presenting problem?
Q2: What further questions would you like to ask to help you differentiate between your hypotheses?
Q3: What investigations would be most helpful to you and why?
Q4: In the light of the clinical presentation, how would you interpret the laboratory test results?
Q5: What is your final hypothesis?
Q6: What issues in the given history, examination and laboratory tests support your final hypothesis?

Clinical cases

● CASE 8.1 – I have never had trouble with my driving.

Neill Roitt, a 51-year-old taxi driver, comes in to see Dr Celia Kemp because of tiredness and infrequent headaches of a few months' duration. He has also noticed that he wakes up at night two or three times to pass urine and is always thirsty. His colleagues have noticed that his voice has changed and become deeper. Over the last 8–12 months, several customers with whom he chatted have commented on his taxi ID photo saying, 'Your face has changed a lot. When did you take this photo?'. Three months ago, he had trouble with his driving and nearly hit two pedestrians who were crossing the road while he was turning into another street. He also has had an accident where he did not see a car on his side and hit it while changing lanes. He exclaimed, 'I've never had trouble with my driving!'.

● CASE 8.2 – I became very slow and unable to finish tasks at work.

Jane Marcus, a 48-year-old shop assistant, comes in to see the local GP, Dr Mary March, because of decreased energy, gradual weight gain, and becoming slow and unable to finish tasks at work. Jane migrated from Italy to Australia 2 years ago. She speaks little English. Her girlfriend Lisa, who joins her, helps in translation. Over the last 8 months, Jane has also noticed progressive changes in her bowel habits. Now she passes hard stools, once only every 3 or 4 days. Previously, she used to open her bowels once or twice a day. Her appetite is good and she has not made any changes to the type of food she eats. Over the last 2 years, her menstrual periods have become irregular and infrequent. Her husband left her 7 months after their arrival in Australia. She faces financial difficulties after her separation from her husband. She has one daughter, Leah, who is working with her in a small local factory.

On examination, she looks unhappy and her skin looks dry and rough. Her body mass index (BMI) is 30 (it used to be 25). Her vital signs are shown in Table 8.1.

Table 8.1 Vital signs for Case 8.2

Vital signs	Jane's results	Normal range
Blood pressure (mmHg)	130/80	100/60–135/85
Pulse rate (/min)	60, regular	60–100
Respiratory rate (/min)	12	12–16
Temperature (°C)	36.5	36.6–37.2

● CASE 8.3 – I am very tired and started vomiting again.

Eva Sheridan, an 82-year-old retired midwife, comes in to see her GP, Dr James Webster, because of repeated vomiting, nausea and generalized tiredness for the last few days. She gives a history of similar problems when she was interstate, visiting her sister, about 2 months ago. Hospital investigations at that time, including gastrointestinal endoscopy, showed no abnormality except for low serum sodium level (121 mmol/L), low blood glucose level (3.5 mmol/L) and relatively elevated serum potassium level (5 mmol/L). Further history questions reveal that Ms Sheridan has no abdominal pain and no changes in her bowel movements. She is not on any medication and gives no history of allergies. She used to work as a missionary in Africa a long time ago. On examination, she looks unwell and drowsy. Her BMI is 22 and her vital signs are shown in Table 8.2.

Table 8.2 Vital signs for Case 8.3

Vital signs	Eva's results	Normal range
Blood pressure (mmHg)	90/65	100/60–135/85
Pulse rate (/min)	100	60–100
Respiratory rate (/min)	19	12–16
Temperature (°C)	37.2	36.6–37.2

Abdominal examination

- Abdomen is soft and not tender or rigid
- Intestinal sounds are normal
- No abdominal masses or organomegaly
- Old appendectomy scar is pigmented.

Cardiovascular and respiratory examinations are normal.

Neurological examination

- Cranial nerves normal
- No signs of meningitis or signs suggesting increased intracranial tension.

Ear examination is normal.

Integrated medical sciences questions

CASE 8.1 – Briefly discuss the hormones secreted from the anterior pituitary, their cell source, regulating mechanisms, their functions and target organs.

CASE 8.2 – What are the metabolic functions of thyroxine?

CASE 8.3 – What are the causes of Cushing's syndrome? Discuss the mechanisms underlying each cause and associated changes.

Key concepts

In order to work through the core clinical cases in this chapter, you will need to understand the following key concepts.

What is a hormone?

- A hormone is a substance released by an endocrine gland and transported through the bloodstream to another tissue where it acts to regulate the function of the target tissue.

- The action of a hormone may be mediated by the binding of a hormone to receptor molecules.

- Hormones are either proteins (glycoproteins) or derived from glycoproteins, amino acids or lipids.

- The polypeptide hormones are derived from larger precursor proteins, the catecholamines, and thyroid hormones are derivatives of amino acids; the steroid hormones and vitamin D are derived from cholesterol.

- Prostaglandins, prostacyclins and leukotrienes are related to hormones and are derived from fatty acids.

The causes of adrenal insufficiency

- Adrenal enzyme defects, e.g. 21-hydroxylase deficiency

- Congenital adrenal hyperplasia

- Infections, e.g. tuberculosis (TB), histoplasmosis, HIV infection

- Autoimmune disorders

- Meningococcal septicaemia and haemorrhage

- Thrombosis, e.g. adrenal vein thrombosis

- Neoplastic, e.g. secondary carcinoma

- Drugs, e.g. ketoconazole

- Secondary adrenal insufficiency, e.g. hypopituitarism, isolated adrenocorticotrophic hormone (ACTH) deficiency.

The hormones produced by the different cells of the adrenal gland

Table 8.3 The main functions of each hormone and the mechanisms controlling their secretion

Area/zone	Cells	Hormones secreted	Function	Controlling mechanisms
The adrenal cortex Zona glomerulosa (outer zone)	Thin, subcapsular cells	Secrete mineralocorticoids, mainly aldosterone and deoxycorticosterone	Contribute to sodium, potassium and water homoeostasis Maintain cardiac output and blood pressure Aldosterone controls the synthesis of sodium pump in several cells including salivary glands, gastric mucosa and sweat glands	Angiotensin II
Zona fasciculata (middle zone)	Cells are large, rectangular cells, containing cholesterol and their cytoplasm appears clear	Secret glucocorticoids, mainly cortisol and corticosterone, and small amounts of the adrenergic steroid DHA	Raise plasma glucose levels (gluconeogenesis in liver) Immunosuppressive effects Anti-inflammatory activity Behavioural effects on the CNS Effects on calcium and bone metabolism Lipolysis and metabolism of fat In acute stress, glucocorticoids maintain endothelial integrity and vascular permeability	ACTH
Zona reticularis (the inner zone)	Inner zone cells Cells have eosinophilic cytoplasm	Secrete androgenic hormones (DHA and androstenedione) and some glucocorticoids	These are weak androgens of limited physiological value under normal conditions	ACTH
The adrenal medulla	Cells appear brown in colour when exposed to air (amines are oxidized and appear brown)	Adrenaline and noradrenaline	Vasoconstriction, increased heart rate, rises of blood pressure	Drop of blood pressure, hypovolaemia, sympathetic stimulation

CNS, central nervous system; DHA, dehydroepiandrosterone.

The main symptoms and signs of hypothyroidism

Table 8.4 Symptoms and signs of thyroidism

Organ/body system	Symptoms	Signs
Metabolic changes	Cold intolerance	Weight gain
Neuropsychiatric changes	Fatigue	Psychosis
	Depression	
	Impaired concentration	
	Tasks take more time to finish	
Skin	Dryness, rough	Loss of the outer third of brows and scalp hair. Skin is yellowish (carotenaemic)
Cardiovascular system	Shortness of breath	Bradycardia
		Pericardial effusion
		Cardiomegaly
		Heart failure
		Cardiac rub
Gastrointestinal system	Decreased appetite	Small intestine ileus
	Constipation	Increased BMI
	Increased weight	
Musculoskeletal system	Arthralgia	Muscle stiffness
	Myalgia	
	Cramps	
Haematological	Pallor	Anaemia
Genitourinary	Decreased libido	Galactorrhoea
	Menorrhagia or oliguria	

BMI, Body mass index

The causes of hypothyroidism and the mechanisms underlying each cause

● Autoimmune thyroiditis (e.g. Hashimoto's disease): mechanism – anti-thyroid antibodies attack the thyroid cells and cause inflammation and decreased thyroid function.

● Thyroiditis (e.g. subacute or lymphatic thyroiditis): mechanism – transient inflammation of the thyroid gland → interference with its function.

● Drug-induced hypothyroidism (e.g. lithium): mechanism – blockade of organification and hormone release from the thyroid gland.

● Secondary hypothyroidism: mechanism – lack of stimulation of the thyroid gland by thyroid-stimulating hormone (TSH).

Answers

 CASE 8.1 – I have never had trouble with my driving.

 Q1: What are the possible causes for the presenting problem?

A1

The following are possible causes (hypotheses) for Neill's presentation:

● Pituitary adenoma secreting growth hormone (GH)

● GH-releasing hormone (GHRH) excess (rare)

● Visual field defect secondary to the pituitary adenoma

● Secondary diabetes mellitus (possibly caused by excessive secretion of GH).

Q2: What further questions would you like to ask to help you differentiate between your hypotheses?

A2

Table 8.5 Further history questions for Case 8.1

History questions	In what way answers can help
Characteristics of the patient's headache: site of pain, frequency, duration, severity, radiation, any associated symptoms such as dizziness, photophobia, fatigue mood changes. What improves the headache and any precipitating factors?	Headache may be present because of increased intracranial pressure
Any increased sweating, muscle weakness, facial appearance or breast enlargement (gynaecomastia)? You may ask the patient to show you a photo taken of him 3–5 years ago	Increased GH may be associated with increased sweating and warmth of the palms (as a result of increased metabolic rate). The skin may be thickened and proximal muscle weakness may be present. Facial changes are characteristic, such as frontal bossing, large supraorbital ridge and protrusion of the lower jaw
Medications, recent investigations, eye examinations, use of spectacles	Visual field defect (bilateral hemianopia) may occur if the pituitary tumour is large

Q3: What investigations would be most helpful to you and why?

A3

Further investigations

- GH level
- Insulin-like growth factor I (IGF-I), also known as somatomedin C
- Magnetic resonance imaging (MRI) of pituitary
- Serum prolactin (PRL)
- Glucose tolerance test.

 CASE 8.2 – I became very slow and unable to finish tasks at work.

 Q1: What are the possible causes for the presenting problem?

A1

The following are possible causes (hypotheses) for Jane's presentation:

- Primary hypothyroidism (thyroid failure, e.g. resulting from an autoimmune disease)
- Secondary hypothyroidism (pituitary TSH deficiency)
- Tertiary hypothyroidism (caused by hypothalamic deficiency of thyroid-releasing hormone or TRH, rare)
- Subacute thyroiditis
- Drug-induced hypothyroidism (e.g. drugs that block the biosynthesis of thyroid hormones)
- Peripheral resistance to the action of thyroid hormones
- Depression.

 Q2: What further questions would you like to ask to help you differentiate between your hypotheses?

A2

Table 8.6 Further history questions for Case 8.2

History questions	In what way answers can help
Other symptoms suggestive of hypothyroidism, e.g. menstrual irregularities, cold intolerance and hoarseness of voice	Hypothyroidism impairs the conversion of peripheral metabolism of oestrogen precursors to oestrogen, resulting in altered FSH and LH secretion and anovulatory cycles. This may be associated with severe menorrhagia. Thyroxine (T_4) regulates energy utilization and heat production. Thus, its deficiency is usually associated with cold intolerance

Any medications, e.g. lithium carbonate, propylthiouracil or methimazole	Drugs interfering with the biosynthesis of thyroid hormones may cause hypothyroidism
Any cardiovascular symptoms, e.g. decreased cardiac output, shortness of breath, chest pain, palpitations and symptoms suggestive of anaemia	T_4 enhances the contraction of the heart muscle via direct stimulation of SA node and cardiac muscle. Its deficiency results in bradycardia and poor contraction of cardiac muscle
	Anaemia in patients with hypothyroidism may be caused by: impaired Hb synthesis because of T_4 deficiency; iron deficiency because of menorrhagia; folate deficiency because of impaired intestinal absorption of folate; or vitamin B_{12} deficiency resulting from an autoimmune disorder as part of the autoimmune thyroiditis
Any neuromuscular symptoms, e.g. muscle cramps, paraesthesiae and muscle weakness	Hypothyroidism may be associated with a goitre. Hypothyroidism may, however, occur without any enlargement of the thyroid gland
Has the patient noticed any masses in front of her neck (goitre)	To assess her for the support needed for her and whether she needs any treatment for depression

FSH, follicle-stimulating hormone; LH, luteinizing hormone; SA, sinoatrial.

 Q3: What investigations would be most helpful to you and why?

A3

Further investigations

- Full blood examination and blood film

- Thyroid function tests (thyroxine or T_4, triiodothyronine or T_3 and TSH)

- Electrocardiogram (ECG)

- Chest radiograph and echocardiography

- Thyroid scan

- Ultrasound with high resolution

- Thyroid antibodies.

CASE 8.3 – I am very tired and started vomiting again.

Q1: What are the possible causes for the presenting problem?

A1

The following are the possible causes (hypotheses) for Eva's presentation:

- Chronic infections of the adrenal glands (e.g. TB, histoplasmosis, opportunistic bacteria as in HIV-infected patients)

- Autoimmune disorders affecting the adrenal glands

- Acute bleeding/infarction of the adrenal glands (e.g. meningococcal septicaemia and haemorrhage in the gland – less likely)

- Secondary adrenal insufficiency (e.g. hypopituitarism, isolated ACTH deficiency)

- Drug-induced adrenal failure (less likely).

Q2: What further questions would you like to ask to help you differentiate between your hypotheses?

A2

Table 8.7 Further history questions for Case 8.3

History questions	In what way answers can help
Past history of treatment for tuberculosis (TB), cough, expectoration, haemoptysis, exposure to TB or other chronic infections	Infection of the adrenal glands with tubercle bacilli is one of the causes of adrenal insufficiency
	Other causes of adrenal insufficiency are fungal infections, infection with opportunistic bacteria as in HIV-infected patients or autoimmune disorders of the adrenal glands
Past investigations, e.g. CT of adrenals, CT of the pituitary or chest radiograph	These investigations might help in assessing the progress of the adrenal lesion and the possible causes
Detailed history of medications and allergy	Some medications such as ketoconazole (an antifungal drug used in the treatment of fungal diseases such as candidiasis, histoplasmosis and blastomycosis) could cause adrenal failure
Any other signs of autoimmunity, e.g. vitiligo	Patients with adrenal insufficiency as a result of autoimmune disorders might have other signs related to autoimmune disorders, e.g. vitiligo (a skin disorder characterized by smooth white spots on various parts of the body)

A3

Further investigations

- Serum sodium and potassium

- Blood urea and creatinine

- Plasma ACTH and random blood cortisol

- Short ACTH stimulation test

- CT of the adrenal glands

- CT of the thorax

- Adrenocortical autoantibodies.

Further progress

CASE 8.1 – I have never had trouble with my driving.

Dr Kemp arranges for some tests for Neill. The results are shown in Table 8.8.

Table 8.8 Test results for Case 8.1

Test	Neill's results	Normal range
Serum GH (µg/L)	7	0–4
IGF-I level (somatomedin C) (units/mL)	2.9	<1.4
Serum PRL (µg/L)	17	3–14.7
Glucose tolerance test (mmol/L):		
– fasting	8.9	3.9–5.8
– 60 min	12	6.7–9.4
– 90 min	12	5.6–7.8
– 120 min	10	3.9–6.7
Pituitary MRI	Enlarged pituitary gland and its fossa. A pituitary adenoma, about 17 mm in diameter, is present within the gland	–

CASE 8.2 – I became very slow and unable to finish tasks at work.

Dr March arranges for some tests for Jane. The results are shown in Table 8.9.

Table 8.9 Test results for Case 8.2

Test	Jane's results	Normal range
Haemoglobin (Hb) (g/L)	90	115–160
White blood cell count (WCC) ($\times 10^9$/L)	3.3	4.0–11.0
Platelet count ($\times 10^9$/L)	290	150–400
Free T_4 (pmol/L)	5.3	9–26
T_3 (nmol/L)	0.7	0.9–2.6
TSH (mU/L)	9	0.5–5.0

Thyroid nuclear scan and ultrasound with high resolution: mild enlargement of the gland; no cysts or solid masses.

ECG: bradycardia.

Echocardiography: normal, no evidence of heart failure; no pericardial effusion.

Thyroid antibodies: not detected.

● CASE 8.3 – I am very tired and started vomiting again.

Dr Webster arranges for some tests for Eva. The results are shown in Table 8.10.

Table 8.10 Test results for Case 8.3

Test	Eva's results	Normal range
Serum sodium (mmol/L)	123	135–145
Serum potassium (mmol/L)	5.8	3.5–5.0
Blood urea (mmol/L)	32	2.5–8.3
Serum creatinine (mmol/L)	0.15	0.05–0.11
Plasma ACTH (ng/L)	842	5–36
Random serum cortisol (nmol/L)	142	Various depending on the time of blood sampling. A sample at 8am with a concentration < 100 clearly favours the diagnosis of adrenal insufficiency
Short ACTH stimulation test:		Normally, a significant rise in the serum cortisol level (> 600 nmol/L) should be observed 30 min after the injection of ACTH (tetracosactide 250 µg i.v.)
– cortisol at 0 min (nmol/L)	102	
– cortisol at 30 min (nmol/L)	117	
CT of the adrenal gland		The adrenal glands are small and atrophic; some calcification of both glands is noticed
CT of the thorax		Bilateral apical fibrotic changes; some calcification of the right apex
Adrenocortical autoantibodies		Cannot be detected

Further questions

 CASE 8.1 – I have never had trouble with my driving.

Q4: In the light of the clinical presentation, how would you interpret the laboratory test results?

A4

Table 8.11 Interpretation of lab test results for Case 8.1

Test	Change	Interpretation
Serum GH	Raised	GH is a single polypeptide with a molecular mass of 22 000. The release of GH is controlled by the release of the hypothalamic factor GHRH. The GH inhibitory factor is known as somatostatin. The secretion of GH is stimulated by several physiological factors such as sleep, stress, exercise, hypoglycaemia, protein ingestion (rise of amino acid concentration in blood, particularly arginine) and oestrogen. A high blood level as in this patient is consistent with the presence of a pituitary adenoma secreting GH
IGF-I level (somatomedin C)	Raised	Some of the effects of GH are not exerted directly and are mediated indirectly by secreting a second hormonal messenger known as IGF-I (somatomedin C). The liver is the main source of IGF-I, which has a chemical structure very similar to that of proinsulin, hence its name. IGF-I is always raised in acromegaly and its level usually reflects the GH level over 24 h. IGF-I is less useful in following patients after therapy
Serum PRL	Raised	Mild rise in PRL level occurs in 30–40 per cent of patients
Glucose tolerance test: – fasting – 60 min – 90 min – 120 min	Impaired blood glucose test (diabetic glucose tolerance test)	GH opposes insulin action and decreases glucose utilization (about 25 per cent of patients with acromegaly have a diabetic glucose tolerance test). Other actions of GH include: increased amino acid uptake by cells, increased fat mobilization and inhibition of protein breakdown In young people, GH stimulates the epiphyseal bone growth
Pituitary MRI	Enlarged pituitary gland and its fossa. A pituitary adenoma, about 17 mm in diameter, is present within the gland	Very useful in providing information about tumour size, location and planning for the therapeutic approach

Q5: What is your final hypothesis?

A5

The clinical picture and laboratory results are suggestive of a pituitary adenoma with excessive secretion of GH causing diabetes mellitus (acromegaly). The adenoma mass compresses the chiasma causing a field defect (bitemporal hemianopia).

 Q6: What issues in the given history, examination and laboratory tests support your final hypothesis?

A6

Supportive evidence

History and examination

- Tiredness and infrequent headaches of a few months' duration
- Wakes up at night to pass urine two to three times
- Facial changes
- ? visual field defects (lateral field).

Investigations

- Raised blood GH level
- Diabetic glucose tolerance curve
- PRL level: moderately raised
- Pituitary MRI: reveals a 17 mm pituitary adenoma within the gland.

 CASE 8.2 – I became very slow and unable to finish tasks at work.

 Q4: In the light of the clinical presentation, how would you interpret the laboratory test results?

A4

Table 8.12 Interpretation of lab test results for Case 8.2

Test	Change	Interpretation
Hb	Low	Anaemia in patients with hypothyroidism may be the reuslt of: impaired Hb synthesis because of thyroxine deficiency; iron deficiency because of menorrhagia; folate deficiency because of impaired intestinal absorption of folate; and vitamin B_{12} deficiency caused by an autoimmune disorder as part of the autoimmune thyroiditis

Free T$_4$ T$_3$	Low	Low FT$_4$ and T$_3$ levels together with high TSH concentration indicate primary hypothyroidism
TSH	Raised	The concentration of plasma TSH is measured by radioimmuno-assay. In primary hypothyroidism, anterior pituitary secretion of TSH is increased because of the low concentration of circulating T$_4$ and T$_3$
Thyroid nuclear scan and ultrasound with high resolution	Mild enlargement of the gland. No cystic or solid masses	The findings suggest the presence of goitre
ECG	Bradycardia	T$_4$ seems to have a direct effect on cardiac excitability, which in turn increases the heart rate. Low thyroid hormone is associated with decreased cardiac excitability and heart rate (bradycardia)
Echocardiography	Normal, no evidence of heart failure. No pericardial effusion	Hypothyroid patients have reduced cardiac output, stroke volume and blood volume. Circulation time is prolonged but right and left heart filling pressures are within normal ranges, unless they are elevated by pericardial effusion
Thyroid antibodies	Not detected	Autoimmune causes of hypothyroidism are less likely

 Q5: What is your final hypothesis?

A5

The clinical picture and laboratory results are suggestive of primary hypothyroidism.

 Q6: What issues in the given history, examination and laboratory tests support your final hypothesis?

A6

Supportive evidence

History

- Decreased energy and gradual weight gain.

- Becoming slow and unable to finish tasks at work.

- The patient migrated from Italy to Australia 2 years ago and speaks little English.

- Progressive changes in her bowel habits with a tendency for constipation.

- Her appetite is good and she has not made any changes to the types of food she eats.

- Over the last 2 years, her menstrual periods have become irregular and infrequent.

- Her husband left her 7 months after their arrival in Australia.

- She faces financial difficulties after her separation from her husband.

Examination

- She looks depressed.

- Her skin looks dry and rough.

- Her BMI is 30 (used to be 25).

- Her pulse is only 60/min (bradycardia).

Investigations

- Hb: low

- FT_4: low

- T_3: low

- TSH: raised

- Thyroid nuclear scan and ultrasound with high resolution: mild enlargement of the gland; no cystic or solid masses

- ECG: bradycardia

- Echocardiography: normal; no pericardial effusion

- Thyroid antibodies: not detected.

● CASE 8.3 – I am very tired and started vomiting again.

 Q4: In the light of the clinical presentation, how would you interpret the laboratory test results?

A4

Table 8.13 Interpretation of lab test results for Case 8.3

Test	Change	Interpretation
Serum sodium	Low	Hyponatraemia is a common electrolyte disturbance in elderly people. However, the presence of hyponatraemia in this patient's condition, together with decrease in blood pressure, low blood glucose, high potassium, low random serum cortisol and high plasma ACTH, should highlight the diagnosis of adrenal insufficiency.
		Inappropriate secretion of ADH should be excluded and it is not the cause of her hyponatraemia. Inappropriate ADH secretion is characterized by the following: hyponatraemia resulting from excessive water retention; urinary sodium > 35 mmol/L; no hypokalaemia or hypotension; normal renal and adrenal function; or urine osmolality higher compared with plasma osmolality

		The main causes of inappropriate ADH secretion are tumours, e.g. small cell lung cancer, pancreatic, prostate and thymus tumours; pulmonary lesions, e.g. TB, pneumonia; CNS disorders, e.g. head injury or meningitis; and drugs, e.g. chlorpropamide and phenothiazines. Thus, her hyponatraemia is not the result of inappropriate secretion of ADH
Serum potassium	Raised	Hyperkalaemia may be caused by: decreased renal excretion as in acute renal failure; drugs, e.g. amiloride, triamterene, spironolactone, ACE inhibitors; Addison's disease and aldosterone deficiency; increased release of potassium resulting from inhibition of the Na^+/K^+ ATPase function, e.g. acidosis, digoxin poisoning; increased release of potassium from muscles, e.g. tissue trauma and rhabdomyolysis; and other causes, e.g. sample haemolysis
Blood urea	Raised	This should also make inappropriate secretion of ADH less likely. It reflects hypovolaemia and decreased renal perfusion
Plasma ACTH	Very high	Raised blood ACTH level is diagnostic of primary adrenal failure
Random serum cortisol	Low	Measurement of random serum cortisol can be a useful screening test to exclude or confirm renal insufficiency. However, the interpretation of results should be made in relation to blood level and time of blood sampling, e.g. a morning sample at 8am with a blood cortisol concentration > 500 nmol/L clearly excludes the possibility of adrenal insufficiency, whereas a morning sample at 8am with a concentration < 100 nmol/l clearly confirms adrenal insufficiency
Short ACTH stimulation test – cortisol at 0 min – cortisol at 30 min	Blunted response	This is diagnostic of primary adrenal insufficiency because there is no increase in blood cortisol 30 min after the injection of ACTH
CT of the adrenal gland	The adrenal glands are small and atrophic; some calcification of both glands is noticed	These changes suggest chronic adrenal infection. Calcification of the gland is consistent with TB
CT of the thorax	Bilateral apical fibrotic changes; some calcification of the right apex	These changes are consistent with old pulmonary TB
Adrenocortical autoantibodies	Cannot be detected	Although destruction of the adrenal gland is usually caused by autoimmune diseases, particularly in industrialized western countries, adrenal insufficiency may occur as a result of infection with a wide range of organisms that cause infections including: TB, fungal infections, and opportunistic bacteria in immunodeficient individuals. The absence of adrenocortical autoantibodies and the adrenal calcification might indicate infection with TB as the cause

Q5: What is your final hypothesis?

A5

The clinical picture and laboratory results are suggestive of adrenal insufficiency (Addison's disease) caused by infection with *Mycobacterium tuberculosis*.

 Q6: What issues in the given history, examination and laboratory tests support your final hypothesis?

A6

Supportive evidence

History

- Repeated vomiting, nausea and generalized tiredness for the last few days

- A history of similar problems about 2 months ago

- Hospital investigations at that time, including gastrointestinal endoscopy, showed no abnormality except for low serum sodium level (121 mmol/L), low blood glucose level (3.5 mmol/L) and relatively elevated serum potassium level (5 mmol/L)

- No abdominal pain and no changes in her bowel movements

- Not on any medication and no history of allergies

- Worked in Africa a long time ago.

Examination

- Looks unwell and drowsy

- BMI 22

- Low blood pressure, afebrile

- Abdomen soft and not tender or rigid

- Intestinal sounds normal

- No abdominal masses or organomegaly

- An old appendectomy scar is pigmented

- Cardiovascular and respiratory examinations normal

- Cranial nerves normal

- No signs of meningitis or signs suggesting increased intracranial tension

- Ear examination is normal.

Investigations

- Serum sodium: low
- Serum potassium: raised.
- Blood urea: raised
- Plasma ACTH very raised
- Short ACTH stimulation test: blunted response
- CT of the adrenal gland: the adrenal glands are small and atrophic, some calcification of both glands is noticed
- CT of the thorax: bilateral apical fibrotic changes, some calcification of the right apex
- Adrenocortical autoantibodies: cannot be detected.

👥 Integrated medical sciences questions

● CASE 8.1 – Briefly discuss the hormones secreted from the anterior pituitary, their cell of origin, regulating mechanisms, their functions and target organs.

Table 8.14 Pituitary hormones and their functions

Anterior pituitary hormone	Cell	Stimulation	Inhibition	Target	Function
GH	Somatotrophs	Hypothalmic releasing factor: GHRH	Somatostatin IGF-I Cortisol	Receptors on the surface of various body cells	GH promotes lipolysis and hyperglycaemia GH promotes the uptake of amino acids and increases protein synthesis GH stimulates RNA and protein synthesis Part of its action is mediated by somatomedins
TSH	Thyrotrophs	Thyrotrophin-releasing hormone (TRH)	Thyroid hormone feedback on both the hypothalamus and the pituitary gland inhibiting TSH release – somatostatin	Specific receptors of TSH are present on the basal surface of the thyroid follicular cells	TSH induces proliferation of the thyroid follicular cells TSH promotes synthesis of T_4 and T_3 and their secretion into the circulation
PRL	Lactotrophs	TRH Estradiol	Dopamine	Breast epithelium	Hypertrophy of breast epithelium during pregnancy Essential for lactation PRL and progesterone promote the growth of breast lobules and alveoli
LH	Gonadotrophs	Gonadotrophin-releasing hormone (GnRH) Estradiol level in females differentially reduces FSH and promotes LH release (positive feedback)	Progesterone Testosterone (in males)	Male and female gonad receptors	Action on the testes: LH stimulates Leydig cells to produce testosterone, which has local and systemic effects Action on the ovary: LH stimulates thecal cell androgen secretion; LH induces ovulation and luteinization; LH sustains the corpus luteum

FSH	Gonadotrophs	GnRH	Inhibin	Males and female gonads	Action on the testes: FSH stimulates Sertoli cells, with local testosterone, regulates spermatogenesis
			Estradiol		
			Progesterone		
			Testosterone (in males)		Action on the ovary: stimulates ovarian follicles and prepares new crop of follicles for next cycle
ACTH	Corticotrophs	Corticotrophin-releasing hormone (CRH) Vasopressin (ADH) Interleukin-1 (IL-1)	Excessive glucocorticoids feedback on both the pituitary and the hypothalamus	Cells mainly of zona fasciculata of the adrenal cortex	ACTH stimulates cortisol secretion from the zona fasciculate cells and the growth of adrenal cells

CASE 8.2 – What are the metabolic functions of thyroxine?

- Increased metabolic rate: T_4 increases O_2 consumption and metabolic rate of metabolically active tissues. It stimulates glucose absorption from the intestine.

- T_4 lowers blood cholesterol level and converts carotene to vitamin A.

- Effects of thyroid hormones on the cardiovascular system: increased blood flow and increased cardiac output; increased metabolism of tissues and more rapid utilization of O_2; vasodilatation in most body tissues; increased cardiac output, heart rate and cardiac excitability; increased systolic blood pressure as in hyperthyroidism; and thyroid hormones potentiate the actions of catecholamines on the heart (T_4 upregulates the β-receptors).

- Increased respiration: mainly because of increased utilization of O_2 and formation of CO_2.

- Effects on the gastrointestinal system: increased appetite; increased rate of secretion of the digestive secretions; and increased gastrointestinal motility (diarrhoea often occurs in hyperthyroidism).

- Effects on the CNS: T_4 is important for the process of cerebration and essential for brain development and function.

- Effects on the muscles: thyroid hormones make the skeletal muscles contract vigorously. However, prolonged excessive secretion of thyroid hormones will make muscles weaker as a result of excess protein catabolism.

CASE 8.3 – What are the causes of Cushing's syndrome? Discuss the mechanisms underlying each cause and associated changes.

Table 8.15 Mechanisms underlying causes of Cushing's syndrome

Cause	Mechanism	Associated changes
Pituitary tumour	Excessive ACTH secretion by pituitary tumour cells → stimulation of the adrenal cells to grow and secrete excessive amounts of glucocorticoids	Elevated serum ACTH Hyperplasia of the adrenal cortex Elevated serum cortisol
A tumour secreting ACTH (e.g. small cell lung cancer, islet cell tumour of the pancreas)	Excessive ACTH secretion by the tumour cells → stimulation of the adrenal cells to grow and increase and secrete excessive amounts of glucocorticoids	Elevated serum ACTH Hyperplasia of the adrenal cortex Elevated serum cortisol

Adrenal tumour	Excessive secretion of cortisol by the tumour cells → increased blood cortisol levels → feedback suppression of ACTH secretion	Increased cortisol
		Decreased serum ACTH
		Atrophy of other parts of the adrenal cortex
Excessive intake of cortisol medication	Excessive cortisol intake → increased blood cortisol → feedback suppression of ACTH secretion	Increased serum cortisol
		Decreased serum ACTH
		Atrophy of the adrenal cortex

Further reading

Ackerman MJ, Clapham DE. Ion channels– basic sciences and clinical disease. *New England Journal of Medicine* 1997;**336**:1575–1586.

Arlt W, Allolio B. Adrenal insufficiency. *Lancet* 2003;**361**:1881–1893.

Brent GA. Mechanisms of disease: the molecular basis of thyroid hormone action. *New England Journal of Medicine* 1994;**331**:847–853.

Cooper DS. Drug therapy: antithyroid drugs. *New England Journal of Medicine* 2005;**352**:905–917.

Dayan CM, Daniels GH. Medical progress: chronic autoimmune thyroiditis. *New England Journal of Medicine* 1996;**335**:99–107.

Dorin RI, Qualls CR, Crapo LM. Diagnosis of adrenal insufficiency. *Annals of Internal Medicine* 2003;**139**:194–204.

Levy A, Lightman SL. Fortnightly review: diagnosis and management of pituitary tumours. *British Medical Journal* 1994;**308**:1087–1091.

Oelkers W. Current concepts: adrenal insufficiency. *New England Journal of Medicine* 1996;**335**:1206–1212.

Perazella MA. Drug-induced hyperkalemia: old culprits and new offenders. *American Journal of Medicine* 2000;**109**:307–314.

Vance ML. Medical progress: hypopituitarism. *New England Journal of Medicine* 1994;**330**:1651–1662.

Weetman AP. Medical progress: Graves' disease. *New England Journal of Medicine* 2000;**343**:1236–1248.

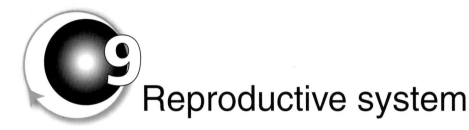

Reproductive system

Clinical cases

● CASE 9.1 – **We have been together for about 2 years.**

Kevin Fleming, a 32-year-old professional photographer, comes in with his girlfriend Regina to see the local GP, Dr Robert Fredrick. Kevin and Regina have been together for about 2 years and she wants to have his child. Kevin has been married twice before meeting Regina but has never had children. Regina has two children, aged 5 and 3, from a previous relationship. Regina is a 27-year-old primary school teacher. The couple do not use contraception and they do not smoke or drink.

Kevin has a history of maldescended testes when he was a child. He is able to ejaculate and he is able to carry out successful relationships with women. Recently he has gained some body weight and also noticed a decrease in his libido. On examination, Kevin's height is 181 cm, body weight 89 kg and his body mass index (BMI) is 27. His arm span is 181 cm. Both his testes are small and firm. Gynaecomastia is present on both sides. His urine glucose is + .

Cardiovascular and respiratory examinations are normal.

● CASE 9.2 – **What is wrong with me?**

Fiona Hull, a 28-year-old music teacher, comes in to see the local GP, Dr Samuel Derek, because of progressive generalized fatigue and occasional dizziness over the last 12 months. Fiona always feels tired, even after light activities. She has not had her period for about 18 months following an abortion. At that time she felt down but did not care to seek medical advice. Since that time, she has started to feel weak and lacking in energy. She is currently on no medication and has no history of ear troubles. On examination, her skin is fine, pale and smooth with fine wrinkling of the face. Her vital signs are shown in Table 9.1.

Table 9.1 Vital signs for Case 9.2

Vital signs	Fiona's results	Normal range
Blood pressure (mmHg)	90/60	100/60–135/85
Pulse rate (/min)	60	60–100
Respiratory rate (/min)	12	12–16
Temperature (°C)	36.5	36.6–37.2

● She has no body, axillary or pubic hair (lost about 4–5 months after the miscarriage).

● She has no goitre.

- Cardiovascular examination: bradycardia and weak heart sounds.

- Respiratory and neurological examinations are normal.

- Abdominal examination: normal.

- Urinalysis: negative for sugar.

CASE 9.3 – So what is the gender of my baby?

Mary and Mark Johnston, a couple aged 25 and 28 years respectively, have had their first child, Michael, who was born by normal delivery at term. On the third day after delivery, Michael and Mary were discharged from hospital. Over the next 2 days, Mary notices that Michael is always lethargic and sleeping most of the time. On the fifth day he vomits repeatedly and looks ill. They contact their GP who arranges an urgent transfer to the hospital. The paediatric registrar examines Michael and finds no obvious cause for his vomiting. He asks the consultant to have a look at Michael's genitalia. He believes that Michael has ambiguous genitalia and what is thought to be a penis could be an enlarged clitoris.

Integrated medical sciences questions

● **CASE 9.1 –** Briefly discuss the causes of subfertility, investigations recommended and scientific bases behind these investigations.

● **CASE 9.2 –** Discuss the physiological and hormonal changes during the menstrual cycle.

● **CASE 9.3 –** Discuss the mechanisms underlying the pathogenesis of Michael's condition.

🔑 Key concepts

In order to work through the core clinical cases in this chapter, you will need to understand the following key concepts.

The causes of panhypopituitarism

- Pituitary tumours
- Surgery, irradiation of the pituitary region
- Pituitary infarction (apoplexia)
- Peripituitary tumours
- Meningiomas, gliomas
- Metastases to the pituitary region
- Trauma, infection, abscess
- Haemochromatosis
- Granulomatous disease
- Histocytosis.

The causes of primary amenorrhoea

- Hypothalamic causes: stress, anorexia nervosa, obesity, drugs, e.g. phenothiazines
- Pituitary: tumours
- Adrenal: congenital adrenal hyperplasia
- Ovary: ovarian tumours, ovarian failure, gonadal dysgenesis
- Uterus: agenesis, testicular feminization syndrome
- Vagina: imperforated hymen, agenesis.

The secondary male sex characteristics

- Penis has increased in length and width.
- Scrotum becomes pigmented.
- Voice deepens.
- Beard appears.
- Pubic hair grows and hair appears in axilla, on chest and around anus.
- General body hair increases.
- Interest in opposite sex develops.
- Shoulders broaden and muscles enlarge.

Hormones involved in breast development

- Oestrogen
- Progesterone
- Prolactin
- Placental lactogen
- Glucocorticoids
- Thyroxine (T_4)
- Insulin.

During puberty, increased levels of oestrogen cause the stimulation of breast growth (as part of secondary sexual characteristics). Progesterone, prolactin and placental lactogen play an important role during pregnancy but the secretion of milk occurs only after the delivery of the placenta. Glucocorticoids, T_4 and insulin are important in facilitating the action of oestrogen and progesterone on the breast tissue.

Breast development involves: (1) proliferation of lactiferous ducts, (2) branching of lactiferous ducts, and (3) accumulation of adipose tissue and connective tissue.

Why does breast milk secretion occur only after parturition and not during pregnancy?

During pregnancy, the blood levels of progesterone and oestrogen levels are high. These two hormones are able to block the action of prolactin on the breast. Subsequent to the delivery of the placenta, the levels of oestrogen and progesterone drop significantly, allowing prolactin to act on the breast tissue and secrete milk.

The characteristics of a normal semen analysis

- Semen volume: >2 mL
- Sperm:
    - total count > 40×10^6/ejaculate
    - motility: > 50 per cent motile
    - morphology: > 30 per cent normal
    - vitality (live): > 75 per cent
- Leukocytes: <1 million/mL
- Red blood cells: absent.

Answers

● CASE 9.1 – We have been together for about 2 years.

Q1: What are the possible causes for the presenting problem?

A1

The following are possible causes (hypotheses) for Kevin's presentation:

- Hypothalamic–pituitary failure
- Testicular failure
- Testicular obstruction
- Systemic disorders, e.g. chronic illnesses.

The testicular causes are the result of the following:

- Azoospermia (caused by hyalinizing fibrosis of the seminiferous tubules and absence of spermatogenesis as in Klinefelter's syndrome; about 80 per cent of cases are the result of congenital numerical chromosome aberration: 47,XXY)
- Decreased number of normal sperms
- Increased number of dysfunctional spermatozoa
- Reduced fertility capacity of sperms
- Abnormal sperm morphology.

Testicular problems may be a result of drugs, trauma, surgery or radiotherapy.

Drugs affecting testes may include sulfasalazine, methotrexate, chemotherapy (less likely).

Chemicals and radiation may affect the testicular function, such as pesticides, herbicides and radiation at work.

Testicular obstruction or congenital bilateral absence of vas deferens (CBAVD): the latter is more common in cystic fibrosis patients (less likely in this patient's condition because there are no respiratory symptoms).

Systemic disorders: less likely in this case.

Q2: What further questions would you like to ask to help you differentiate between your hypotheses?

A2

Table 9.2 Further history questions for Case 9.1

History questions	In what way answers can help
Frequency of coitus, erectile function, ejaculation, any congenital problems with the testicles	Within a year of regular intercourse, more than 90 per cent of fertile couples should become pregnant. After 2 years, this rises to over 95 per cent. Thus, only 5–10 per cent of normal fertile couples take more than a year or two to conceive. From the case scenario it seems as though Kevin's girlfriend, Regina, has no apparent problem and it might be useful to start by assessing frequency of coitus and Kevin's medical history. The testes are normally located in the scrotum where they are maintained at a temperature 1–2°C below that of body core temperature. This lower temperature is essential for normal spermatogenesis
Scrotal/testicular disorders, testicular torsion, inguinal hernia repair and trauma to the testes	About 80 per cent of the testis is made up of the seminiferous tubules, which are responsible for the production of sperm (approximately 100×10^6–180×10^6 sperm are normally produced daily). They also contain the Leydig cells, which are responsible for the production of testosterone. Damage to the testicles can affect the function of the seminiferous tubules and the production of normal sperm
Urinary symptoms, e.g. dysuria, passing blood or pus in urine and past illness of sexually transmitted infection	Recurrent urinary tract infections may cause inflammation of the epididymis. The epididymis is the main place for storage and maturation of spermatozoa. Chronic epididymo-orchitis (chronic inflammation of the epididymis and testes) may be responsible for infertility
Lifestyle factors and occupational risks	Exposure to chemicals such as pesticides, herbicides and radiation at work may affect the testicular functions and the production of sperm
Medication	Drugs may affect the testicles and cause subfertility by different mechanisms: impair spermatogenesis, e.g. sulfasalazine, methotrexate, chemotherapy; antiandrogenic effects, e.g. cimetidine, spironolactone; failure to ejaculate, e.g. α blockers; and erectile dysfunction, e.g. β blockers, thiazide diuretics and metoclopramide

Q3: What investigations would be most helpful to you and why?

A3

Further investigations

- Semen analysis
- Levels of follicle-stimulating hormone (FSH), luteinizing hormone (LH), testosterone, free testosterone, sex hormone-binding globulin (SHBG), estradiol
- Chromosomal analysis.

CASE 9.2 – **What is wrong with me?**

 Q1: What are the possible causes for the presenting problem?

A1

The following are possible causes (hypotheses) for Fiona's presentation:

- Pituitary–hypothalamic failure

- Panhypopituitarism

- Invasive lesions of pituitary (e.g. large tumours)

- Infarction (post-miscarriage infarction)

- Infiltration (e.g. sarcoidosis infiltrating pituitary region)

- Injury (trauma to pituitary–hypothalamus region)

- Idiopathic causes.

Q2: What further questions would you like to ask to help you differentiate between your hypotheses?

A2

Table 9.3 Further history questions for Case 9.2

History questions	In what way answers can help
Symptoms of thyroid deficiency, e.g. cold intolerance, mental dullness, hoarseness of voice	Symptoms suggestive of hypothyroidism, similar to but of a lesser severity to those caused by primary hypothyroidism may be present. Also hypothyroidism occurs because of TSH deficiency. This is called 'secondary hypothyroidism'
Symptoms of adrenal insufficiency, e.g. weakness, nausea, vomiting, anorexia, postural hypotension	ACTH deficiency is less evident than primary adrenal deficiency, because in most cases mineralocorticoid secretion remains intact. It can be severe and sometimes life threatening, however, because the patient's body fails to respond to stress, especially during infectious illness, or after trauma or surgery. Hyponatraemia, malaise, somnolence and poor response to stress may be the result of lack of ACTH and cortisol
Symptoms suggestive of hypoglycaemia	Hypoglcaemia may occur because of lack of cortisol, ACTH and GH
Symptoms suggestive of hyperprolactinaemia	Hyperprolactinaemia may occur because of interference with the production or delivery of dopamine to the pituitary lactotrophs. Dopamine normally suppresses the production of prolactin and lack of dopamine causes high blood prolactin levels. Hyperprolactinaemia may also have contributed to her amenorrhoea

Changes in the skin, e.g. diminished tanning as a result of ACTH insufficiency	This might explain the 'waxen doll' appearance of the skin. The patient might not be anaemic. The thin skin and pallor might also be the result of lack of GH
Any other symptoms associated with gonadal insufficiency	Gonadotrophin deficiency in premenopausal women will result in menstrual disturbances and symptoms suggestive of oestrogen deficiency (amenorrhoea, oligomenorrhoea, infertility, loss of libido, osteoporosis). Lack of gonadal sex hormones might also explain breast atrophy and loss of sex drive. Loss of secondary sexual hair is much more common in panhypopituitarism than in any other condition associated with only lack of gonadal sex hormones
Circumstances and more history about her last abortion	During pregnancy, the pituitary gland normally enlarges under the action of oestrogen on the lactotrophs. However, the blood supply to the pituitary does not increase, making the gland vulnerable to a fall in blood pressure, e.g. because of excessive bleeding during abortion. This might result in the development of infarction of the pituitary gland and panhypopituitarism. The aetiology of hypopituitarism may, however, be obscure or the result of an autoimmune process

ACTH, adrenocorticotrophic hormone; GH, growth hormone.

 Q3: What investigations would be most helpful to you and why?

A3

Further investigations

- Full blood examination and blood film
- Fasting blood glucose
- Serum sodium
- FSH, LH, prolactin, estradiol.
- Thyroid function tests (thyroxine or T_4, triiodothyronine or T_3 and thyroid-stimulating hormone or TSH)
- ACTH and blood cortisol
- ECG.

CASE 9.3 – So what is the gender of my baby?

 Q1: What are the possible causes for the presenting problem?

A1

The following are possible causes (hypotheses) for Michael's presentation:

- Congenital adrenal hyperplasia

- Defect(s) in synthesis of cortisol by adrenal glands

- Ambiguous genitalia because of exposure to high levels of androgens *in utero*

- Lethargy, vomiting and excessive sleeping as a result of excessive loss of sodium.

Q2: What further questions would you like to ask to help you differentiate between your hypotheses?

A2

Table 9.4 Further history questions for Case 9.3

History questions	In what way answers can help
History of similar conditions in siblings, previous neonatal deaths, giving birth to children with ambiguous genitalia, parental consanguinity	Congenital adrenal hyperplasia (CAH), caused by 21-hydroxylase deficiency, is inherited as an autosomal recessive disorder. The disease usually presents with virilization in females beginning *in utero* and incorrect sex assignment at birth. The disease occurs in 1 in 15 000 live births. CAH has been reported in families of consanguineous parents. There are numerous causes for ambiguous genitalia: under-virilized male (XY karyotype) as a result of androgen resistance, testicular feminization or defects in androgen synthesis; virilized female (XX karyotype) caused by excess androgen as in CAH or maternal androgen exposure, e.g. medication, virilizing adrenal tumour; intersex (mosaic karyotypes XO/XY); and structural abnormalities
Any history of vomiting, lethargy (duration and frequency)?	These non-specific symptoms may be the result of low serum sodium (hyponatraemia), which may progress to hypovolaemic shock, also known as 'adrenal crisis', and may prove fatal if not treated immediately. The presence of genital ambiguity should alert the treating doctor to consider the diagnosis of CAH
Family ethnicity/race	CAH is less common in black compared with white individuals. Its incidence is particularly high in two geographically isolated populations: Yupik Eskimos of western Alaska and France, La Reunion in the Indian Ocean. It has also been reported in other countries including Sweden, the USA and Japan

Bodyweight at birth	This may help in establishment of the cut-off point for the normal level of 17-hydroxyprogesterone (17-OHP) and also for follow-up of bodyweight and growth
Antenatal care, any hormonal use, alcohol intake, fever, medication during pregnancy	Antenatal intake of hormones (e.g. for treatment of infertility or endometriosis); excessive alcohol intake during pregnancy may have caused ambiguous genitalia

Q3: What investigations would be most helpful to you and why?

A3

Further investigations

- Full blood count
- Serum ACTH
- Serum sodium and serum potassium
- Plasma 17-hydroxyprogesterone (17-OHP) levels
- Urinary pregnanetriol and 17-oxosteroids
- Plasma renin activity
- Buccal smear for Barr bodies or karyotyping
- Ultrasonography (to help identify internal structures, particularly the uterus and occasionally the ovaries)
- Genetic analysis: molecular studies including polymerase chain reaction (PCR) and Southern blot studies.

Further progress

CASE 9.1 – We have been together for about 2 years.

Dr Fredrick arranges for some tests for Kevin. The results are shown in Table 9.5.

Table 9.5 Semen analysis: azoospermia

Test	Kevin's results	Normal range
FSH (IU/L)	33.9	3–15
LH (IU/L)	18.7	3–13
Testosterone (nmol/L)	10.8	12–40
Free testosterone (pmol/L)	180	> 250
SHBG (nmol/L)	80.5	11–71
Estradiol (pmol/L)	82.5	73–184
Chromosome analysis	47, XXY	46, XY

● CASE 9.2 – What is wrong with me?

Dr Derek arranges for some tests for Fiona. The results are shown in Table 9.6.

Table 9.6 Blood test results for Case 9.2

Blood test	Fiona's results	Normal range
Haemoglobin (Hb) (g/L)	112	115–160
White blood cell count (WCC) ($\times 10^9$/L)	3.3	4.0–11.0
Platelet count ($\times 10^9$/L)	270	150–400
Free thyroxine (FT$_4$) (pmol/L)	5.1	9–26
Triiodothyronine (T$_3$) (nmol/L)	1.7	0.9–2.6
TSH (mU/L)	0.3	0.5–5.0
Serum FSH (IU/L)	3	3–15
Serum LH (IU/L)	3	3–13
Serum estradiol (pmol/L)	77	145–1870
Serum prolactin (mU/L)	1110	50–750
Plasma ACTH (ng/L)	Decreased	5–36
Random serum cortisol (nmol/L)	150	Various depending on the time of blood sampling. A sample at 8am with a concentration < 250 clearly favours the diagnosis of moderate-to-severe ACTH deficiency
Fasting blood glucose (mmol/L)	3.5	3.6–5.3
Serum sodium (mmol/L)	132	136–145
Serum potassium (mmol/L)	3.8	3.5–5.0

ECG: bradycardia.

● CASE 9.3 – So what is the gender of my baby?

The treating doctor arranges for some tests for Michael. The results are shown in Table 9.7.

Table 9.7 Blood test results for Case 9.3

Blood test	Michael's results	Normal range
Hb (g/L)	130	125–205
PCV	0.55	0.39–0.63
WCC ($\times 10^9$/L)	10.6	5.0–19.5
Platelet count ($\times 10^9$/L)	230	150–400
Random serum cortisol (nmol/L)	15	193–690
Plasma ACTH (pmol/L)	155	< 13
Serum sodium (mmol/L)	125	135–145
Serum potassium (mmol/L)	6.1	3.5–5.5
Plasma 17-OHP (nmol/L)	38	Normal birthweight: 0.9–6.6
		Low birthweight: < 9
Serum androstenedione (nmol/L)	47	3.1–5.9
Serum testosterone (nmol/L)	7	1.3–3.8

Urinary pregnanetriol and 17-oxosteroid concentrations: both raised.

Plasma renin activity: raised.

Karyotype: 46,XX.

Genetic analysis: evidence of mutations in the *CYP21* (*CYP21A2*) gene, which is located in the highly polymorphic HLA histocompatibility complex on chromosome 6p21.3. Mutations identified in the patient were assigned by family studies.

Further questions

● **CASE 9.1 –** **We have been together for about 2 years.**

(?) Q4: **In the light of the clinical presentation, how would you interpret the laboratory test results?**

A4

Table 9.8 Interpretation of lab test results for Case 9.1

Test	Change	Interpretation
Semen analysis	Azoospermia	Semen analysis is the main method for assessing male fertility. If the semen analysis shows normospermia, examination of the male patient has no added prognostic value for the couples. According to the WHO criteria, a normal semen should show a sperm count of 20×10^6/ml, and the spermatozoa should show 50 per cent progressive motility and 30 per cent healthy morphology
		Azoospermia (absence of sperm from semen) can be caused by: hypothalamic–pituitary failure; testicular failure; or testicular obstruction. A small testicular size and increased FSH and LH levels indicate testicular failure and failure of the seminiferous tubular cells to respond to pituitary FSH and LH. Serum testosterone in these patients is usually low. These changes (azoospermia, small testes, increased FSH and LH, and decreased testosterone) are characteristic of Klinefelter's syndrome (47,XXY). Klinefelter's syndrome is an example of diseases causing non-obstructive azoospermia. Other examples of non-obstructive azoospermia are Y chromosome deletions after chemotherapy and radiotherapy, and many of the cases are idiopathic
		Men with obstructive azoospermia have normal spermatogenesis, normal size of testes, normal concentration of serum FSH and LH, and they are normally virilized
		Obstructive azoospermia may also occur: in congenital bilateral absence of the vas deferens (in patients with cystic fibrosis); after vasectomy; or as epididymal obstruction after chlamydial or gonorrhoea infections
FSH	Raised	FSH shows the most discrimination between normal patients and those with testicular failure (e.g. Klinefelter's syndrome because of damage of seminiferous tubules)
LH	Raised	LH is raised in testicular failure. The androgen sensitivity index (LH concentration multiplied by testosterone concentration) is high because the LH concentration is very high

Testosterone	Low	In Klinefelter's syndrome, serum testosterone concentrations begin to decrease by 15 years of age, being lower than normal in 80 per cent of patients with the 47,XXY karyotype
		The exact mechanism of low testosterone is not known and the degree of Leydig cell dysfunction is variable (the Leydig cell is responsible for the production of testosterone)
Free testosterone	Low	Low free testosterone may be related to high SHBG
SHBG	Raised	SHBG concentration is high, causing a further decrease in biologically active free testosterone
Chromosome analysis		Approximately, 80 per cent of Klinefelter's syndrome are the result of the congenital numerical chromosome aberration (47,XXY), the remaining 20 per cent having high-grade chromosome aneuploidies (48,XXXY, 48 XXYY, 49,XXXXY or structurally abnormal X chromosome)

FSH, follicle-stimulating hormone; LH, luteinizing hormone; SHBG, sex-hormone-binding globulin

 Q5: What is your final hypothesis?

A5

The clinical picture and laboratory results are suggestive of infertility as a result of Klinefelter's syndrome.

 Q6: What issues in the given history, examination and laboratory tests support your final hypothesis?

A6

Supportive evidence

History

● Kevin and Regina have been together for about 2 years.

● Kevin married twice before meeting Regina but he never had children.

● Regina has two children, 5 and 3 years old, from a previous relationship.

● Regina is a 27-year-old primary school teacher and Kevin is a 32-year-old professional photographer.

● The couple use no contraception and do not smoke or drink.

● History of maldescended testes when Kevin was a child.

● He is able to ejaculate and carry out successful relationships with women.

● He gained some bodyweight recently.

● He has noticed a decrease in his libido.

Examination

- Kevin's height is 181 cm, bodyweight 89 kg and BMI 27

- His arm span is 181 cm

- Both his testes are small and firm

- Gynaecomastia is present on both sides

- His urine glucose ++

- Cardiovascular and respiratory examinations normal.

Investigations

- Semen analysis: azoospermia

- FSH and LH both high

- Serum testosterone: low

- SHBG: raised

- Free testosterone: low

- Chromosome analysis: 47,XXY.

CASE 9.2 – What is wrong with me?

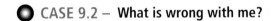

Q4: In the light of the clinical presentation, how would you interpret the laboratory test results?

A4

Table 9.9 Interpretation of test results for Case 9.2

Blood test	Change	Interpretation
Hb	Lower limit of normal	Anaemia may be absent in patients with panhypopituitarism, although the lack of T_4 might contribute to the development of anaemia
Free T_4	Low	The presence of low serum free or total T_4 concentration together with inappropriately normal serum TSH clearly indicates the presence of secondary hypothyroidism (pituitary problem). This combination usually requires assessment of pituitary function
T_3	Normal	T_3 may be normal in panhypopituitarism. It is less helpful in patients with panhypopituitarism. It may be within normal range despite very low T_4 concentration

TSH	Within normal	TSH is not a useful tool in assessment of secondary hypopituitarism. It may be normal or slightly raised
Serum FSH, LH and estradiol	All low	Low serum gonadotrophins in premenopausal women may explain her amenorrhoea and associated symptoms caused by low oestrogen. The presence of low serum estradiol concentrations in the presence of normal or low concentration of FSH are the main clue to diagnosing hypogonadotrophic hypogonadism
Serum prolactin	Raised	Hyperprolactinaemia may be responsible for gonadotrophin deficiency
Plasma ACTH and random serum cortisol	Low	The plasma ACTH together with low serum cortisol support the diagnosis of pituitary problem such as panhypopituitarism
Fasting blood glucose	Low	Low fasting blood glucose is a result of lack of cortisol, GH and ACTH
Serum sodium	Low	Low serum sodium may be the result of lack of mineralocorticoids
ECG	Bradycardia	This is mainly caused by a lack of T_4 – 'hypothyroidism'

 Q5: What is your final hypothesis?

A5

The clinical picture and laboratory results are suggestive of panhypopituitarism.

 Q6: What issues in the given history, examination and laboratory tests support your final hypothesis?

A6

Supportive evidence

History

- Progressive generalized fatigue

- Increased bodyweight and occasional dizziness over the last 14 months

- Always feels tired, even after light activities

- Has not had a period for about 18 months following an abortion

- At that time she felt down and did not care to seek medical advice

- Since that time, she started to feel weak and lacking in energy

- She is not on any medications

- No history of ear troubles.

Examination

- Skin is fine, pale and smooth with fine wrinkling of the face.

- Her vital signs show low blood pressure, bradycardia and low body temperature.

- She has no body, axillary or pubic hair (lost about 4–5 months after the miscarriage).

- Respiratory, cardiovascular and neurological examinations are all normal.

- Urinalysis negative for glucose.

Investigations

- Hb: normal

- Free T_4: low

- T_3 and TSH: within normal

- Serum FSH, LH and estradiol: low

- Serum prolactin: raised

- Plasma ACTH and random serum cortisol: low

- Fasting blood glucose: low

- Serum sodium: low

- ECG: bradycardia.

● CASE 9.3 – So what is the gender of my baby?

 Q4: In the light of the clinical presentation, how would you interpret the laboratory test results?

A4

The treating doctor arranges for some tests for Michael. The results are shown in Table 9.10.

Table 9.10 Interpretation of lab test results for Case 9.3

Test	Change	Interpretation
PCV	Raised	Raised PCV reflects hypovolaemia and excessive loss of fluids (e.g. vomiting)
Random serum cortisol	Low	The possible sources of ACTH are: pituitary gland or malignant cells such as small cell carcinoma or islet cell tumours. The last is less likely. The presence of high serum cortisol indicates that ACTH is secreted in excess because of feedback mechanism and stimulation of pituitary by low blood cortisol levels. These changes are consistent with CAH. ACTH acts through a specific G-protein-coupled receptor to increase levels of cAMP, which has short-term effects on cholesterol transport into mitochondria and long-term effects on transcription of genes, encoding the enzymes required to synthesize cortisol. Other actions of ACTH are: it influences the remaining steps of steroidogenesis; it stimulates the uptake of cholesterol from plasma lipoproteins; it maintains the size of the adrenal gland (excessive secretion of ACTH is responsible for adrenal hyperplasia); and it stimulates melanocytes and results in hyperpigmentation when secreted in excess (as in Addison's disease)
Plasma ACTH	Raised	
Plasma 17-OHP	Raised	
		CAH is caused by 21-hydroxylase deficiency → deficiency of glucocorticoid and other mineralocorticoids → increased secretion of ACTH by the anterior pituitary → adrenal hyperplasia and increased production of androgens and steroid precursors for which 21-hydroxylase is not necessary → high levels of 17-OHP in serum
Serum sodium	Low	Excessive salt loss in babies with CAH may occur resulting in low serum sodium or inappropriately raised urinary sodium
		Excessive salt wasting is responsible for symptoms such as poor appetite, vomiting and lethargy. It may also result in hypotension, shock and death if untreated
Serum potassium	Raised	The serum levels of aldosterone and other mineralocorticoids are low, resulting in low serum sodium and high serum potassium
		Three-quarters of patients with CAH cannot synthesize adequate amounts of aldosterone because pf severely impaired 21-hydroxylation of progesterone. Aldosterone is essential for normal sodium and potassium homoeostasis
Serum androstenedione	Raised	In CAH, serum levels of androstenedione are raised in girls and boys

Serum testosterone	Raised	In CAH, serum levels of testosterone are raised in girls → virilization in females starting *in utero* (e.g. clitoral enlargement) and incorrect sex assignment at birth
Urinary pregnanetriol and 17-oxosteroid concentrations	Raised	These are the metabolites of 17-OHP. Raised urinary levels are consistent with raised 17-OHP levels and the diagnosis of CAH
Karyotyping and genetic analysis	46,XX Evidence of mutations in the *CYP21* (*CYP21A2*) gene. Mutations identified in the patient were assigned by family studies	Karyotyping indicates a female newborn with virilization. The genetic analysis confirms the presence of mutations in *CYP21*, confirming the diagnosis of CAH

 Q5: What is your final hypothesis?

A5

The clinical picture and laboratory results are suggestive of CAH resulting from 21-hydroxylase deficiency (caused by mutations on the *CYP21* gene located on the short arm of chromosome 6).

 Q6: What issues in the given history, examination and laboratory tests support your final hypothesis?

A6

Supportive evidence

History

- Michael is born by normal delivery at term.
- Michael is always lethargic and sleeping most of the time.
- On the fifth day he vomited repeatedly and looked ill.

Examination

- The paediatric registrar examines Michael and finds no obvious cause for Michael's vomiting.
- Michael could have ambiguous genitalia and what is thought to be a penis could be an enlarged clitoris.

Investigations

- PCV: raised

- Serum cortisol: low

- Serum ACTH: raised

- Serum sodium: low

- Serum potassium: raised

- Serum androstenedione and testosterone: both raised

- 17-OHP: raised

- Urinary pregnanetriol and 17-oxosteroid concentrations: both raised

- Karyotyping: 46,XX

- Genetic studies: evidence of mutations in the *CYP21* (*CYP21A2*) gene, which is located in the highly polymorphic HLA histocompatibility complex on chromosome 6p21.3. Mutations identified in the patient were assigned by family studies.

⚕ Integrated medical sciences questions

◉ CASE 9.1 – Briefly discuss the causes of subfertility, investigations recommended and scientific basis behind these investigations.

Table 9.11 Causes of subfertility

Causes of subfertility	Investigations	Scientific basis
Male causes		
Hypothalamic–pituitary failure	FSH, LH, testosterone, prolactin, CT of the pituitary and hypothalamic region	Rare cause for male infertility
Sperm dysfunction	Semen analysis Normally volume > 2.5 mL, sperm count > 20 million/mL, > 50 per cent motile, > 15 per cent normal sperm morphology	Several hormones play a role in spermatogenesis: LH secreted by anterior pituitary; testosterone, secreted by the interstitial cells of Leydig; prolactin and inhibin facilitate the stimulation of Leydig cells; FSH, secreted by anterior pituitary; and GH, secreted by anterior pituitary
	Semen should be analysed after 3 days' abstinence from ejaculation. If the results are suboptimal, the test should be repeated after 4–6 weeks. For abnormal results, LH, FSH and testosterone should be measured	The role of testosterone in spermatogenesis are: active form of testosterone, dihydrotestosterone, is essential for the growth and division of spermatogonia; testosterone stimulates the formation of FSH receptors in Sertoli cells; and testosterone and FSH work synergistically stimulating the synthesis of the androgen-binding protein which transports oestrogen and testosterone into the seminiferous tubular fluid to support spermatogenesis and maturation of sperm
	Calculate as motile normal sperm concentration = count × percentage motile × (percentage normal/mL)	
	Normal > 1 million/mL	In the Sertoli cells, testosterone is converted to oestrogen, which is believed to be involved in the process of spermatogenesis
		GH provides a physiological metabolic environment for normal spermatogenesis
Testicular obstruction, e.g. congenital bilateral absence of the vas deferens (as in cystic fibrosis), after vasectomy, epididymal obstruction after chlamydial infection or gonorrhoea	History, examination, urethral swabs for microbiological studies, chlamydia serology	

Female causes

Ovarian disorders	Progesterone (about 7 days after ovulation), FSH, LH, SHBG, thyroid function tests, prolactin	Ovulatory functions depend on a surge of LH secreted by the anterior pituitary
	Ultrasonography can be used to monitor follicular growth and formation of the corpus luteum	Other hormones important for normal ovarian function are: FSH; gonadotrophin-releasing hormone (GnRH), as the secretion of FSH and LH are dependent on changes in hypothalamic GnRH secretion; and gonadal steroids and inhibin, as both regulate GnRH secretion
	Laparoscopic direct visualization of the corpus luteum in the second half of the cycle	
		Polycystic ovary syndrome is associated with amenorrhoea, hyperoestrogenism, dyslipidaemia, obesity, multiple follicular cysts of the ovary and impairment of glucose metabolism. The syndrome is an important cause of infertility and endometrial hyperplasia
Fallopian tube damage/blockage	Chlamydial serology, ultrasonography, contrast salpingography, laparoscopy	Endometritis resulting from chlamydial infection and tuberculosis may result in severe inflammation, lymphocytic infiltration and obstruction of the fallopian tubes
		Inflammation interferes with the normal function of cilia responsible for movement of oocyte into the oviduct
Endometriosis	Laparoscopy and dye	Endometriosis is the presence of endometrial glands in sites other than the uterine corpus. Endometriosis may result in pelvic inflammation, infertility and pain
		The main sites of endometriosis are: the pouch of Douglas; the pelvic peritoneum; the ovary; the serosal surface of the uterus, cervix, vulva and vagina; and possibly in extragenital sites such as urinary bladder, small and large intestine
Uterine abnormalities	Ultrasound examination	The majority of congenital abnormalities result from a partial or complete failure of müllerian (paramesonephric) ducts to fuse
Others such as: increased age, extreme bodyweight loss or obesity, chronic diseases, smoking, medication, occupation, exposure to chemicals and radiation	Clinical examination, BMI, full blood examination, hepatitis B and C and HIV serology, blood glucose, rubella serology	These factors should be considered in assessment of patients presenting with subfertility

Other causes

Cervical mucus disorders	Postcoital test (aspiration of a sample of cervical mucus around the time of ovulation, within 6 hours of intercourse). The test is controversial and there are a number of factors interfering with its interpretation
Coital failure or inadequacy	

● CASE 9.2 – Discuss the physiological and hormonal changes during the menstrual cycle.

The normal cyclical changes in the endometrium are normally controlled by the hypothalamic–pituitary–ovarian axis, mainly the FSH and LH, which control ovulation and hence ovarian hormones.

The physiological events in the endometrium are determined by the blood concentrations of the ovarian hormones.

During the days preceding ovulation, the endometrium increases in thickness and the endometrial glands proliferate (proliferative phase).

After ovulation, the endometrium undergoes secondary changes (secretory phase) because of the effect of progesterone produced by the corpus luteum. These changes aim at the preparation of the endometrium to receive and implement a fertilized ovum (an embryo).

If the blood progesterone levels are not maintained (as is the case when there is no pregnancy and degeneration of the corpus luteum occurs), progesterone blood levels gradually decrease → spasm of the endometrial arterioles in the basal layer → shedding of the superficial layer of the endometrium → menstruation (usually continues for 5 days).

The whole menstrual cycle is about 28 days; ovulation occurs approximately on day 14 and menstruation continues for about 5 days. However, these times varies from cycle to cycle in the same woman.

● CASE 9.3 – Discuss the mechanisms underlying the pathogenesis of Michael's condition.

Congenital deficiency in 21-hydroxylase enzyme, resulting from mutations in CYP21 (CYP21A2), which is located in the highly polymorphic HLA histocompatibility complex on chromosome 6p21.3 → (1) cortisol deficiency, (2) aldosterone deficiency, (3) increased plasma levels of 17-OHP and (4) increased synthesis of adrenal androgens.

Decreased cortisol production → feedback → stimulation of the anterior pituitary → increased ACTH production → excessive stimulation of the adrenal → hyperplasia of the adrenal gland without any increase in cortisol production (because of 21-hydroxylase deficiency). As the process continuous → more hyperplasia of the adrenal.

Aldosterone deficiency → mineralocorticoid deficiency syndrome → hyperkalaemia + renal salt loss (hyponatraemia) + dehydration + hypovolaemia (may progress to shock, called 'adrenal crisis') if not treated immediately.

Increased production of 17-OHP and its urinary metabolites → increased urinary pregnanetriol and 17-oxosteroid concentrations. 17-OHP does not normally require 21-hydroxylase for its synthesis.

Increased synthesis of adrenal androgens → masculinization in newborn and virilization (e.g. enlargement of clitoris in girls).

Further reading

Baird DT. Amenorrhoea. *Lancet* 1997;**350**:275–279.

Constine LS, Woolf PD, Cann D *et al*. Hypothalamic–pituitary dysfunction after radiation for brain tumours. *New England Journal of Medicine* 1993;**328**:87–94.

Evers JLH. Female subfertility. *Lancet* 2002;**360**:151–159.

Gruber CJ, Tschugguel W, Schneeberger C, Huber JC. Mechanisms of disease: production and actions of estrogens. *New England Journal of Medicine* 2002;**346**:340–352.

Kamischke A, Baumgardt A, Horst J, Nieschlag E. Clinical and diagnostic features of patients with suspected Klinefelter syndrome. *Journal of Andrology* 2003;**24**:41–48.

Lamberts SWJ, de Herder WW, Jan der Lely AJ. Pituitary insufficiency. *Lancet* 1998;**352**:127–134.

Merke DP, Bernstein SR, Avila NA, Chrousos GP. NIH conference: Future directions in the study and management of congenital adrenal hyperplasia due to 21-hydroxylase deficiency. *Annals of Internal Medicine* 2002;**136**:320–334.

New MI, Carlson A, Obeid J. *et al*. Update on prenatal diagnosis for congenital adrenal hyperplasia in 532 pregnancies. *Journal of Clinical Endocrinology and Metabolism* 2001;**86**:5651–5657.

Norwitz ER, Schust DJ, Fisher SJ. Mechanisms of disease: implementation and survival of early pregnancy. *New England Journal of Medicine* 2001;**345**:1400–1408.

Speiser PW, White PC. Medical progress: congenital adrenal hyperplasia. *New England Journal of Medicine* 2003;**349**:776–788.

Taylor A. ABC of subfertility. Making a diagnosis. *British Medical Journal* 2003;**327**:494–497.

Vance ML. Medical progress: hypopituitarism. *New England Journal of Medicine* 1994;**330**:1651–1662.

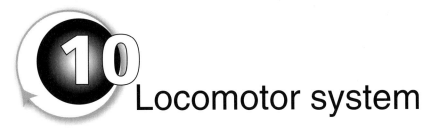

Locomotor system

Q1: What are the possible causes for the presenting problem?
Q2: What further questions would you like to ask to help you differentiate between your hypotheses?
Q3: What investigations would be most helpful to you and why?
Q4: In the light of the clinical presentation, how would you interpret the laboratory test results?
Q5: What is your final hypothesis?
Q6: What issues in the given history, examination and laboratory tests support your final hypothesis?

Clinical cases

● CASE 10.1 – My right knee is red, warm and sore.

Mr Bush Lloyd-Jones, a 48-year-old fisherman, comes in to see his GP, Dr Amanda Marshall, because of pain in his right knee. He says, 'I woke up at about 3am with pain in my right knee. The next morning, I noticed that my knee was swollen and red. The paracetamol tablets I took last night did not help with the pain.' Bush enjoys eating and usually drinks about four cans of full-strength beer every day. He has been treated for over 3 years with a thiazide diuretic and an angiotensin-converting enzyme (ACE) inhibitor (lisinopril) for high blood pressure. His older brother and mother had joint problems and his father died at the age of 58 because of a heart attack.

On examination, his body mass index (BMI) is 31. His vital signs are shown in Table 10.1.

Table 10.1 Vital signs for Case 10.1

Vital signs	Bush's results	Normal range
Blood pressure (mmHg)	180/90	100/60–135/85
Pulse rate (/min)	90	60–100
Respiratory rate (/min)	16	12–16
Temperature (°C)	37	36.6–37.2

● His right knee swollen, red, warm to touch and tender.

● No other joint involvement

● Respiratory and cardiovascular examinations: normal

● Abdominal examination normal

● Urinalysis: normal.

● CASE 10.2 – I can't get out of my chair.

Mr Joshua Backdoor, a 43-year-old cleaner, comes in to see his GP, Dr Hansen Wales, because of weakness in both legs when getting out of a low chair. He has noticed difficulty walking up and down the stairs over the last four weeks. The muscles of his legs and arms are painful, particularly after exercise. He has also noticed progressive tiredness over the last few months. Joshua also gives a history of muscle cramps in both legs. He has been treated with a hydroxyglutaryl-coenzyme A (HMG-CoA) reductase inhibitor (simvastatin) over the last 3 years. His father has type 2 diabetes. There is no family history of muscle disease.

On examination, his vital signs are as shown in Table 10.2.

Table 10.2 Vital signs for Case 10.2

Vital signs	Joshua's results	Normal range
Blood pressure (mmHg)	120/80	100/60–135/85
Pulse rate (/min)	79	60–100
Respiratory rate (/min)	16	12–16
Temperature (°C)	37	36.6–37.2

- Neurological examination: no neurological abnormality affecting spinal cord or peripheral nerves. No sensory loss.

- Weakness mainly of the shoulder girdle muscles and thigh muscles. Muscles are tender.

- Unable to get out of a chair and needs assistance.

- No signs of hypo- or hyperthyroidism.

● CASE 10.3 – I have pins and needles in both hands.

Mrs Maria Sharp, a 30-year-old factory worker, comes in to see her GP, Dr Ray Rodman, because of pins and needles in both hands. The pain wakes her up at night at about 3am. She also has the pain after using a vibrating machine at work. Sometimes, Maria feels pins and needles during driving. Her hands are slightly puffy in the morning. She gives a past history of falling from a swing at the age of 13 and she had to wear a collar for about 2 weeks. No neurological damage occurred because of the fall and she has had no neck or arm pain since then. She is 3 months' pregnant and on insulin for gestational diabetes.

On examination:

- Hands: are slightly puffy. Joints: normal range of movement. Thenar eminence is wasted bilaterally.

- Sensory examination: touch sensation in the thumb, index and middle finger of both hands is altered.

- Sustained wrist flexion, for about 1 minute, reproduces her symptoms of numbness of the hands.

⚭ Integrated medical sciences questions

● CASE 10.1 – Briefly discuss uric acid metabolism using a flow diagram. Discuss causes of hyperuricaemia.

● CASE 10.2 – Discuss the function and structure of dystrophin and its relationship with other sarcolemma-associated proteins. Briefly discuss the pathogenesis and the genetic basis of Duchenne muscle dystrophy. You may use diagrams to outline your answer.

● CASE 10.3 – Briefly discuss the anatomy of the carpal tunnel and the main structures of the wrist. Briefly discuss the motor and sensory supply of the median nerve and the effects of median nerve damage at the elbow and the wrist.

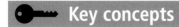

Key concepts

In order to work through the core clinical cases in this chapter, you will need to understand the following key concepts.

What is a motor unit?

A motor nerve fibre, including its cell body, and all the muscle fibres innervated by it are called a motor unit. The muscle fibres of a single motor unit are not all clustered together but are dispersed throughout a muscle.

The types of muscle fibres?

Muscle fibres may be divided on the basis of their morphology and physiochemical characteristics into types 1 and 2 as shown in Table 10.3.

Table 10.3 Characteristics of type 1 and 2 muscle fibres

Type 1	Type 2
Contracts at a slow speed	Contracts at a much faster rate
High resistance to fatigue	Low resistance to fatigue
High myoglobin content (smaller diameter, red in colour)	Low myoglobin content (larger diameter, white, pale in colour)
Increased capacity to hold O_2	Low capacity to hold O_2
Increased number of mitochondria	Fewer mitochondria
Aerobic metabolism	Anaerobic metabolism (uses glycogen as the source of energy)
Greater blood supply (abundant capillaries)	Less blood supply (fewer capillaries)
Usually in deeper planes near the trunk and limb axis	Usually in superficial planes and away from the trunk

The main physiological mechanisms of muscle contraction

1. Excitation: the process in which action potentials in the nerve fibre lead to action potentials in the muscle fibre.

2. This process includes stimulation of voltage-gated calcium channels at the neuromuscular synapse → release of calcium ions → stimulation of the release of acetylcholine (ACh) from ACh-gated channels into the synaptic cleft → ACh diffusing across the synaptic cleft and binding to specific receptor proteins on the sarcolemma → these receptors changing shape and an ion channel opening through the middle of the receptor protein → Na^+ diffusing into the cell and K^+ out → sarcolemma reversing polarity (resulting in rapid fluctuation in membrane voltage at the motor end-plate, known as end-plate potential) → creation of action potential.

3. Excitation–contraction coupling: this process involves the events that link the action potentials to activate the myofilaments. The action potential travels along the muscle fibre membrane → release of calcium ions from the sarcoplasmic reticulum into the myofibrils → calcium ions initiating forces between the actin and myosin filaments.

4. Contraction: muscle fibre develops tension with or without shortening. This process involves the sliding of the actin filaments inwards along the myosin filaments, using ATP present in the myosin head. Hydrolysis of ATP to produce energy needed is carried out by 'myosin ATPase', an enzyme in the myosin head → formation of a myosin–actin cross-bridge + the release of ADP and phosphate. The process repeats.

5. Relaxation: a muscle fibre relaxes and returns to its resting length.

The molecular mechanisms of muscle contraction

1. Filaments slide alongside each other: chemical bonds are generated (interaction of myosin cross-bridges with actin filaments), causing actin filaments to slide inwards along the myosin filaments. At rest, the interaction between actin and myosin is prevented by the proteins tropomyosin and troponin. During muscle rest, the calcium ion levels are low.

2. With the start of muscle contraction, an action potential travels over the muscle fibre membrane and large quantities of calcium ions are released from the sarcoplasmic reticulum → (1) activation of the chemical bonds between myosin and actin filaments, (2) stopping troponin and tropomyosin from blocking the interaction between actin and myosin → start of muscle contraction.

3. The myosin molecules are composed of a myosin tail and head. The myosin head functions as an ATPase enzyme → cleavage of ATP and energization of the formation of myosin–actin cross-bridge and muscle contraction.

4. The myosin head attached to an active site automatically tilts towards the tail that is dragging along the actin filament. This tilt of the head is called 'the power stroke'. Immediately after head tilting, the head breaks away from the active site and returns to its normal perpendicular position. The head immediately combines with a new active site further along the actin filament. As this process repeats, the ends of the actin filaments are pulled towards the centre of the myosin filament.

Answers

 CASE 10.1 – **My right knee is red, warm and sore.**

 Q1: What are the possible causes for the presenting problem?

A1

The following are possible causes (hypotheses) for Bush's presentation:

- Trauma/haemarthrosis – but there is no history of knee trauma.
- Inflammation of the knee joint, e.g. rheumatoid arthritis.
- Bacterial infection.
- Acute gout (crystal-induced inflammation, e.g. monosodium urate deposition): most likely because of (1) the clinical presentation: red, swollen, warm, and tender right knee and (2) the presence of a number of predisposing factors, e.g. treated with a thiazide diuretic for over 3 years, excessive alcohol intake, excessive ingestion of food containing high levels of purine, obesity, vascular disease and high blood pressure, and decreased fluid intake. Hypertension and vascular diseases may be genetically associated with gout rather than complications of hyperuricaemia.
- Pseudo-gout (calcium pyrophosphate deposition).
- Osteoarthritis – less likely.

 Q2: What further questions would you like to ask to help you differentiate between your hypotheses?

A2

Table 10.4 Further history questions for Case 10.1

History questions	In what way answers can help
Any history of trauma to the right knee?	Trauma to the knee may produce haemarthrosis (red, hot, warm, tender knee), which is usually the result of a tear of the anterior or posterior cruciate ligaments, medial or lateral meniscal tears, or trauma to collateral ligaments. Isolated soft tissue injuries may occur
Details of dietary intake	Gout is an abnormality of uric acid metabolism that results in the deposition of sodium urate crystals in the joints. Excessive ingestion of food rich in purines may be a contributing factor
Any history of recent operation?	Tissue damage, as with trauma and surgery, may result in excessive production of xanthine and uric acid
Any history of renal troubles?	Uric acid is completely filtered by the glomeruli; 100 per cent is then reabsorbed in the proximal tubule and 75 per cent is secreted in the distal tubule. Renal troubles could interfere with uric acid secretion. Patients may give a history of urate stones

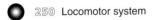
Past history of similar attacks	Most patients have had previous attacks of acute gout
Any joint affected other than his right knee?	Most patients have one joint affected at a time. The first metatarsophalangeal joint is commonly involved at presentation but other commonly affected joints are the ankle, knee and tarsal areas. Any joint including the spine may be affected
Any family history of gout?	One-third of patients with gout have a positive family history

 Q3: What investigations would be most helpful to you and why?

A3

Further investigations

- Radiograph of right knee

- Full blood examination and C-reactive protein (CRP)

- Serum uric acid level

- Blood urea, creatinine, sodium and potassium

- Synovial fluid examination.

 CASE 10.2 – I can't get out of my chair.

 Q1: What are the possible causes for the presenting problem?

A1

The fact that there is no neurological abnormality affecting the spinal cord or peripheral nerves indicates that the patient's proximal weakness is the result of a muscle problem or a neuromuscular junction problem. The duration of his illness is only a few weeks, indicating that inherited myopathies (e.g. Duchenne type dystrophy) are less likely. Joshua most probably has an acute illness affecting his proximal muscles.

The following are possible causes (hypotheses) for Joshua's presentation:

- Idiopathic inflammatory myopathy (e.g. polymyositis, dermatomyositis) – symmetrical weakness over weeks of proximal muscles, muscle pain and tenderness

- Drug-induced and toxic myopathies

- Infectious myositis (e.g. acute viral myositis)

- Metabolic myopathies, e.g. glucose and glycogen metabolism disorders; lipid metabolism disorders; and mitochondrial disorders – less likely

- Inherited muscular dystrophies (e.g. Duchenne-type dystrophy) – less likely because: Duchenne muscle dystrophy usually presents as early as age 2–3 years; it usually presents as delays in motor milestones and difficulty running; and most patients die of respiratory complications in their 20s

- Channelopathies (e.g. chloride channelopathies, sodium channelopathies and calcium channelopathies) – less likely

- Myopathies caused by endocrine and systemic disorders, e.g. Cushing's disease, hypo- or hyperthyroidism, diabetes-related myopathy – less likely

- Neuromuscular junction disease (e.g. myasthenia gravis) – less likely because there is no ocular muscle involvement (ptosis and diplopia), weakness of other muscles innervated by cranial nerves (facial muscles, slurred or nasal speech or jaw drop).

 Q2: What further questions would you like to ask to help you differentiate between your hypotheses?

A2

Table 10.5 Further history questions for Case 10.2

History questions	In what way answers can help
History of numbness, pins and needles, and cranial nerve involvement	Absence of numbness, pins and needles, and cranial nerve involvement helps in determining whether the weakness is a primary muscle disorder or secondary to a peripheral nerve problem
History of difficulty squatting, going up stairs, rising from a chair or dysphagia	Polymyositis/dermatomyositis are characterized by proximal muscle weakness. Dysphagia caused by oesophageal muscle involvement occurs in 50 per cent of patients
Skin rash	Skin rash in dermatomyositis may accompany or precede the onset of muscle weakness. The rash may be a heliotrope rash (purplish discoloration of the eyelids often associated with periorbital oedema); popular erythematous, scaly lesion over the knuckles; or sun-sensitive rash on the face, neck, anterior chest, shoulders and elbows
Symptoms suggestive of Cushing's disease, hypo- or hyperthyroidism	To exclude myopathies caused by endocrine diseases
History of shortness of breath, palpitations or heart failure	Some myopathies may be associated with cardiac failure and arrhythmias. Interstitial lung disease may develop in patients with dermatomyositis and polymyositis
Medication	Toxic myopathies may be caused by any of these drugs: cimetidine, D-pencillamine, cholesterol-lowering drugs, alcohol, cocaine, halothane, glucocorticoids and zidovudine
Family history	Some myopathies are inherited, e.g. Duchenne-type dystrophy is an X-linked disorder resulting from mutations of the large dystrophin gene located at Xp21. Myotonic dystrophy is an autosomal dominant disorder

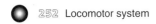 **Q3: What investigations would be most helpful to you and why?**

A3

Further investigations

- Serum creatine kinase.

- Chest radiograph

- Muscle biopsy

- Full blood examination and erythrocyte sedimentation rate (ESR)

- Elecromyography (EMG)

- Thyroid function tests

- Autoimmune screen.

 CASE 10.3 – I have pins and needles in both hands.

Q1: What are the possible causes for the presenting problem?

A1

The following are possible causes (hypotheses) for Marla's presentation:

- Cervical spondylosis

- Cervical disc prolapse

- Cervical trauma

- Injury to the median nerve at the elbow

- Injury to the median nerve at the wrist (e.g. carpal tunnel compression of the median nerve)

- Metabolic disorders that may cause arthropathy of the small joints of the hand (e.g. haemochromatosis).

Q2: What further questions would you like to ask to help you differentiate between your hypotheses?

A2

Table 10.6 Further history questions for Case 10.3

History questions	In what way answers can help
What triggers her hand pain?	In carpal tunnel syndrome, hand pain may be triggered by vibrating machines and holding a newspaper or telephone for a prolonged time

Any history of arthritis, skin rash, muscle weakness or symptoms suggestive of hypothyroidism?	Carpal tunnel syndrome may occur in rheumatoid arthritis (disease process involving the synovial sheaths of the flexor tendons) → contents of the tunnel increasing in bulk → compression of the median nerve. Other conditions associated with carpal tunnel syndrome are pregnancy and myxoedema
What relieves her hand pains?	In carpal tunnel syndrome, pain may be relieved by night splints, or hanging hands over the edge of the bed
Distribution of pain/discomfort in her hands	In carpal tunnel syndrome pain may be felt anywhere in the arm. This poor localization of pain may make the diagnosis difficult. It may be confused with cervical spondylosis

 Q3: What investigations would be most helpful to you and why?

A3

Further investigations

- Full blood examination

- Serum iron and ferritin levels

- Nerve conduction tests

- EMG.

Further progress

 CASE 10.1 – **My right knee is red, warm and sore.**

Dr Amanda Marshall arranges some tests for Bush. The results are shown in Table 10.7.

Table 10.7 Test results for Case 10.1

Test	Bush's results	Normal range
Haemoglobin (Hb) level (g/L)	120	115–160
White blood cell count (WCC) ($\times 10^9$/L)	13.5	4.0–11.0
Platelet count ($\times 10^9$/L)	210	150–450
C-reactive protein (CRP) (mg/L)	> 300	< 10
Serum uric acid (μmol/L)	890	150–450
Blood urea (mmol/L)	13.6	2.5–8.3
Serum creatinine (mmol/L)	1.2	0.05–0.11
Serum sodium (mmol/L)	132	135–145

Serum potassium (mmol/L)	3.8	3.5–5.0
Radiograph of right knee	No evidence of joint or bone disease	–
Synovial fluid examination	Fluid is opaque, creamy yellow, of reduced viscosity. WCC 23 × 10⁹/L (all neutrophils). Polarized microscopy: numerous negatively birefringent crystals typical of monosodium urate monohydrate crystals (both extracellular and within neutrophils) Gram staining and culture: negative	

CASE 10.2 – I can't get out of my chair.

Dr Hansen Wales arranges some tests for Joshua. The results are shown in Table 10.8.

Table 10.8 Test results for Case 10.2

Test	Joshua's results	Normal range
Hb level (g/L)	10	115–160
WCC (× 10⁹/L)	5.0	4.0 –11.0
Platelet count (× 10⁹/L)	330	150–450
Erythrocyte sedimentation rate (ESR) (mm/h)	29	< 20
Blood film	A picture suggestive of normocytic/normochromic anaemia	
Serum creatine kinase (CK) (IU/L)	3600	40–300
Chest radiograph (PA and lateral views)	Normal	
Needle muscle biopsy	Type 2 fibre atrophy with perivascular inflammatory changes and mononuclear cell infiltration. Muscle fibres are irregular in size and shape. Necrotic fibres are seen	–
Electromyography	Myopathic changes. No evidence of nerve lesion	

PA, posteroanterior.

Thyroid function tests: normal.

Autoimmune screen: negative.

CASE 10.3 – I have pins and needles in both hands.

Dr Ray Rodman arranges some tests for Maria. The results are shown in Table 10.9.

Table 10.9 Test results for Case 10.3

Test	Maria's results	Normal range
Hb level (g/L)	120	115–160
WCC ($\times 10^9$/L)	5.0	4.0 –11.0
Platelet count ($\times 10^9$/L)	330	150–450
ESR (mm/h)	45	< 20
Serum iron (μmol/L)	15	9–30
Serum ferritin (μg/L)	87	10–120

- CT of cervical spine: normal.

- Electromyography: no motor axonal degeneration. No evidence of myopathy.

- Nerve conduction test (median nerve): a delay in conduction velocities bilaterally. Prolonged motor and sensory latencies bilaterally.

- Nerve conduction studies of radial and ulnar nerves are normal.

Further questions

 CASE 10.1 — **My right knee is red, warm and sore.**

Q4: **In the light of the clinical presentation, how would you interpret the laboratory test results?**

A4

Table 10.10 Interpretation of lab test results for Case 10.1

Test	Change	Interpretation
WCC	Raised	WCC may be raised in the presence of infection (joint sepsis) or acute inflammation such as acute gout or pseudo-gout
CRP	Raised	CRP is so called because it reacts with the C-polysaccharide of pneumococci. It is one of the acute phase reaction proteins and is increased in conditions associated with tissue damage (trauma, infection, inflammation, malignancy)
Serum uric acid	Raised	Humans convert the major purine nucleosides adenosine and guanosine to uric acid via a number of biochemical reactions. In these reactions, hypoxanthine and guanine form xanthine, catalysed by xanthine oxidase and guanase, respectively. In a second reaction, xanthine is oxidized to uric acid, catalysed by xanthine oxidase
		The serum uric acid may be raised or remains within the normal range at the time of presentation of acute gout. The diagnosis of acute gout should not be rejected when a normal serum uric value is found. The supportive findings from medical history and clinical examination should be considered in making the correct diagnosis. Hyperuricaemia may result from: overproduction (e.g. idiopathic, haematological disorders, treatment of malignancy by chemotherapy or irradiation, non-malignant increase in cell turnover as in psoriasis), but is more usually the result of poor excretion of urate by the kidney (e.g. renal failure, ethanol intake, ketoacidosis, lactic acidosis, severe hypothyroidism, hyperparathyroidism, intake of diuretics 'thiazides', 'low-dose' salicylate, ethambutol, pyrazinamine)
Blood urea and serum creatinine	Raised	Raised blood urea and creatinine may indicate renal impairment. It is difficult to decide, from the information provided in the case scenario, whether the patient's renal impairment has resulted in high blood pressure or is a complication of his high blood pressure
		The following factors might have contributed to the patient's hyperuricaemia: renal impairment, use of diuretics and thiazides, alcohol intake, obesity and possibly hyperlipidaemia, and possibly family history

Serum sodium	Low	Thiazide diuretics may result in a number of side effects including: abnormalities of fluid and electrolyte balance, hypovolaemia, hypokalaemia, hyponatraemia, hypochloraemia, metabolic alkalosis, hypomagnesaemia, hypercalcaemia and hyperuricaemia; possible decrease in glucose tolerance and cause of latent diabetes mellitus, and hyperglycaemia may be related to potassium depletion; thiazide diuretics may also increase plasma lipids LDL-cholesterol, total cholesterol and total acylglycerols. Other side effects include: vertigo, headache, weakness, anorexia, nausea, vomiting, cramping, changes in bowel motions, skin rash, photosensitivity and sexual dysfunction (erectile problems)
Serum potassium	Normal	The patient is on a thiazide diuretic and an ACE inhibitor (lisinopril); although hypokalaemia is expected to occur as a result of thiazide diuretic use, an ACE inhibitor such as lisinopril may cause hyperkalaemia, particularly in patients with renal insufficiency. It is possible that the normal serum potassium level is the outcome of the effect of the thiazide diuretic and ACE inhibitor
		ACE inhibitors do not alter plasma concentration of uric acid or calcium. They may improve insulin sensitivity in patients with insulin resistance and decrease cholesterol and lipoprotein (a) levels
Radiograph of right knee	No evidence of joint or bone disease	In acute gout there is usually no evidence of joint or bone changes
Synovial fluid examination	Fluid is opaque, creamy yellow, of reduced viscosity. WCC 23×10^9/L (all neutrophils)	The synovial fluid may contain a number of crystals and particles including: MSUM, CPPD crystals, cholesterol, BCPs and fibrin
		Both MSUM and CPPD are pathogenic. CPPD are positively birefringent rods/rhomboids, 1–20 μm, and can form a 'beachball'. The presence of CPPD in synovial fluids and high polymorphonuclear count may support the diagnosis of pseudo-gout
	Polarized microscopy: numerous negatively birefringent crystals typical of MSUM crystals (both extracellular and within neutrophils)	MSUM crystals are very birefringent needles of size 1–20 μm. They can form in a 'beachball' array. The presence of a high polymorphonuclear cell count (indicative of acute inflammation) is essential for the diagnosis of acute gout attack
		The results of Gram staining and synovial fluid culture exclude joint infection
	Gram staining and culture: negative	

ACE, angiotensin-converting enzyme; BCP, basic calcium phosphate; CPPD, calcium pyrophosphate dehydrate; LDL, low-density lipoprotein; MSUM, monosodium urate monohydrate

Q5: What is your final hypothesis?

A5

The clinical picture and laboratory results are suggestive of acute gout of right knee.

Q6: What issues in the given history, examination and laboratory tests support your final hypothesis?

A6

Supportive evidence

History

- The patient presents with pain in his right knee.
- His knee is swollen, painful and red.
- He enjoys eating and usually drinks about four cans of full-strength beer every day.
- He has been treated for over 3 years with a thiazide diuretic and an ACE inhibitor (lisinopril) for high blood pressure.
- His older brother and mother had joint problems and his father died at the age of 58 because of a heart attack.

Examination

- He is obese (BMI 31).
- Blood pressure is 180/90 mmHg and afebrile.
- His right knee is swollen, red, warm to touch and tender.
- Urinalysis is normal.

Investigations

- WCC: raised
- CRP: raised
- Serum uric acid: raised
- Blood urea and creatinine: raised
- Serum sodium: low
- Radiograph of right knee: normal
- Synovial fluid examination: fluid is opaque, creamy yellow, of reduced viscosity. WCC 23×10^9/L (all neutrophils). Polarized microscopy: numerous negatively birefringent crystals typical of monosodium urate monohydrate crystals (both extracellular and within neutrophils)
- Gram staining and culture: negative.

CASE 10.2 – I can't get out of my chair.

Q4: In the light of the clinical presentation, how would you interpret the laboratory test results?

A4

Table 10.11 Interpretation of lab test results for Case 10.2

Test	Change	Interpretation
Hb level	Low	Anaemia may be caused by impaired proliferation of erythroid progenitor cells, blunted erythropoietin response, dysregulation of the reticuloendothelial system or autoimmune related
ESR	Raised	In polymyositis ESR may be raised in 5–10 per cent of patients
Blood film	A picture suggestive of normocytic/ normochromic anaemia	This picture may be present in polymyositis
Serum CK	Raised	CK is a muscle enzyme that phosphorylates creatinine and is important in the energy metabolism of muscle. Measurement of serum enzymes such as CK helps to differentiate myopathic from neurogenic diseases. In polymyositis, serum level of muscle-derived enzymes, particularly CK, transaminases, lactate dehydrogenase and aldolase, are elevated. CK is the most sensitive. The levels of CK correlate with disease activity
		The patient is taking a HMG-CoA reductase inhibitor (simvastatin) and it is known that this drug may cause a number of side effects including: elevation of serum transferase activity and liver dysfunction, elevation of serum CK activity and the development of myopathy. Simvastatin is catabolized mainly through the hepatic cytochrome P-450 3A4 system. The serum levels of simvastatin may be significantly raised in the presence of drugs that inhibit or compete for 3A4 cytochrome (e.g. macrolide antibiotics, ciclosporin, ketoconazole or verapamil). It is important to note that the side effects of simvastatin may occur in some individuals when treated with simvastatin at normal doses and in the absence of drug interaction
Chest radiograph (PA and lateral views)	Normal	Polymyositis may be associated with malignancy. However, there are no specific clinical features that differentiate it from polymyositis alone. Chest radiograph may be ordered as a screening test for lung cancer. Extensive radiological screening, faecal occult blood tests, sigmoidoscopy and gastroscopy may be recommended depending on the clinical presentation and laboratory findings

		Several factors are thought to influence the incidence of coexisting malignancy. Increasing age, female sex, normal CK levels, and refractory or recurrent disease are all thought to increase the likelihood of occult malignancy
Needle muscle biopsy	Type 2 fibre atrophy with perivascular inflammatory changes and mononuclear cell infiltration. Muscle fibres are irregular in size and shape. Necrotic fibres are seen	In polymyositis, muscle biopsy is characterized by: degeneration or atrophy of individual fibres ± vacuolation; necrosis of muscle fibres; sarcoplasmic basophilia, large nuclei, prominent nucleoli; variation in fibre size; mononuclear cell infiltration; interstitial mononuclear cell infiltration; and interstitial fibrosis These changes may vary from patient to patient and not all these changes are necessarily present in all biopsies
Electromyography (EMG)	Myopathic changes. No evidence of nerve lesion	EMG in muscle diseases such as dermatomyositis is characterized by the following changes: no activity in the muscle at rest; no changes in the number of motor units firing during a contraction; and the potentials are of shorter duration and smaller in amplitude (this is mainly because of fewer surviving muscle fibres in each motor unit)
Thyroid function tests	Normal	Both hypo- and hyperthyroidism may cause proximal muscle weakness. In hypothyroidism, serum CK may reach high levels
Autoimmune screen	Negative	A number of autoantibodies have been detected in patients with dermatomyositis including Jo-1 (antibodies to histidyl-tRNA synthase), antinuclear antibody and rheumatoid factor

HMG-CoA, hydroxymethylglutaryl-coenzyme A.

Q5: What is your final hypothesis?

A5

The clinical picture and laboratory results are suggestive of polymyositis, most likely caused by cholesterol-lowering drug (HMG-CoA reductase inhibitor).

> **Q6: What issues in the given history, examination and laboratory tests support your final hypothesis?**

A6

Supportive evidence

History

- The patient presents with proximal muscle weakness.
- He has noticed difficulty walking up and down the stairs over the last 4 weeks.
- The muscles of his legs and arms are painful, particularly after exercise.
- He has also noticed progressive tiredness over the last few months.
- He has been treated with a HMG-CoA reductase inhibitor (simvastatin) over the last 3 years.
- His father has type 2 diabetes.
- No family history of muscle disease.

Examination

- His vital signs are normal.
- There is no evidence of neurological abnormality affecting the spinal cord or peripheral nerves.
- He has no sensory loss.
- He has weakness mainly of the shoulder girdle muscles and thigh muscles.
- Muscles are tender.
- There are no signs of hypo- or hyperthyroidism.

Investigations

- Hb: low.
- Blood film: normocytic/normochromic anaemia.
- Serum CK: raised.
- Chest radiograph: normal.
- Muscle biopsy: type 2 fibre atrophy with perivascular inflammatory changes and mononuclear cell infiltration; muscle fibres irregular in size and shape; necrotic fibres seen.
- EMG: myopathic changes; no evidence of nerve lesion.
- Thyroid function tests: normal.
- Autoimmune screen: negative.

CASE 10.3 – I have pins and needles in both hands.

> **Q4: In the light of the clinical presentation, how would you interpret the laboratory test results?**

A4

Table 10.12 Interpretation of lab test results for Case 10.3

Test	Change	Interpretation
Serum iron and serum ferritin	Normal	Normal studies help to exclude haemochromatosis. Haemochromatosis is an autosomal recessive disease, characterized by: bronze skin pigmentation caused by melanin deposition; hepatomegaly; diabetes mellitus; hypogonadism secondary to pituitary–gonadal axis dysfunction; cardiac failure and arrhythmias; and arthropathy and small joint pains
		Biochemically, haemochromatosis is characterized by high serum iron (> 30 µmol/L) and serum ferritin (> 500 µg/L)
		These results exclude haemochromatosis as a possible cause
CT of cervical spine	Normal	CT of the cervical spine helps in assessment of these conditions: degenerative arthritis particularly of C5/C6, C6/C7 and C7/T1; intervertebral disc spaces and foraminal spaces; and osteophytes or narrowing of the intervertebral foramina
		Normal studies help in exclusion of cervical spondylosis, cervical disc prolapse and cervical trauma as a cause for her presentation
EMG	No motor axonal degeneration. No evidence of myopathy	EMG allows physiological evaluation of the motor unit, including the anterior horn cell, peripheral nerve and muscle. Thus, it can help in the assessment of the following: to determine whether the weakness is the result of anterior horn cell lesion, nerve root injury, peripheral neuropathy or intrinsic muscle disease; to differentiate acute denervation from chronic denervation; to determine whether the neuropathy is the result of a lesion of a nerve root, individual peripheral nerve or multiple peripheral nerves (polyneuropathy); and to differentiate active myopathies from chronic myopathies
		There is no axonal damage of the motor nerve (median nerve). Her presentation is possibly related to compression of the median nerve at the carpal tunnel. No evidence of myopathy

Nerve conduction test (median nerve)	A delay in conduction velocities bilaterally. Prolonged motor and sensory latencies bilaterally	These findings are suggestive of carpal tunnel compression of the median nerve. Carpal tunnel is formed by the flexor retinaculum anteriorly and by the distal row of the carpus posteriorly. The median nerve and the flexor tendons pass through it. Any pathological condition causing compression of the median nerve as it passes the carpal tunnel, e.g. pregnancy (oedema under the tunnel because of fluid retention), myxoedema, unknown causes and rheumatoid arthritis, may be responsible.
		The median nerve arises from the medial and lateral cords of the brachial plexus. It gives off no cutaneous or motor branches in the axilla or the arm. In the proximal third of the front of the forearm, it supplies all the muscles except the flexor carpi ulnaris and the medial half of the flexor digitorum profundus
		Just before the wrist, the median nerve gives off the palmar cutaneous branch. In the hand, the median nerve supplies: three thenar muscles; first two lumbricals; and palmar digital branches to the lateral three and a half fingers
Nerve conduction studies of radial and ulnar nerves	Normal studies	Other nerves supplying the hand (radial and ulnar nerves) are not involved

 Q5: What is your final hypothesis?

A5

The clinical picture and laboratory results are suggestive of bilateral carpal tunnel syndrome (compression of the median nerve). Her symptoms may be aggravated by pregnancy and the use of vibrating machines at work.

 Q6: What issues in the given history, examination and laboratory tests support your final hypothesis?

A6

Supportive evidence

History

- The patient presents with pins and needles in both hands.
- The pain wakes her at night at about 3am.
- She has the pain after using a vibrating machine at work.
- Sometimes she feels pins and needles during driving.

- Past history of falling from a swing at the age of 13 and had to wear a collar for about 2 weeks. No neurological damage occurred because of the fall and she has had no neck or arm pain since then. She is 3 months' pregnant and she is on insulin for gestational diabetes.

Examination

- Her hands are slightly puffy.

- Joints: normal range of movement.

- Thenar eminence is wasted bilaterally.

- Sensory examination: touch sensation in the thumb, index and middle finger of both hands is altered.

- Sustained wrist flexion, for about 1 min, reproduces her symptoms of numbness of the hands.

Investigations

- Serum iron and serum ferritin: normal (no haemochromatosis).

- CT of cervical spine: normal

- EMG: no motor axonal degeneration

- Nerve conduction test (median nerve): a delay in conduction velocities bilaterally; prolonged motor and sensory latencies bilaterally

- Nerve conduction studies of radial and ulnar nerves: normal studies.

👥 Integrated medical sciences questions

⬤ CASE 10.1 – Briefly discuss uric acid metabolism using a flow diagram. Discuss causes of hyperuricaemia.

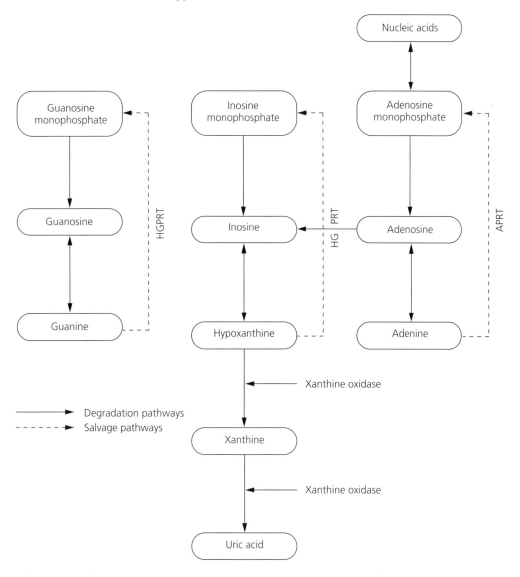

Figure 10.1 Normal purine metabolism and uric acid synthesis. APRT, adenine phosphoribosyltransferase; HGPRT, hypoxanthine–guanine phosphoribosyltransferase.

Causes of hyperuricaemia are:

- Increased production of uric acid:
  - idiopathic.

- polycythaemia vera (increased turn over of purines).

- leukaemia, cancer, psoriasis

- treatment of cancer by chemotherapy or radiotherapy

- increased synthesis of new purines

● Decreased excretion of uric acid:

- idiopathic.

- chronic renal disease.

- medication, e.g. thiazide diuretics, low-dose aspirin

- excessive alcohol intake.

- hypertension

- lead toxicity.

● **CASE 10.2 – Discuss the function and structure of dystrophin and its relationship with other sarcolemma-associated proteins. Briefly discuss the pathogenesis and the genetic basis of Duchenne muscle dystrophy. You may use diagrams to outline your answer.**

Dystrophin is a cytoplasmic 427-kDa protein located adjacent to the sarcolemmal membrane in myocytes. It is mainly present over Z-bands, where it forms a strong mechanical link to cytoplasmic actin. The dystrophin molecules and dystrophin-associated protein complexes, such as dystroglycans and sarcoglycans, form an interface between the intracellular contractile apparatus and the extracellular connective tissue matrix. It has been proposed that, as these protein complexes are responsible for the transfer of the force of contraction to connective tissue, they are also the basis for the myocyte degeneration that occurs in the absence of dystrophin or other proteins which interact with it (Figures 10.2 and 10.3).

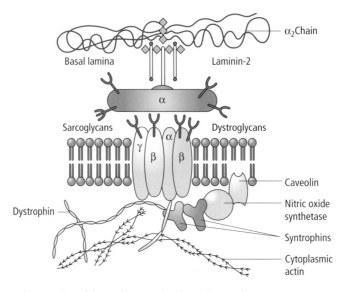

Figure 10.2 The dystrophin protein and dystrophin-associated protein complexes.

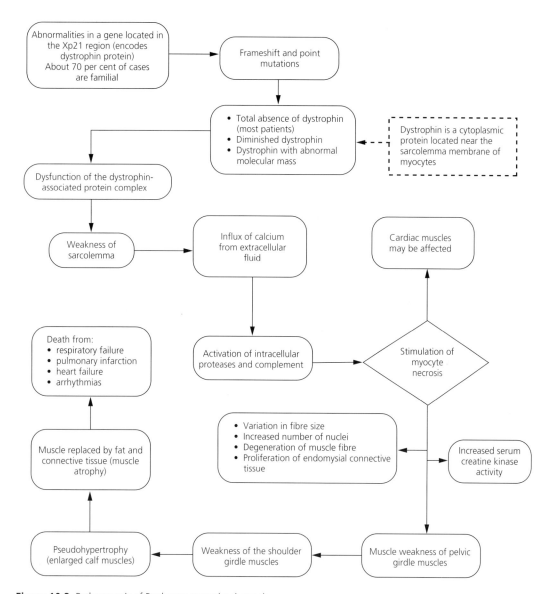

Figure 10.3 Pathogenesis of Duchenne muscular dystrophy.

⬤ CASE 10.3 – **Briefly discuss the anatomy of the carpal tunnel and the main structures at the wrist. Briefly discuss the motor and sensory supply of the median nerve in the hand and the effects of median nerve damage at the wrist.**

The carpal tunnel is formed by the flexor retinaculum anteriorly and by the distal row of carpus posteriorly.

The long flexor tendons to the fingers and thumb pass through the carpal tunnel and are accompanied by the median nerve.

The motor supply of the median nerve supply in the hand

The median nerve usually supply five muscles in the hand (the three thenar muscles and the two lateral lumbrical muscles). These muscles are supplied by two main branches:

1. The recurrent branch which supplies:

   – abductor pollicis brevis

   – opponens pollicis

   – flexor pollicis brevis

2. The palmar digital branches which supplies:

   – first lumbrical muscle

   – second lumbrical muscle.

The effects of damage of the median nerve at the wrist:

● Paralysis and wasting of the thenar muscles

● Paralysis of opponens pollicis

● Loss of sensory sensation:

   – dorsum of the hand: the distal parts of the lateral three and a half digits

   – palm of the hand: the lateral three and a half digits, the lateral part of the hand including the skin overlying the thenar muscles.

Further reading

Bannwarth B. Drug-induced myopathies. *Expert Opinion on Drug Safety* 2002;**1**:65–70.

Burke FD, Lawson IJ, McGeoch KL, Miles JN, Proud G. Carpal tunnel syndrome in association with hand–arm vibration syndrome: A review of claimants seeking compensation in the mining industry. *Journal of Hand Surgery* 2005;**30**:199–203.

Christopher-Stine L, Plotz PH. Myositis: an update on pathogenesis. *Current Opinion in Rheumatology* 2004;**16**:700–706.

Dalakas MC. Inflammatory disorders of muscle: progress in polymyositis, dermatomyositis and inclusion body myositis. *Current Opinion in Neurology* 2004:**17**;561–567.

Dalakas MC, Hohlfeld R. Polymyositis and dermatomyositis. *Lancet* 2003;**362**:971–982.

Drake RL, Vogl W, Mitchell AWM. *Gray's Anatomy for Students*. Philadelphia: Elsevier Churchill Livingstone, 2005.

Harris MD, Siegel LB, Alloway JA. Gout and hyperuricemia. *American Family Physician* 1999;**59**:925–934.

Jordan R, Carter T, Cummins C. A systematic review of the utility of electrodiagnostic testing in carpal tunnel syndrome. *British Journal of General Practice* 2002;**52**:670–673.

Kandel ER, Schwartz JH, Jessell TM. *Principles of Neural Science*, 4th edn. New York: McGraw-Hill, 2000.

Kao SY. Carpal tunnel syndrome as an occupational disease. *Journal of the American Board of Family Practice* 2003;**16**:533–542.

Mackinnon SE. Pathophysiology of nerve compression. *Hand Clinics* 2002;**18**:231–241.

Marshall S. Carpal tunnel syndrome. *Clinical Evidence* 2003;**9**:1154–1171.

Moore KL, Dalley AF. *Clinically Oriented Anatomy*, 4th edn. Philadelphia: Lippincott Williams & Wilkins, 1999.

Rotman MB, Donovan JP. Practical anatomy of the carpal tunnel. *Hand Clinics* 2002;18:219–230.

Swan A, Amer H, Dieppe P. The value of synovial fluid assays in the diagnosis of joint disease: a literature survey. *Annals of the Rheumatic Diseases* 2002;**61**:493–498.

Underwood M. Acute gout. *Clinical Evidence* 2003;**10**:1238–1246.

Werner RA, Andary M. Carpal tunnel syndrome: pathophysiology and clinical neurophysiology. *Clinical Neurophysiology* 2002;**113**:1373–1381.

Wortmann RL. Gout and hyperuricemia. *Current Opinion in Rheumatology* 2002;14:281–286.

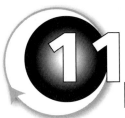

Haematopoietic system

Clinical cases

● CASE 11.1 – I always feel tired.

Mrs Athenia Georgiou, a 65 year old, comes in to see her GP, Dr Anita Maxwell, because of generalized tiredness, palpitation and shortness of breath after minor exercise of a few months' duration. Athenia has always been healthy and over the last 3 years she preferred to become vegetarian and very selective about what she eats. She lost 8 kg in body weight over the last 6 months. She also gives a history of upper abdominal discomfort and recent changes in her bowel motions – a few days of constipation followed by a loose bowel motion. On examination, both conjunctivae are pale. Her body mass index (BMI) is 27 and her vital signs are normal.

● Abdomen examination: no organomegaly in the abdomen; no lymphadenopathy.

● Rectal examination: no haemorrhoids and no bleeding per rectum. Stools are hard but of normal colour.

● Cardiovascular and respiratory examinations are normal.

● CASE 11.2 – I have sudden bleeding from my nose and gums.

Ms Margo Mufeed, a 24-year-old kindergarten teacher is brought to the accident and emergency department (A&E) of a local hospital because of severe nose and gum bleeding. Margo gives no history of trauma to her head or nose. She also has no history of fever, nausea, vomiting, abdominal pain or joint pain. She had an upper respiratory tract infection about 10 days ago. Her menstrual periods are regular. She has no past history of bleeding from nose or mouth, or easy bruising of the skin. On examination, Margo is alert but anxious. Her vital signs are summarized in Table 11.1.

Table 11.1 Vital signs for Case 11.2

Vital signs	Margo's results	Normal range
Blood pressure (mmHg)	110/80	100/60–135/85
Pulse rate (/min)	95	60–100
Respiratory rate (/min)	18	12–16
Temperature (°C)	37	36.6–37.2

● Red blood oozing from her nose and gums

● No jaundice or conjunctival pallor

- Skin: multiple, 1 mm, flat, reddish spots on her arms, legs and abdomen

- No lymphadenopathy

- Abdominal examination: no organomegaly and rectal examination normal

- The neurological, respiratory and cardiology examinations unremarkable.

CASE 11.3 – I have fever and rigors about a week after chemotherapy.

Michael Murray, a 64-year-old senior citizen, is brought to A&E because of fever and rigors (shaking chills) for the last 12 h. About a week ago, Michael was treated with chemotherapy (cyclophosphamide, doxorubicin [Adriamycin], vincristine and prednisone) for non-Hodgkin's lymphoma. On examination, he looks ill. His skin shows no rash but is warm and sweating. His vital signs are summarized in Table 11.2.

Table 11.2 Vital signs for Case 11.3

Vital signs	Michael's results	Normal range
Blood pressure (mmHg)	110/65	100/60–135/85
Pulse rate (/min)	120	60–100
Respiratory rate (/min)	23	12–16
Temperature (°C)	38.5	36.6–37.2

A tunnelled vascular catheter at the left internal jugular vein is present and there is erythema of the overlying skin. No purulent discharge at the catheter area.

Chest examination and cardiovascular examinations: normal to auscultation.

Abdominal examination: normal.

Rectal examination: normal and no blood on the examining gloved finger.

👥 Integrated medical sciences questions

CASE 11.1 – Discuss the physiological regulation of red blood cell production and the role of erythropoietin in this process.

CASE 11.2 – Discuss the role of platelets and the coagulation cascade in haemostasis after bleeding from a damaged blood vessel. You may use diagrams to outline your answer.

CASE 11.3 – Outline the origin and function of the monocyte–macrophage (reticuloendothelial) system.

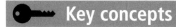 **Key concepts**

In order to work through the core clinical cases in this chapter, you will need to understand the following key concepts.

Table 11.3 The main elements of blood and the functions of each element

Element	Function
Red blood cells (erythrocytes)	Transport of O_2 and CO_2
White blood cells (WBCs; leukocytes)	Defence mechanisms: destroy invading bacteria and viruses, and remove dead particles
Platelets (thrombocytes)	Participate in blood clotting system and first line of defence when blood vessels are damaged
Plasma	Carries nutrients, metabolites, antibodies, hormones, proteins of blood clotting system

The main characteristics of red blood cells

- Contain haemoglobin (Hb)

- Main function: transport of O_2 and CO_2

- Rounded, biconcave shape to maximize surface area/volume ratio and hence enhance capacity for the exchange of gases

- About 6.5–7.5 μm in diameter

- Darker in the periphery and paler in the centre

- Have no nucleus or cell organelles (precursors of red blood cells have nuclei and organelles)

- Drive energy by anaerobic metabolism of glucose and ATP generation by the hexose monophosphate shunt

- Have soluble enzymes in their cytoplasm (e.g. carbonic anhydrase, which facilitates the formation of carbonic acid from CO_2 and water; this enzyme plays a role in CO_2 transport by red blood cells)

- Able to squeeze through small blood vessels

- Cell membrane is braced by an actin/spectrin cytoskeleton which maintains the biconcave shape

- Human erythrocytes have a lifespan of about 120 days

- Old red blood cells are destroyed by macrophages of the spleen, bone marrow and liver.

The main enzymes found in a red blood cell

- Those of the glycolytic pathway.

- Carbonic anhydrase

- Those responsible for the monophosphate shunt.

The structures/organs responsible for red blood cell production

- Early weeks of embryonic life: yolk sac

- Middle trimester of gestation: the liver (mainly) and spleen

- Last month of gestation and after birth: bone marrow (long bones, e.g. femur and tibia; after the age of 20, the bone marrow of the vertebrae, sternum, ribs and pelvis are the main structures responsible for red cell production).

Clinical application: in severe inherited haemolytic diseases such as thalassaemia major, extramedullary haematopoiesis may be re-established in sites of fetal haematopoiesis (e.g. liver and spleen)

What is haemoglobin?

Haemoglobin is a red pigment that gives the red cells their colour; it consists of four protein chains called globins. Two of these are the α chains and the other two the β chains. Each chain is conjugated with a non-protein moiety called the haem group. The haem is able to bind O_2 to a ferrous ion at its centre, and the Hb molecule is able to carry up to four O_2 molecules. Hb exists in several forms with slight differences in the globin chains. Table 11.4 summarizes the different types of Hb.

Table 11.4 Different types of Hb

Hb type	Structure	Function
A	α_2, β_2	Comprises over 93 per cent of normal adult Hb
A_2	α_2, δ_2	Comprises over 2 per cent of normal adult Hb, elevated in β-thalassaemia.
F	α_2, γ_2	Normal fetal haemoglobin, increased in β-thalassaemia.
H	β_4	Found in α thalassaemia
S	α_2, β_2	Present in sickle-cell anaemia

What are the causes of anaemia and the main mechanisms underlying each type?

For anaemia associated with low reticulocytic count, see Table 11.5.

Table 11.5 Anaemia associated with low reticulocytic count

Type of anaemia	Examples	Underlying mechanism
Microcytic (MCV < 80 fL)	Iron deficiency	Absence of iron to incorporate into the porphyrin ring
	Thalassaemia	Failure of globin synthesis
	Sideroblastic	Failure to synthesize the porphyrin ring (most probably because of inhibition of the haem synthetic pathway enzymes)
	Lead poisoning	Lead blocks the incorporation of iron into haem

Macrocytic (MCV > 100 fL)	Megaloblastic anaemia	Folate deficiency (nutritional insufficiency, increased demand, malabsorption)
		Vitamin B$_{12}$ deficiency (pernicious anaemia, partial/total gastrectomy, pancreatic insufficiency, bacterial overgrowth, diseases affecting terminal ileum, resection of terminal ileum)
		Drug-induced megaloblastic anaemia (e.g. methotrexate)
	Non-megaloblastic anaemia	Advanced liver disease (mainly caused by abnormalities in the membrane of red blood cells and abnormal lipid present in red blood cell membrane)
		Hypothyroidism
Normocytic (MCV 80–100 fL)	Anaemia of chronic disease	Depressed erythropoietin and mixed nutritional deficiencies
	Uraemia	Depressed erythropoietin and mixed nutritional deficiencies

MCV, mean corpuscular volume.

Anaemia associated with increased reticulocyte count (reticulocytosis):

- Haemolytic anaemia (premature destruction of red blood cells)
- Acute bleeding
- Clinical implication: blood films are essential in the assessment of patients with anaemia.

The changes that occur in serum iron studies of patients with iron deficiency, chronic disease, chronic haemolysis and haemochromatosis

Table 11.6 Changes in serum iron studies

Disorder	Serum iron	TIBC	Serum ferritin[a]	Iron in bone marrow
Iron deficiency	Decreased	Increased	Decreased	Absent
Chronic disease	Decreased	Decreased	Increased	Present
Chronic haemolysis	Increased	Decreased	Increased	Present
Haemochromatosis	Increased	Decreased	Increased	Increased

[a]The level of serum ferritin reflects the amount of stored iron.
TIBC, total iron-binding capacity

The causes of iron deficiency

- Blood loss, e.g. from the gastrointestinal tract, urinary tract or the uterus
- Decreased absorption of iron, e.g. postgastrectomy and coeliac disease
- Poor intake
- Increased demand, e.g. pregnancy and growth.

The factors influencing iron absorption

- Ferrous iron absorbed better than ferric iron

- Reducing agents, e.g. ascorbic acid

- Low iron stores

- Increased erythropoiesis, e.g. bleeding, haemolysis, high altitude

- Idiopathic haemochromatosis.

The different types of white blood cells

- Neutrophils 40–75 per cent

- Eosinophils 5 per cent

- Basophils 0.5 per cent

- Lymphocytes 20–50 per cent

- Monocytes 1–5 per cent.

The main characteristics of platelets

- Small, disc-shaped, non-nucleated cells

- About 2–4 μm in diameter.

- Formed from megakaryocytes in the bone marrow.

- Contain mitochondria, microtubules, glycogen granules, Golgi apparatus and ribosomes.

- Contain enzymes for aerobic and anaerobic respiration.

- Contain four types of granules:

  – dense granules (contain serotonin)

  – α granules (contain coagulation factors)

  – lysosomes

  – peroxisomes.

- Platelet functions may include: essential in normal haemostasis; secrete procoagulants; secrete vasoconstrictors; form temporary platelet plugs; adhere to the damaged region of the vessel wall (platelet adhesion) and to each other (platelet aggregation); and secrete specific chemicals that attract neutrophils and monocytes to the site of inflammation.

Answers

 CASE 11.1 – I always feel tired.

 Q1: What are the possible causes for the presenting problem?

A1

The following are possible causes (hypotheses) for Athenia's generalized tiredness, palpitation and shortness of breath after minor exercise:

- Iron deficiency anaemia: deceased intake of nutrients rich in iron (vegetarian diet).

- Anaemia caused by malabsorption: problem with absorption in the small intestine.

- Anaemia caused by blood loss: blood loss possibly from a colonic tumour (she gives a history of bodyweight loss, upper abdominal discomfort and changes in her bowel motion). Chronic gastrointestinal blood loss is the most common cause of iron deficiency anaemia in patients aged over 50. The source is upper gastrointestinal bleeding in 20–40 per cent of patients and colonic in 15–30 per cent of patients. In about 20–40 per cent of patients the source is not found.

- Thalassaemia: the patient's name implies that she has a Greek background and her symptoms could be caused by thalassaemia, although β-thalassaemia is less likely in her case because there is no enlargement of the liver or spleen and there is no past history of anaemia or blood transfusion.

- Anaemia: caused by bone marrow problem (e.g. malignancy or leukaemia).

- Anaemia caused by a chronic disease.

 Q2: What further questions would you like to ask to help you differentiate between your hypotheses?

A2

Table 11.7 Further history questions for Case 11.1

History questions	In what way answers can help
Details of dietary intake, type of food and amount	To assess her nutritional intake of iron, vitamin B_{12}, folate and protein
Any history of blood loss, e.g. epistaxis (bleeding from nose), haematemesis (vomiting blood), haematuria (bleeding in urine) or bleeding per rectum?	Evidence of external or internal bleeding will help in the assessment of the cause of her anaemia
History of dyspepsia, upper abdominal pain, nausea and weight loss, past medical history of previous episodes, ulcers, liver disease and the results of past investigations	The source of bleeding from upper gastrointestinal tract may be peptic ulcer disease, gastric ulcer, gastritis and oesophagitis

Ingestion of alcohol, NSAIDs, aspirin, warfarin and corticosteroids	NSAIDs, aspirin and corticosteroids may cause gastric and duodenal erosions, haemorrhage and peptic ulcers. These drugs are a particular problem in patients aged over 60. Warfarin causes the plasma levels of prothrombin and factors VIII, IX and X to fall. It causes this effect by competing with vitamin K for reactive sites in the enzymatic processes needed for the synthesis of prothrombin and the other three clotting factors
History of colicky abdominal pain, constant abdominal pain, anal pain, air and faeces being passed via urethra or vagina. Nature and duration of changes in her bowel motions	Colicky abdominal pain may suggest intestinal obstruction; constant abdominal pain may suggest invasion of the wall of the intestine by a tumour. Passage of air and faeces via urethra or vagina may suggest a fistula. She might be losing blood from a bowel cancer. Anaemia may occur in patients with bowel cancer via a number of mechanisms: blood loss from an ulcerating tumour mass; loss of appetite and decreased food intake; bone marrow suppression; and lymphatic obstruction and malabsorption
Family history of anaemia or colon cancer	Thalassaemia intermedia (both β genes are affected but the clinical course is less severe). The haemoglobin level is usually in the range 60–80 g/L

NSAID, non-steroidal anti-inflammatory drug.

Q3: What investigations would be most helpful to you and why?

A3

Further investigations

- Full blood examination
- Blood film
- Serum iron, transferrin, iron saturation, ferritin
- Red cell folate, serum vitamin B_{12} levels
- Hb electrophoresis
- Colonoscopy.

● CASE 11.2 – I have sudden bleeding from my nose and gums.

Q1: What are the possible causes for the presenting problem?

A1

The following are possible causes (hypotheses) for Margo's presentation:

- Bleeding as a result of a local problem in the nose, gums, pharynx, oesophagus, upper gastrointestinal tract or lungs (this hypothesis cannot explain the purpuric skin changes).

- Bleeding as a result of a systemic problem causing a reduction in the number of circulating platelets (a condition known as thrombocytopenia). The causes of thrombocytopenia may be: decreased production of platelets as a result of bone marrow problems; increased sequestration of platelets by splenomegaly, liver disease and malignancy; and increased destruction of platelets by autoimmune bodies. Purpura and mucosal bleeding usually suggest a platelet disorder.

- Bleeding because of coagulation disorders, e.g. problems with the intrinsic and the extrinsic factors. (Skin bruising and haemarthrosis are more indicative of a coagulation disorder. This hypothesis is less likely.)

 Q2: What further questions would you like to ask to help you differentiate between your hypotheses?

A2

Table 11.8 Further history questions for Case 11.2

History questions	In what way answers can help
Assess how the bleeding started and if there is mucous membrane bleeding or associated bleeding into joints	Assess if the bleeding is a localized problem or the result of a systemic generalized problem
Assess for any associated illness – viral infection a few days before her bleeding disorder or symptoms suggesting collagen vascular diseases (systemic lupus erythematosus [SLE], inflammatory bowel disease and hepatitis)	Viral infections may trigger the process of idiopathic thrombocytopenia (especially in young patients) Collagen vascular diseases are autoimmune in nature and are associated with an autoimmune thrombocytopenia
Drug history (aspirin, NSAIDs, warfarin, quinidine)	Aspirin and NSAIDs may cause bleeding from gastric and duodenal ulcers. Quinidine may serve as heptan and facilitates an immune-associated thrombocytopenia
History of blood transfusion	Transfusion of blood containing platelet A1 antigen (PLA-1) - positive platelets to a PLA-1 negative patients may result in formation of antibodies to PLA-1 antigen and the development of autoimmune thrombocytopenia
Last menstrual period, pregnancy and any current complications	Diseases such as disseminated intravascular coagulation (widespread deposition of fibrin and platelets within the microcirculation and the consumption of coagulation factors and platelets). This is likely to be the case in this patient because there is no history of fever, sepsis or shock

Q3: What investigations would be most helpful to you and why?

A3

Further investigations

- Full blood examination

- Blood film

- Prothrombin time (PT)

- Activated partial thromboplastin time (APTT)

- Thrombin time (TT).

● CASE 11.3 – I have fever and rigors about a week after chemotherapy.

Q1: What are the possible causes for the presenting problem?

A1

The following are possible causes (hypotheses) for Michael's fever and rigors:

- Michael is immunocompromised. He is treated with combination chemotherapy for a haematological malignancy, non-Hodgkin's lymphoma, a condition that results in lymphocyte and granulocyte dysfunction and possibly abnormal immunoglobulin production. Treatment with combination chemotherapy causes further immune suppression and results in bone suppression and neutropenia. Thus, Michael is at high risk for infection, particularly after the chemotherapy. The causative organisms for infection in immunocompromised patients are: bacteria, e.g. Gram-positive (pneumococci), Gram-negative (*Haemophilus influenzae*); viruses (herpes simplex virus, varicella-zoster virus, cytomegalovirus); yeasts (*Candida* spp.); fungi (cryptococci); and protozoa (*Pneumocystis* and *Toxoplasma* spp.). Infection may occur in any of the following forms:

  - abscess (intra-abdominal, pelvic abscess)

  - endovascular infections (infective endocarditis, infected atherosclerotic plaque)

  - infection of the intravascular catheter site – associated with bacteraemia

  - urinary tract infection

  - pneumonia

  - sinusitis and intracranial infection

  - osteomyelitis

  - perirectal infection

  - periodental infection.

- Reactivation of mycobacterial infection.

- Relapse of underlying disease.

- Drug-induced fever.

- Thromboembolic complications.

 Q2: What further questions would you like to ask to help you differentiate between your hypotheses?

A2

Table 11.9 Further history questions for Case 11.3

History questions	In what way answers can help
Cough, expectoration, chest pain	These questions might help in guiding the possible site of infection and provide an idea about the antibiotics you will use after taking the blood, urine and stool samples. However, the information collected may be of limited help
When did the skin changes around the intravenous catheter start?	
Headache, facial pain	
Abdominal pain, nausea, vomiting or loose bowel motions	
Pain in the perianal area	
Pain on passing urine or loin pains	
Skin rash, sweating, lymphadenopathy	
Any pattern for the fever and rigors?	
Past history of tuberculosis or treatment for infective endocarditis, urinary tract infection or any other infections	

 Q3: What investigations would be most helpful to you and why?

A3

Further investigations

- Full blood examination (including differential count and absolute number)

- Blood film

- Chest radiograph (to assess for pneumonia and chest infections)

- Urinalysis

- Culture of blood, urine, stool and the intravenous catheter tip

- Blood urea, creatinine, sodium and potassium

- Ultrasonography or computed tomography (CT) of the abdomen (to assess for intra-abdominal, pelvic abscess)

- Echocardiography (to assess for valvular infection).

The patient was treated immediately after taking the blood, urine and stool samples. He was started on intravenous gentamicin plus piperacillin. As the intravenous catheter is removed, a new one is placed. As his fever continued for more than 48 h despite antibiotic treatment, he was switched to vancomycin.

Further progress

● CASE 11.1 – I always feel tired.

Dr Maxwell arranges some tests for Athenia. The results are shown in Tables 11.10–10.12.

Table 11.10 Full Blood examination for Case 1.1

Test	Athenia's results	Normal range
Haemoglobin (Hb) (g/L)	95	115–160
White blood cell count (WCC) ($\times 10^9$/L)	9.3	4.0–11.0
Platelet count ($\times 10^9$/L)	320	150–400
Red blood cell count ($\times 10^{12}$/L)	4.60	4.40–5.80
Packed cell volume (PCV)	0.34	0.37–0.47
Mean corpuscular volume (MCV) (fL)	68	80.0–100.0
Red cell distribution width (RDW) (per cent)	19.7	11.0–15.0
Neutrophils ($\times 10^9$/L)	6.10	2.00–7.50
Lymphocytes ($\times 10^9$/L)	2.49	1.50–4.00
Monocytes ($\times 10^9$/L)	0.51	0.20–0.80
Eosinophils ($\times 10^9$/L)	0.15	0.04–0.44
Basophils ($\times 10^9$/L)	0.05	0.00–0.10

Blood film report: red blood cells show moderate anisocytosis, poikilocytosis, microcytosis, hypochromia and polychromasia. Both platelets and white blood cells (WBCs) are morphologically normal.

Table 11.11 Iron studies, and red cell folate and serum vitamin B$_{12}$ levels for Case 11.2

Test	Athenia's results	Normal range
Serum iron (μmol/L)	5	9–30
Transferrin (g/L)	4.5	2.0–4.0
Iron saturation (per cent)	6	15–50
Ferritin (μg/L)	4	10–120
Red cell folate (nmol/L packed cells)	912	317–1422
Serum vitamin B$_{12}$ (pmol/L)	316	148–616

Table 11.12 Hb electrophoresis for Case 11.1

Test	Athenia's results	Normal range
HbA$_2$ (per cent)	2.5	1.5–3.5
HbF (per cent)	0.6	< 2.0
HbA (per cent)	96.9	> 95

Colonoscopy: a tumour mass of size 2 cm × 3 cm, infiltrating the wall of the sigmoid colon. Histological studies of the tumour mass show neoplastic epithelial cells invading the muscle layer of the wall of the colon. The invading cells passed through the submucosa layer.

● CASE 11.2 – I have sudden bleeding from my nose and gums.

The treating doctor arranges some tests for Margo. The results are shown in Tables 11.13 and 11.14.

Table 11.13 Full blood examination for Case 11.2

Test	Margo's results	Normal range
Hb (g/L)	133	115–160
WCC (× 10^9/L)	9.51	4.0–11.0
Platelet count (× 10^9/L)	20	150–400
Red blood cell count (× 10^{12}/L)	4.88	4.40–5.80
PCV	0.39	0.37–0.47
MCV (fL)	92	80.0–100.0
RDW (per cent)	13.4	11.0–15.0
Neutrophils (× 10^9/L)	5.60	2.00–7.50
Lymphocytes (× 10^9/L)	3.5	1.50–4.00
Monocytes (× 10^9/L)	0.23	0.20–0.80
Eosinophils (× 10^9/L)	0.10	0.04–0.44
Basophils (× 10^9/L)	0.08	0.00–0.10

Blood film report: a few platelets are seen, platelets vary in size and some are of large size (> 4 μm) in diameter. Both red blood cells and WBCs are morphologically normal.

Table 11.14 Coagulation studies for Case 11.2

Test	Margo's results	Normal range
PT (s)	Normal	10–14
APTT (s)	Normal	30–40
TT (s)	Normal	Time of control 25 when control is 9–13

CASE 11.3 – I have fever and rigors about a week after chemotherapy.

The treating doctor arranges some tests for Michael. The results are shown in Tables 11.15 and 11.16.

Table 11.15 Full blood examination for Case 11.3

Test	Michael's results	Normal range
Hb (g/L)	120	115–160
WCC ($\times 10^9$/L)	2.93	4.0–11.0
Platelet count ($\times 10^9$/L)	290	150–400
Red blood cell count ($\times 10^{12}$/L)	4.2	4.40–5.80
PCV	0.39	0.37–0.47
MCV (fL)	82.0	80.0–100.0
RDW (per cent)	15.0	11.0–15.0
Neutrophils ($\times 10^9$/L)	0.57	2.00–7.50
Lymphocytes ($\times 10^9$/L)	2.02	1.50–4.00
Monocytes ($\times 10^9$/L)	0.24	0.20–0.80
Eosinophils ($\times 10^9$/L)	0.05	0.04–0.44
Basophils ($\times 10^9$/l)	0.05	0.00–0.10

Blood film report: low number of leukocytes, particularly neutrophils.

Red blood cells and platelets are normal.

Chest radiograph: normal.

Urinalysis: normal; no white or red blood cells; no casts or epithelial cells.

Table 11.16 Culture results for Case 11.3

Test	Michael's results
Blood culture	*Staphylococcus aureus* and *S. epidermidis* are isolated; both are sensitive to vancomycin and resistant to methicillin
Urine culture	No growth
Stool culture	No growth
Intravenous catheter tip culture	*S. aureus* and *S. epidermidis* are isolated ;both are sensitive to vancomycin and resistant to methicillin.

Blood urea, creatinine, sodium and potassium: within normal range.

Ultrasonography or CT of the abdomen: no intra-abdominal or pelvic abscess.

Echocardiography: normal; no evidence of valvular vegetations.

Further questions

 CASE 11.1 – I always feel tired.

 Q4: In the light of the clinical presentation, how would you interpret the laboratory test results?

A4

Table 11.17 Interpretation of lab test results for Case 11.1

Test	Results	Interpretation
Hb	Low	The fact that only Hb is low whereas WCC and platelet counts are normal excludes bone marrow pathology as a cause for Athenia's problem. The findings of the blood film 'microcytosis, hypochromia, anisocytosis and poikilocytosis' and the low MCV support the diagnosis of a microcytic anaemia. The main causes of microcytic anaemia are: iron deficiency anaemia; thalassaemia; chronic disease; and sideroblastic anaemia
WCC	Normal	
Platelet count	Normal	
Red blood cell count	Normal	
PCV	Normal	An increased RDW indicates that red blood cells are of a wide range of sizes (anisocytosis)
MCV	< 80.0 fL (microcytic red cells)	
RDW	Raised	The results of the iron studies (low serum iron, increased transferrin, low iron saturation and low ferritin) together with normal Hb electrophoresis studies support the diagnosis of iron deficiency anaemia
Blood film report	Red blood cells show moderate anisocytosis, poikilocytosis, microcytosis, hypochromia and polychromasia. Both platelets and WBCs are morphologically normal	In pure iron deficiency anaemia, serum vitamin B_{12} and folate are expected to be normal. Deficiency of either vitamin B_{12} or folate is associated with macrocytic anaemia
Serum iron	Low	
Transferrin	Raised	
Iron saturation	Low	
Ferritin	Low	
Red cell folate	Normal	
Serum B_{12}	Normal	

Table 11.18 Colonoscopy results for Case 11.1

Test	Results	Interpretation
Colonoscopy	A tumour mass of 2 cm × 3 cm infiltrating the wall of the sigmoid colon. Histological studies of the tumour mass show neoplastic epithelial cells invading the muscle layer of the wall of the colon. The invading cells passed through the submucosa layer	The cause of the patient's iron deficiency anaemia is chronic loss of blood from a colorectal carcinoma. Chronic gastrointestinal blood loss is the most common cause of iron deficiency anaemia in patients aged over 60. The source is the upper gastrointestinal tract in 20–40 per cent of patients and colonic in 15–30 per cent of patients. Athenia needs further assessment of her colorectal carcinoma including chest radiograph, liver function tests, pelvic and abdominal CT scans to look for any metastatic spread. She will also need to undergo a laparotomy for staging and therapeutic options. In her case, invasion of the submucosa is classified as T1. Further investigations will help in assessment of lymph node spread (N) and distant metastatic (M) assessment

 Q5: What is your final hypothesis?

A5

Iron deficiency anaemia as a result of chronic blood loss from a colorectal carcinoma. Further studies are needed to assess the stage of her malignancy and the plan of her management.

 Q6: What issues in the given history, examination and laboratory tests support your final hypothesis?

A6

Supportive evidence

History

- The patient presented with generalized tiredness, palpitation and shortness of breath
- She has always been healthy
- Vegetarian diet for 3 years
- Lost 8 kg in bodyweight in 6 months
- History of changes in her bowel motions.

Examination

- Pale conjunctivae
- No lymphadenopathy; no organomegaly
- No fresh blood per rectum.

Investigations

- Low Hb

- Blood film: microcytic/hypochromic anaemia

- Iron studies: low serum iron, high transferrin, low ferritin

- Colonoscopy and histological studies: colorectal carcinoma invading submucosa (T1).

- Further studies are needed to assess the stage of her malignancy and the plan of her management.

● CASE 11.2 – I have sudden bleeding from my nose and gums.

 Q4: In the light of the clinical presentation, how would you interpret the laboratory test results?

A4

Table 11.19 Interpretation of lab test results for Case 11.2

Test	Results	Interpretation
Hb	Normal	The presence of thrombocytopenia (low platelet count) without significant changes in red blood cell count and WCC excludes pancytopenia and bone marrow suppression as a cause for low platelets
WCC	Normal	
Platelet count	Very low	
Red blood cell count	Normal	The results of the patient's PT, APPT and TT are normal, supporting the hypothesis that her skin purpura and bleeding from nose and gums (mucous membrane) is the result of low platelets rather than a disorder affecting extrinsic, intrinsic, common coagulation cascades or the clot formation process
PCV	Normal	
MCV	Normal	
RDW	Normal	PT: examines the extrinsic and common pathway. The normal range is 10–14 s. Prolongation of the PT by more than 2 s compared with control suggests a defect in any of these factors (VII, X, V, II) or the presence of inhibitor for these factors
Blood film report	Few platelets are seen, they vary in size and some are large (> 4 μm) in diameter. Both red blood cells and WBCs are morphologically normal	
		APTT: examines the intrinsic coagulation cascade and the common pathway. The normal range is 30–40 s. Abnormal results indicate deficiency in any of these factors: I, II, V, X, VIII, IX, XI, XII or the presence of inhibitors
PT	Normal	TT: measures the time for clot formation (i.e. the thrombin–fibrinogen reaction). The TT is prolonged in:
APTT	Normal	
TT	Normal	– heparin treatment
		– presence of inhibitor such as fibrin degradation product (in disseminated intravascular coagulation)
		– liver disease

Q5: What is your final hypothesis?

A5

Immune thrombocytopenic purpura; the cause is unknown, possibly related to the patient's upper respiratory tract infection.

Q6: What issues in the given history, examination and laboratory tests support your final hypothesis?

A6

Supportive evidence

History

- Patient presented with severe nose and gum bleeding
- No history of nose/head trauma
- No history of fever, nausea, vomiting, or joint disease (collagen vascular disease)
- History of upper respiratory tract infection
- No past history of epistaxis or easy skin bruising.

Examination

- Haemodynamically stable
- Bleeding from nose and gums
- No jaundice or conjunctival pallor
- Purpuric rash on her arms, legs and abdomen
- No organomegaly.

Investigations

- Low platelet count
- Normal red blood cell count and WCC
- Normal PT, APTT and TT.

CASE 11.3 – I have fever and rigors about a week after chemotherapy.

Q4: In the light of the clinical presentation, how would you interpret the laboratory test results?

A4

Table 11.20 Interpretation of lab test results for Case 11.3

Test	Results	Interpretation
Hb	Normal	Leukopenia (a total WCC $< 4.0 \times 10^9$/L). Differential blood cell count shows that only neutrophils are low, whereas all other WBCs (lymphocytes, monocytes, eosinophils and basophils) are normal. A low peripheral neutrophil count ($< 2 \times 10^9$/L) is called neutropenia
WCC	Low (leukopenia)	
Platelet count	Normal	
Red blood cell count	Normal	
PCV	Normal	A drop in neutrophil count below 0.5×10^9/L is associated with life-threatening and recurrent infection
MCV	Normal	
RDW	Normal	
Neutrophils	Very low ($< 2 \times 10^9$/L)	
Lymphocytes	Normal	
Monocytes	Normal	
Eosinophils	Normal	
Basophils	Normal	

Table 11.21 Culture results for Case 11.3

Test	Results	Interpretation
Blood culture	*S. aureus* and *S. epidermidis* are isolated and both are sensitive to vancomycin and resistant to methicillin	The results of the blood culture suggest that the systemic infection is most probably related to infection of the intravenous line. The two organisms isolated, *S. aureus* and *S. epidermidis*, are normally found in the skin and support this notion
Intravenous catheter tip culture	*S. aureus* and *S. epidermidis* are isolated and both are sensitive to vancomycin and resistant to methicillin	

Q5: What is your final hypothesis?

A5

Bacteraemia/septicaemia in a neutopenic patient after combination therapy for non-Hodgkin's lymphoma. The clinical picture and laboratory results indicate that the source of the infection is the intravenous catheter tip.

Q6: What issues in the given history, examination and laboratory tests support your final hypothesis?

A6

Supportive evidence

History

- Patient presented with fever and rigors: 12 h (possibly indicate bacteraemia/septicaemia)
- History of chemotherapy for non-Hodgkin's lymphoma – about a week earlier.

Examination

- Looks ill
- Feverish: 38.5°C
- A tunnelled intravenous catheter at the left internal jugular vein – erythema of the overlying skin
- No purulent discharge from the catheter end
- Cardiovascular, respiratory and abdominal examinations all normal.

Investigations

- Leukopenia (neutropenia)
- Normal red blood cell and platelet counts
- Blood culture: *S. aureus* and *S. epidermidis* are isolated and both are sensitive to vancomycin and resistant to methicillin
- Intravenous tip catheter culture: *S. aureus* and *S. epidermidis* are isolated and both are sensitive to vancomycin and resistant to methicillin
- Chest radiograph: normal
- Urinalysis: normal
- Blood urea, creatinine, sodium and potassium: within normal range
- Ultrasonography or CT of the abdomen: no intra-abdominal or pelvic abscess
- Echocardiography: normal; no evidence of valvular vegetations (valvular infection).

♟ Integrated medical sciences questions

⬤ CASE 11.1 – Discuss the physiological regulation of red blood cell production and the role of erythropoietin in this process.

Site of blood cell formation (haematopoiesis)

The site of blood cell formation (including red blood cells) changes several times during fetal development:

- Early weeks of embryonic life: yolk sac
- Middle trimester of gestation: the liver (mainly) and spleen
- Last trimester of gestation and after birth: bone marrow of long bones, e.g. femur and tibia
- After the age of 20: the bone marrow of the vertebrae, sternum, ribs and pelvis.

Red blood cell production

The blood cells originate from a common pluripotential progenitor stem cell (haematopoietic stem cell). The growth factors (secreted systemically or locally) are responsible for modulation of these processes:

- proliferation
- differentiation
- maturation.

Growth factors

Table 11.22 summarizes the main cells of origin and their role in red blood cell production.

Table 11.22 Cells of origin

Growth factor	Cell of origin	Function
Erythropoietin	Endothelial cells of kidney and liver	Proliferation of erythroid precursors
Stem cell factor	Stromal cells of bone marrow	Proliferation of early progenitor cells together with the growth factors

The process of erythropoiesis

In the bone marrow, red blood cells are developed from a dividing population of erythropoietic cells. These cellular changes may be summarized as: proerythroblast (nucleated) → basophilic erythroblast → polychromatic erythroblast → orthochromic erythroblast → reticulocyte (containing residual ribosomal RNA and still able to synthesize Hb) → mature red blood cell (non-nucleated and biconcave discs)

During this differentiation, the following morphological and functional changes occur:

- Decrease in cell size
- Hb production

- Gradual loss of cell organelles

- Eventual loss of nucleus and organelles in the mature red blood cell.

Role of erythropoietin

The process of erythropoiesis is controlled by the hormone erythropoietin. Erythropoietin is produced in the peritubular cells (endothelial cells), the kidney (90 per cent) and the liver (10 per cent). The stimuli for the production of erythropoietin are:

- Hypoxia

- Cardiopulmonary disease

- Anaemia

- Increased erythropoietin → stimulation of bone marrow precursor cells committed to produce red blood cells.

CASE 11.2 – **Discuss the role of platelets and the coagulation cascade in haemostasis following bleeding from a damaged blood vessel. You may use diagrams to outline your answer.**

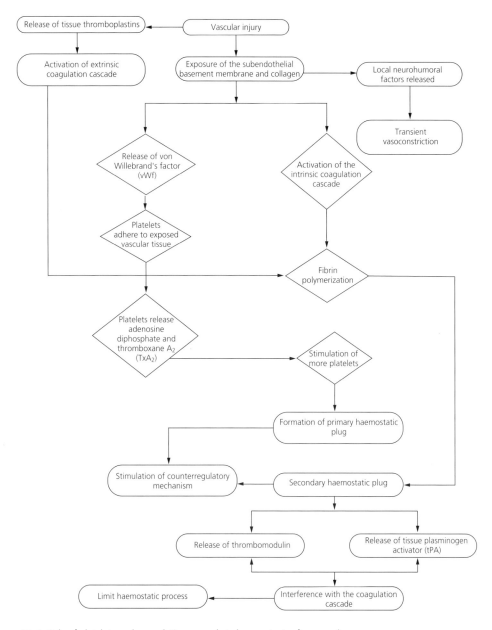

Figure 11.1 Role of platelets and coagulation cascade in haemostasis after vascular surgery.

CASE 11.3 – Outline the origin and function of the monocyte–macrophage system (reticuloendothelial system).

Blood monocytes and tissue macrophages are involved in body defence mechanisms. The functions of these cells may be summarized as follows:

- Defending the body against the invasion of pathogenic organisms by engulfment and phagocytosis

- Activation of acquired immune response

- Macrophages function as scavenger cells (removing dead cells and necrotic tissues)

- Monocytes and macrophages produce large number of monokines, including many growth factors. They play a role in the development and differentiation of other blood cells.

Macrophages (mobile cells) are capable of wandering through the tissues. They can become attached to the tissues for several months/years (called monocytes). Monocytes may be involved in local protective functions.

Fixed tissues macrophages may leave the tissues → becoming mobile macrophages → release into bloodstream. This change is a continuous process. The name monocyte–macrophage system reflects the process. However, the term 'reticuloendothelial system' is still widely used in textbooks and research papers.

The following are examples of fixed tissue macrophages:

- Alveolar macrophages (lung)

- Kupffer cells (liver)

- Macrophages (spleen and lymphoid tissues)

- Microglia cells (brain)

- Osteoclasts (bone)

- Serosal macrophages (pleural and peritoneal cavities).

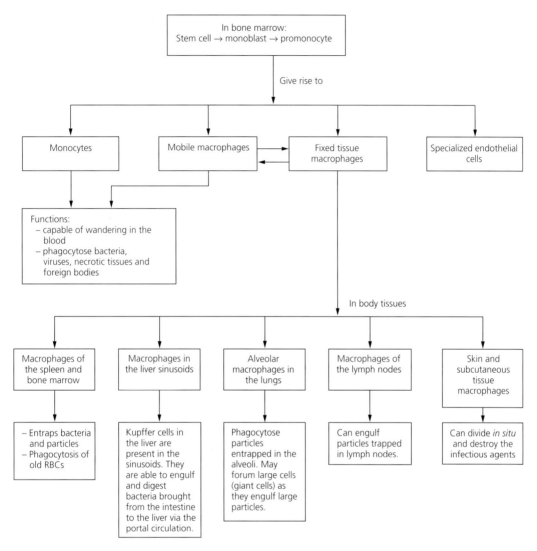

Figure 11.2 The origin and function of the monocyte–macrophage system.

Further reading

Campbell K. Pathophysiology of anemia. *Nursing Times* 2004;**100**:40–43.

Clark BE, Thein SL. Molecular diagnosis of haemoglobin disorders. *Clinical and Laboratory Haematology* 2004;**26**:159–176.

Dhaliwal G, Cornett PA, Tierney LM Jr. Hemolytic anemia. *American Family Physician* 2004;**69**:2599–2606.

Fleming RE. Advances in understanding the molecular basis for the regulation of dietary iron absorption. *Current Opinion in Gastroenterology* 2005;**21**:201–206.

Fleming RE, Bacon BR. Orchestration of iron homeostasis. *New England Journal of Medicine* 2005;**352**:1741–1744.

GuX, Zeng Y. A review of the molecular diagnosis of thalassemia. *Hematology* 2002;**7**:203–209.

Hamidi M, Tajerzadeh H. Carrier erythrocyte: an overview. *Drug Delivery* 2003;**10**:9–20.

Knutson M, Wessling-Resnick M. Iron metabolism in the reticuloendothelial system. *Critical Reviews in Biochemistry and Molecular Biology* 2003;**38**:61–88.

Meremikwu M. Sickle cell disease. *Clinical Evidence* 2003;**10**:21–36.

Provan D, Newland A. Idiopathic thrombocytopenia purpura in adults. *Journal of Pediatric Hematology Oncology* 2003;**23**(suppl):S34–38.

Semple JW. Immune pathophysiology of autoimmune thrombocytopenic purpura. *Blood Reviews* 2002;**16**:9–12.

Sharma N, Butterworth J, Cooper BT, Tselepis C, Iqbal TH. The emerging role of the liver in iron metabolism. *American Journal of Gastroenterology* 2005;**100**:201–206.

Silverberg DS, Iaina A, Wexler D, Blum M. The pathological consequences of anaemia. *Clinical and Laboratory Haematology* 2001;**23**:1–6.

Toh BH, Alderuccio F. Pernicious anaemia. *Autoimmunity* 2004;**37**:357–361.

Umbreit J. Iron deficiency: a concise review. *American Journal of Hematology* 2005;**78**:225–231.

Weiss G, Goodnough LT. Medical progress: Anemia of chronic disease. *New England Journal of Medicine* 2005;**325**:1011–1023.

Woodman R, Ferrucci L, Guralnik J. Anemia in older adults. *Current Opinion in Hematology* 2005;**12**:123–128.

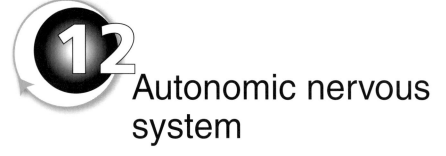

Autonomic nervous system

Q1: What are the possible causes for the presenting problem?
Q2: What further questions would you like to ask to help you differentiate between your hypotheses?
Q3: What investigations would be most helpful to you and why?
Q4: In the light of the clinical presentation, how would you interpret the laboratory test results?
Q5: What is your final hypothesis?
Q6: What issues in the given history, examination and laboratory tests support your final hypothesis?

Clinical cases

● CASE 12.1 – My left eyelid droops.

Linda Michael, a 28-year-old singer, is brought by ambulance to the accident and emergency department (A&E) after a motor-car accident. On admission, she is conscious and oriented, and clinical examination including vital signs is normal. The next morning, the consultant examines Linda and notices ptosis of her left eyelid with ipsilateral miosis (constriction of her left eye pupil). She is able to move her eyes in all directions and there is no nystagmus. No other neurological abnormalities are found. There is no evidence of eye trauma, and cardiovascular and respiratory examinations are normal.

● CASE 12.2 – This is the first time I've experienced such an illness while working on my farm.

Mr Jack Masson, a 53-year-old farmer, is brought to the A&E of a local rural hospital by his son, Bill. Jack spent most of the day working on the farm. He had his lunch there and completed the crop spraying, which he had been doing for the last few days. Jack says: 'I was well in the morning. About an hour ago, I noticed sweating all over my body and I started feeling unwell and a little dizzy.' His son Bill adds: 'Just before driving my dad to the hospital, he vomited about three times and again on our way here.' Jack has loose bowel motions and feels weak all over. On examination, Jack's mouth is full of saliva and he is drooling. His skin is wet all over because of excessive sweating. Several muscles of his upper and lower limbs are twitching (muscle fasciculation). His vital signs are shown in Table 12.1.

Table 12.1 Vital signs for Case 12.2

Vital signs	Jack's results	Normal range
Blood pressure (mmHg)	100/60	100/60–135/85
Pulse rate (/min)	60	60–100
Respiratory rate (/min)	15	12–16
Temperature (°C)	36.5	36.6–37.2

Eye examination: both pupils are pinpoint and unreactive to light.

Lacrimation of both eyes is noticed.

His consciousness gradually deteriorated.

⬤ CASE 12.3 – It all happened immediately after she finished her meal.

Ruth Gleich, a 68-year-old resident of a local nursing home, is brought by ambulance to a local hospital because of dizziness and syncope. The nurse at the nursing home says to the ambulance officers: 'Mrs Gleich suddenly lost consciousness for about 2 minutes. This is the third time she has lost consciousness over the last 4 weeks. It all happened immediately after she finished her meal. This time, I measured her blood pressure immediately after she lost her consciousness, it was 100/70 mmHg. Her blood pressure is usually in the range of 160/85 mmHg.' Ruth says: 'As I finished my lunch, I felt dizzy, weak and lightheaded, I cannot remember what happened next. For the last 3 months, I have felt unable to stand or walk immediately after I complete my meals and I usually prefer to lie down for some time.' Further questions reveal that Ruth has been diabetic and hypertensive for over 20 years. Her medication includes gliclazide (an oral hypoglycaemic agent) for diabetes and lisinopril (an angiotensin-converting enzyme or ACE inhibitor) for hypertension. Both her blood pressure and blood glucose levels are under control. She does not drink or smoke. On examination, about 2 hours after her loss of consciousness, she looks a bit anxious and pale.

Table 12.2 Vital signs for Case 12.3

Vital signs	Ruth's results	Normal range
Blood pressure (mmHg)	145/75 (sitting)	100/60–135/85
	150/80 (lying)	
Pulse rate (/min)	75	60–100
Respiratory rate (/min)	18	12–16
Temperature (°C)	36.6	36.6–37.2

Cardiovascular examination: jugular venous pressure (JVP) not raised. No evidence of heart failure or murmur.

Respiratory system: normal.

Neurological examination: normal except for loss of pain sensation in both upper and lower limbs (polyneuropathy pattern).

Abdominal examination: normal.

No clinical evidence of hypothyroidism or adrenal failure.

Integrated medical sciences questions

CASE 12.1 – Discuss the sympathetic input to the pupil. Briefly discuss the mechanisms underlying the different causes of Horner's syndrome.

CASE 12.2 – Discuss the mechanism of action of organophosphate cholinesterase inhibitors. Explain in your mechanism the pathogenesis of the clinical findings (loose bowel motions, excessive sweating and low blood pressure) found in patients with organophosphate poisoning.

CASE 12.3 – Discuss, using flow diagrams, the physiological mechanisms responsible for blood pressure control. What are the mechanisms underlying Ruth's presentation?

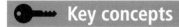 **Key concepts**

In order to work through the core clinical cases in this chapter, you will need to understand the following key concepts.

What is the autonomic nervous system?

The autonomic nervous system (ANS) is also known as the visceral or involuntary nervous system. It is a reflex system analogous to the reflex arcs of the somatic sensory and motor systems. The main difference is that, in the ANS, the afferent fibres are generally from internal body organs and the efferent fibres typically go to the heart, blood vessels, glands, smooth muscle and other visceral organs. Thus, the functions of the ANS include control of the blood pressure, heart rate, gastrointestinal motility and secretion, urinary bladder function, body temperature, blood biochemistry, sweating and body immune response, so the ANS is the neural part of the functional system responsible for homoeostasis.

What are the two major subdivisions of the ANS?

The two divisions are the sympathetic nervous system and the parasympathetic nervous system. The enteric nervous system of the gastrointestinal tract is sometimes considered to be a third subdivision.

The main differences between the sympathetic and parasympathetic nervous system

Table 12.3 Differences between the sympathetic and parasympathetic nervous systems

	Sympathetic nervous system	Parasympathetic nervous system
The ganglia	Generally occur close to the spinal cord	Generally close to the target organ (in the wall of the organ innervated)
Preganglionic neurons	Most of the preganglionic neurons release acetylcholine	Most of them release acetylcholine
Postganglionic neurons	Noradrenaline is the postganglionic neurotransmitter (the only exceptions are postganglionic sympathetic nerve fibres innervating sweat glands, the piloerector muscles and some blood vessels; they use acetylcholine)	Acetylcholine is the postganglionic neurotransmitter
Effects of stimulation	Contraction of the radial muscle of the iris (mydriasis), increased heart rate, increased atrial contractility, constriction of the blood vessels in the skin, bronchial muscle relaxation, decreased motility and tone of the intestine, inhibition of gastrointestinal secretion, relaxation of the detrusor muscle of the urinary bladder and contraction of the urinary bladder sphincter	Contraction of the sphincter muscle of the iris (miosis), decreased heart rate, decreased atrial contractility, dilatation of the blood vessels in the skin, dilatation of pulmonary and cerebral blood vessels, increased salivary secretion, increased motility and tone of the gastrointestinal tract, relaxation of sphincters and increased gastrointestinal secretions, contraction of the detrusor muscle of the urinary bladder and relaxation of the urinary bladder sphincter

The differences between nicotinic and muscarinic acetylcholine receptors

The acetylcholine receptors may be subdivided into nicotinic and muscarinic receptors. The acetylcholine is released by the preganglionic fibres acts through the nicotinic receptors whereas the acetylcholine is released by postganglionic fibres acts through muscarinic receptors.

Answers

 CASE 12.1 – **My left eyelid droops.**

 Q1: What are the possible causes for the presenting problem?

A1

Possible causes (hypotheses) of Linda's left eye ptosis and ipsilateral papillary constriction:

- Horner's syndrome (oculosympathetic paresis) is most likely (ptosis, ipsilateral miosis, no nystagmus).
- Cranial nerve III palsy is less likely (in isolated paralysis of cranial nerve III, the globe is turned out and slightly down, and the pupil is dilated and unreactive to direct and consensual light stimuli).
- Ocular trauma: this may result in ptosis and a large pupil (Linda has no evidence of direct eye trauma).

 Q2: What further questions would you like to ask to help you differentiate between your hypotheses?

A2

Table 12.4 Further history questions for Case 12.1

History questions	In what way answers can help
Did the patient notice any droop of her left eyelid before the accident? Was she aware of the droop of her left eyelid or eye changes before her accident?	To assess if her ptosis is congenital or acquired because of obstetric trauma, old neck trauma or lung problems, or related to her motor-car accident
Does she have any pain along the left side of the neck and around her left eye?	Traumatic carotid dissection in the neck may be associated with such pain
Past history of smoking, coughing or expectoration	Lung cancer associated with apical or mediastinal lesions may interfere with second-order neurons of the sympathetic supply to the eye and produce ptosis
Past history of left ear trouble/surgery or oral cavity surgery	Ear troubles/surgery and oral cavity surgery may result in neurological damage and ptosis

 Q3: What investigations would be most helpful to you and why?

A3

Further investigations

- Computed tomography (CT) of the neck and the skull base
- Ultrasonography of the neck region (carotid artery)
- Chest radiograph (posteroanterior or PA and lateral views).

● CASE 12.2 – **This is the first time I've experienced such an illness while working on my farm.**

Q1: What are the possible causes for the presenting problem?

A1

The following are possible causes (hypotheses) for Jack's presentation:

● Food contaminated with the chemicals used in crop spraying (excessive sweating, excessive salivation, vomiting, loose bowel motions, muscle twitching/fasciculation, low pulse rate, low blood pressure and deterioration in his conscious state). Most probably the result of systemic effects, e.g. cholinomimetic effects or excessive effects of acetylcholine on the ANS, excessive parasympathetic stimulation. Intoxication also may occur via inhalation of organophosphate insecticides, skin absorption and absorption from the conjunctivae and ingestion.

● Low pulse rate and low blood pressure: these findings confirm parasympathetic stimulation. If Jack's problem is only the result of fluid loss we would expect a drop in his blood pressure and an increase in his pulse rate. The drop of his pulse rate despite fluid loss, via vomiting, sweating and loose bowel motions, supports parasympathetic stimulation possibly caused by crop-spraying chemicals (organophosphate cholinesterase inhibitors).

● Acute catastrophic illness such as acute massive myocardial infarction, meningitis, encephalitis, brain haemorrhage, cerebral malaria or heat stroke (but he is not feverish).

Q2: What further questions would you like to ask to help you differentiate between your hypotheses?

A2

Table 12.5 Further history questions for Case 12.2

History questions	In what way answers can help
What type of chemicals did Jack use in crop spraying? Has he used the same chemicals before? Did he wear protective clothing and follow the instructions and preventive measures provided by the manufacturer?	Assess the possibility of organophosphate cholinesterase inhibitors and exposure to toxic chemicals. Most organophosphate cholinesterase inhibitors are well absorbed from the skin, lung, gut and conjunctiva
Who helped him in crop spraying? Did they show similar illnesses? Did they share the same food with him?	To assess the extent of the problem
	To assess the possibility of food contamination by chemicals used in crop spraying. Organophosphate pesticides are well absorbed from the gut
Did he take any medication?	Medications such as neostigmine, pyridostigmine and physostigmine are cholinesterase inhibitors and toxicity with any of these drugs produces similar symptoms

Q3: What investigations would be most helpful to you and why?

A3

Further investigations

- Red cell acetylcholinesterase
- Plasma cholinesterase.

 CASE 12.3 – It all happened immediately after she finished her meal.

 Q1: What are the possible causes for the presenting problem?

A1

The following are possible causes (hypotheses) for Ruth's presentation:

- Dysautonomia: disorders of the ANS, e.g. postprandial hypotension, postural hypotension; postural hypotension or orthostatic hypotension is defined as a fall in blood pressure of over 20 mmHg systolic or 10 mmHg diastolic, on standing or during head-up tilt to at least 60°; this hypothesis is less likely because there are no significant changes in her blood pressure readings when measured while lying and after standing

- Vasovagal syncope

- Cerebral ischaemia, decreased cerebral perfusion, decreased cerebral oxygenation

- Hypoglycaemia

- Cardiac dysfunction, e.g. aortic stenosis (less likely in her case)

- Arrhythmias, e.g. asystole, heart block (less likely in her case)

- Peripheral vasodilatation caused by drugs such as levodopa or glyceryl trinitrate (less likely in her case)

- Intravascular volume depletion, e.g. Addison's disease.

Postprandial hypotension is the most likely hypothesis. There are a number of predisposing factors for postprandial hypotension including: elderly patients with hypertension; autonomic insufficiency/autonomic failure; diabetes mellitus; peripheral neuropathy caused by diabetes mellitus or other disorders; ingestion of food particularly carbohydrates and glucose; and intake of medications such as levodopa. The patient usually presents with the following:

- Dizziness, blurred vision, angina, nausea, light-headedness and black spots in the visual field after the meal

- Marked postprandial decrease in sitting systolic blood pressure

- Decrease in the mean sitting postprandial arterial blood pressure

- Multiple systemic failure may be present (the Shy–Drager syndrome).

Q2: What further questions would you like to ask to help you differentiate between your hypotheses?

A2

Table 12.6 Further history questions for Case 12.3

History questions	In what way answers can help
Intake of any other prescribed medications or over-counter-drugs	Hypotension is a common side effect of a number of drugs
Symptoms or past investigations supporting renal failure	Postprandial hypotension may occur in uraemic patients with autonomic dysfunction
Prolonged sitting	Prolonged sitting may contribute to the pathogenesis of postprandial decrease in blood pressure
History of chest pain, cardiac ischaemia, heart failure, arrhythmias, palpitations	Patients with low cardiac output may develop postprandial hypotension and decreased cerebral perfusion (e.g. patients with heart failure, aortic stenosis or arrhythmias)
Nutritional composition and temperature of the meal	The nutritional composition may affect the magnitude of postprandial hypotension, e.g. carbohydrates, particularly glucose, have been shown to precipitate postprandial hypoglycaemia. Glucose solutions served warm or at room temperature cause a decrease in blood pressure
Time of loss of consciousness	Postprandial hypotension usually occurs during or immediately after a meal, within 5–15 min
Past history of fall, syncope or epilepsy	Postprandial hypotension is common in patients who fall and have syncope. They usually cannot stand or walk after a meal (meal-induced hypotension)
Complications for her diabetes and high blood pressure	The presence of polyneuropathy is possibly related to her diabetes mellitus. Autonomic dysfunction (dysautonomia) is likely to be present and has contributed to her presentation

Q3: What investigations would be most helpful to you and why?

A3

Further investigations

- ECG and echocardiogram
- Full blood examination
- Blood urea, creatinine, sodium, potassium and blood sugar.

Further progress

● CASE 12.1 – My left eyelid droops.

Linda gives no past history of ptosis or troubles with her eyes before the motor-car accident. She does not smoke and has had no past history of chest or neck problems. The treating consultant arranges for some tests for Linda, with the following results:

- Chest radiograph (PA and lateral views) are normal; no evidence of apical lesion.

- Ultrasonography of the neck (left carotid artery): normal lumen and walls.

- CT of the neck and the base of the skull: no evidence of internal haemorrhage or structural changes.

● CASE 12.2 – This is the first time I've experienced such an illness while working on my farm.

The emergency registrar arranges for some tests for Jack, with the following results:

- Red cell acetylcholine: low

- Plasma cholinesterase: low.

● CASE 12.3 – It all happened immediately after she finished her meal.

The A&E registrar arranges for some tests for Ruth, with the following results:

- ECG: regular rhythm, no ischaemic changes, mild left ventricular (LV) hypertrophy.

- Echocardiogram: no evidence of valvular stenosis or regurgitation, no evidence of LV dysfunction, mild LV hypertrophy, no pericardial disease.

- Full blood examination: within the normal range.

- Blood urea, creatinine, sodium, potassium: all results are within the normal range.

- Random blood glucose: 10.8 mmol/L (normal range: 3.6–5.3 mmol/L).

Further questions

● CASE 12.1 – My left eyelid droops.

Q4: In the light of the clinical presentation, how would you interpret the laboratory test results?

A4

Table 12.7 Interpretation of lab test results for Case 12.1

Test	Results	Interpretation
Chest radiograph (PA and lateral views)	Normal; no evidence of apical lesion	This will make the hypothesis that Linda's ptosis is caused by a lesion in her lungs (e.g. apical region) less likely
Ultrasonography of the neck (left carotid artery)	Normal lumen and walls	This will make the hypothesis that Linda's ptosis is caused by dissection of her left carotid artery less likely
CT of the neck and base of skull	Normal and no evidence of structural changes	Although the studies are normal, this does not exclude the presence of minor lesions involving the sympathetic chain. MRI and MRA are recommended

MRA, magnetic resonance angiography; MRI, magnetic resonance imaging; PA, posteroanterior.

Q5: What is your final hypothesis?

A5

Final hypothesis: left-sided Horner's syndrome.

Q6: What issues in the given history, examination and laboratory tests support your final hypothesis?

A6

Supportive evidence

History

- History of a motor-car accident
- Ptosis of left eyelid

- Ipsilateral miosis (constriction of her left eye pupil)
- No past history of ptosis; no history of neck or chest problems.

Examination

- No neurological lesions
- No evidence of eye trauma
- Cardiovascular and respiratory examinations normal.

Investigations

- Normal chest radiograph
- No evidence of carotid dissection
- MRI recommended.

● CASE 12.2 – This is the first time I've experienced such an illness while working on my farm.

 Q4: In the light of the clinical presentation, how would you interpret the laboratory test results?

A4

Table 12.8 Interpretation of lab test results for Case 12.2

Blood test	Results	Interpretation
Red cell acetylcholinesterase	Low levels	The results support the hypothesis of organophosphate intoxication
Plasma cholinesterase	Low levels	

 Q5: What is your final hypothesis?

A5

The history, clinical picture and laboratory results support the diagnosis of organophosphate intoxication.

Q6: What issues in the given history, examination and laboratory tests support your final hypothesis?

A6

Supportive evidence

History

- The patient is a farmer and was recently exposed to chemicals (crop spraying)
- Acute illness
- Sweating all over his body, feeling unwell, excessive salivation, vomiting and loose bowel motions.

Examination

- Lacrimation: both pupils pinpoint and unreactive to light
- Excessive sweating all over his body
- Low pulse rate and low blood pressure
- Muscle fasciculation
- Deterioration of his consciousness state.

Investigations

Decreased plasma and erythrocyte cholinesterase activity confirms the clinical picture.

 CASE 12.3 – It all happened immediately after she finished her meal.

 Q4: In the light of the clinical presentation, how would you interpret the laboratory test results?

A4

Table 12.9 Interpretation of lab test results for Case 12.3

Test	Results	Interpretation
ECG	Regular rhythm, no ischaemic changes, mild LV hypertrophy	This excludes aortic valve stenosis, cardiomyopathy and heart failure as possible causes for her loss of consciousness
Echocardiogram	No evidence of valvular stenosis or regurgitation, no evidence of LV dysfunction, mild LV hypertrophy, no pericardial disease	

Full blood examination	Within normal limits	This excludes anaemia as a possible cause for her loss of consciousness
Blood urea, creatinine, sodium, potassium	Within normal limits	This excludes uraemia and electrolyte imbalance as possible contributing causes
Random blood glucose level	Raised	This excludes hypoglycaemia as a possible cause for her loss of consciousness

 Q5: What is your final hypothesis?

A5

The clinical picture and the investigation results support the diagnosis of postprandial hypotension resulting from autonomic dysfunction.

 Q6: What issues in the given history, examination and laboratory tests support your final hypothesis?

A6

Supportive evidence

History

- The patient presents with dizziness and syncope.

- She suddenly lost her consciousness for the third time over the last 4 weeks.

- It all happened immediately after she finished her meal.

- Her blood pressure is 100/70 mmHg.

- Her blood pressure is usually around 160/85 mmHg.

- For the last 3 months, she felt unable to stand or walk immediately after her meals and preferred to lie down for sometime.

- She has been diabetic and hypertensive for over 20 years.

- Her medication includes gliclazide (an oral hypoglycaemic agent) for diabetes and lisinopril (an ACE inhibitor) for hypertension.

- Both her blood pressure and blood sugar are under control.

- She does not drink or smoke.

Examination

- She looks a bit anxious and pale.

- Her pulse is 75/min (regular), her respiratory rate 18/min and temperature 36.6°C.

- Cardiovascular examination: JVP not raised; no evidence of heart failure or murmur.

- Respiratory system is normal.

- Neurological examination: normal except for loss of pain sensation in both upper and lower limbs (polyneuropathy pattern).

- Abdominal examination is normal.

- No clinical evidence of hypothyroidism or adrenal failure.

Investigations

- ECG: regular rhythm, no ischaemic changes, mild LV hypertrophy.

- Echocardiogram: no evidence of valvular stenosis or regurgitation, no evidence of LV dysfunction, mild LV hypertrophy, no pericardial disease.

- Full blood examination: normal.

- Blood urea, creatinine, sodium, potassium: all normal.

- Random blood glucose: no hypoglycaemia.

🕪 Integrated medical sciences questions

⬤ CASE 12.1 – Discuss the sympathetic input to the pupil. Briefly discuss the mechanisms underlying the different causes of Horner's syndrome.

Sympathetic input to the pupil arises from the hypothalamus → descending through the brain stem → the cervicothoracic spinal cord → fibres ascending along the spine, neck, carotid canal, cavernous sinus → fibres entering the orbit to innervate the iris dilator. The oculosympathetic pathway comprises three neurons:

1. First-order central neurons: these fibres arise in the hypothalamus → neurons descending through reticular formation → the axons of these fibres synapse in the intermediolateral grey column between the eighth cervical and first thoracic segments.

2. Second-order (preganglionic) neurons: these fibres arise in the intermediolateral grey column → exiting via the ventral spinal roots → travelling in the white rami communicants and sympathetic paraspinal chain to synapse in the superior cervical ganglion (this ganglion lies at the level of the angle of the mandible). The second-order fibres, on their way, are closely related to the mediastinum, lung apex, subclavian, jugular veins and brachial plexus.

3. Third-order (postganglionic) neurons: the sympathetic fibres split at the bifurcation of the common carotid artery to: those destined for the eye travelling along the carotid artery (innervate the iris dilator muscle), and those that control facial sweating being distributed along the branches of the facial artery.

The mechanisms underlying Horner's syndrome are:

● Central causes, e.g. dorsolateral medullary infarction: usually Horner's syndrome caused by such an infarction is associated with nystagmus, ataxia, hoarseness or dysphagia. Horner's syndrome is rarely caused by a hypothalamic or thalamic lesion. Other causes may include cervical tumour or cervical trauma (cervicothoracic spinal cord damage).

● Preganglionic Horner's syndrome: the causes may be congenital; difficult forceps deliveries (damage of the sympathetic pathway and the lower brachial plexus). In adults, preganglionic causes include: neck injury (bullet, wounds, surgery) and oral cavity surgery, apical lung cancers (Pancost's syndrome) and mediastinal tumours.

● Postganglionic Horner's syndrome: the causes may include neck trauma, direct damage to the carotid artery wall at skull base, spontaneous and traumatic carotid dissection in the neck, or skull base (usually associated with pain referred to the ipsilateral face and eye). Other causes are neck masses (lymphadenopathy, thyroid tumours, middle-ear surgery and cavernous sinus lesions.)

Horner's syndrome comprises the following:

● Ptosis (never exceeds 2 mm)

● Ipsilateral miosis (small pupil)

● Ipsilateral anhidrosis of the forehead

● Ipsilateral enophthalmos.

CASE 12.2 – **Discuss the mechanism of action of organophosphate cholinesterase inhibitors. Explain in your mechanism the pathogenesis of the clinical findings (loose bowel motions, excessive sweating and low blood pressure) found in patients with organophosphate poisoning.**

Acetylcholineserase is an extremely active enzyme. Acetylcholine binds to the enzyme's active site and is hydrolysed to choline and acetylated enzyme. Acetylcholineserase inhibitors (e.g. organophosphate compounds) are able to compete for the active site of the enzyme and bind to it. This process will result in inhibition of the enzyme and accumulation of endogenous acetylcholine in the vicinity of the cholinoceptors. This inhibition is irreversible and hence it might cause death if not treated at an earlier stage.

The increased acetylcholine in the vicinity of cholinoceptors → amplification of the action of acetylcholine → increased contraction of the smooth muscles of the intestine → short transit time → loose bowel motions.

The increased acetylcholine in the vicinity of cholinoceptors → amplification of the action of acetylcholine → increased vagal nerve activity → negative chronotropic, dromotropic and inotropic effects → decreased cardiac contraction → decreased cardiac output + decreased heart rate → decreased mean arterial blood pressure.

The increased acetylcholine in the vicinity of cholinoceptors → amplification of the action of acetylcholine → stimulation of sweat glands (the chemical transmitter is acetylcholine) → excessive sweating.

CASE 12.3 – **Discuss, using flow diagrams, the physiological mechanisms responsible for blood pressure control. What are the mechanisms underlying Ruth's presentation?**

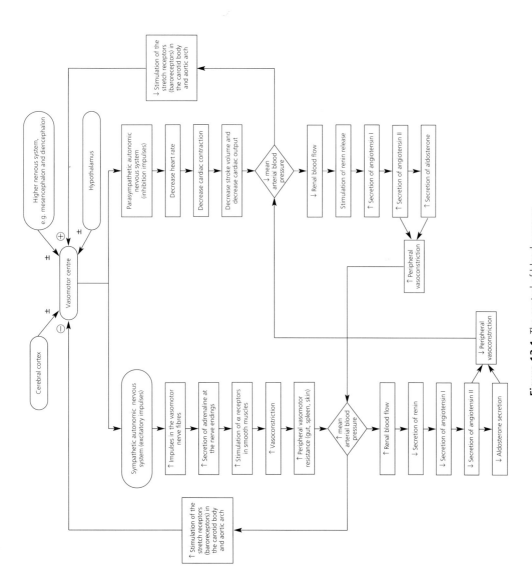

Figure 12.1 The control of blood pressure.

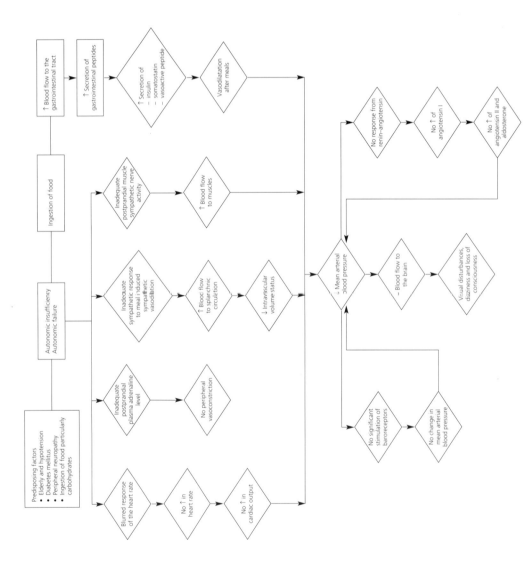

Figure 12.2 The physiological mechanisms underlying postprandial hypotension.

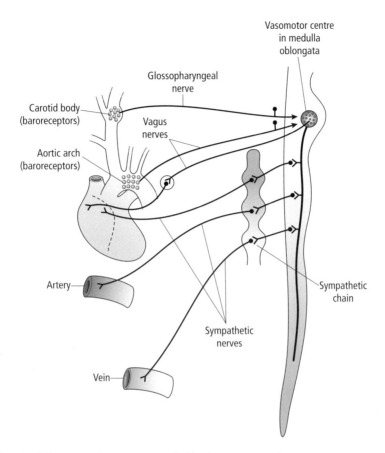

Figure 12.3 The role of the autonomic nervous system in blood pressure control.

Further reading

Appenzeller O, Oribe E. *The Autonomic Nervous System*, 5th edn. Amsterdam: Elsevier, 1997.

Goldstein DS, Robertson D, Ester M, Straus SE. Dysautonomias: clinical disorders of the autonomic nervous system. *Annals of Internal Medicine* 2002;**137**:753–763.

Harpe KG, Roth RN. Horner's syndrome in the emergency treatment. *Journal of Emergency Medicine* 1990;**8**:629–634.

Kwong TC. Organophosphate pesticides: Biochemistry and clinical toxicology. *Therapeutic Drug Monitoring* 2002;**24**:144–149.

Longhurst P. Developmental aspects of bladder function. *Scandinavian Journal of Urology and Nephrology* 2004;**215**(suppl):11–19.

Patel S, Ilsen PF. Acquired Horner's syndrome: clinical review. *Optometry* 2003;**74**:245–256.

Rusyniak DE, Nanagas KA. Organophosphate poisoning. *Seminars in Neurology* 2004;**24**:197–204.

Thrasher TN. Baroreceptors, baroreceptor unloading, and the long-term control of blood pressure. *American Journal of Physiology, Regulatory, Integrative and Comparative Physiology* 2005;**288**:R819–827.

van Leishout JJ, Wieling W, Karemaker JM, Secher NH. Syncope, cerebral perfusion and oxygenation. *Journal of Applied Physiology* 2003;**94**:833–848.

Vinik AI, Mitchell BD, Master RE, Freeman R. Diabetic autonomic neuropathy. *Diabetes Care* 2003;**26**:1553–1579.

Walton KA, Buono LM. Horner syndrome. *Current Opinion in Ophthalmology* 2003;**14**:357–363.

Wilson-Pauwels L, Stewart P, Akesson EJ. *Autonomic Nerves*. Hamilton, BC: Decker Inc, 1997.

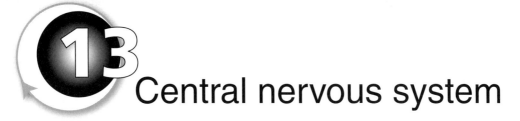

Central nervous system

| ? | **Questions for each of the case scenarios given** |

Q1: What are the possible causes for the presenting problem?
Q2: What further questions would you like to ask to help you differentiate between your hypotheses?
Q3: What investigations would be most helpful to you and why?
Q4: In the light of the clinical presentation, how would you interpret the laboratory test results?
Q5: What is your final hypothesis?
Q6: What issues in the given history, examination and laboratory tests support your final hypothesis?

Clinical cases

● CASE 13.1 – It happened all of a sudden.

Jonathan McRay, a 58-year-old famous magazine editor, is brought by the ambulance because of acute-onset right-sided weakness and inability to speak while in a meeting. His daughter, who rushes to the hospital, says: 'Dad has had two previous episodes of visual disturbances, tingling in arms and mild weakness on two occasions, I cannot remember which side, but he usually recovers in a few minutes.' Jonathan has been on medications to control his high blood pressure, high blood cholesterol and diabetes for over 10 years. He used to smoke 30 cigarettes per day for over 30 years but ceased smoking 3 years ago after the death of his wife as a result of lung cancer; she also used to smoke. Jonathan has not seen his GP for over 6 months because he is always busy at work. His vital signs are summarized in Table 13.1.

Table 13.1 Vital signs for Case 13.1

Vital signs	Jonathan's results	Normal range
Blood pressure (mmHg)	180/95	100/60–135/85
Pulse rate (/min)	95, regular	60–100
Respiratory rate (/min)	18	12–16
Temperature (°C)	37	36.6–37.2

Cardiovascular examination: no cardiac murmurs; a cervical bruit heard over the left carotid artery.

Neurological examination:

● Mild hemiparesis of his right face and saliva is dripping from the right angle of his mouth.

● Weakness of his right arm. Normal power of the left side. Able to flex the right hip and knee but cannot raise his right leg straight from bed.

● Tendon reflexes: reflexes on the right side (biceps, triceps and brachioradialis) are moderately brisk compared with those of left side. The right knee and ankle reflexes are also brisk. Babinski's reflex is present on the right and the plantar response is flexor on left side.

● He is unable to speak but appears to understand.

● Respiratory examination and abdominal examination are both normal.

CASE 13.2 – Her conscious state deteriorated rapidly on the way to hospital.

Rebecca Vines, a 27-year-old primary school teacher, is brought by the ambulance to the accident and emergency department (A&E) because of a 2-day history of headache, fever, rigor and malaise. Rebecca's boyfriend, James, who comes in with her says: 'Rebecca had an upper respiratory tract infection about 3–4 weeks ago.' She is always fit and never ill as such. The ambulance officer notices that Rebecca looks confused and her conscious state rapidly deteriorates on the way to hospital. On examination, Rebecca is drowsy and irritable. Her vital signs are shown in Table 13.2.

Table 13.2 Vital signs for Case 13.2

Vital signs	Rebecca's results	Normal range
Blood pressure (mmHg)	110/70	100/60–135/85
Pulse rate (/min)	120	60–100
Respiratory rate (/min)	24	12–16
Temperature (°C)	39	36.6–37.2

- Her neck is stiff and she is photophobic (unable to open her eyes in light).
- She has a few red blotches on her arms and legs.
- Her pharynx is congested and there are no exudates
- No lymphadenopathy.
- Both pupils reacted to light. Fundus examination was difficult because of her photophobia and irritability.
- Ears: drums look normal, no discharge. Little wax in both ears.
- Cranial nerves: no abnormality found.
- No sensory or motor loss; reflexes are brisk bilaterally.

CASE 13.3 – My congregation wants a new minister – should I resign?

Stewart James, a 59-year-old church minister, comes in to see his GP complaining of clumsiness and stiffness in both arms, but more on the right side. He has noticed tremors in the fingers of both hands and his handwriting has worsened a lot over the last 2 years. On examination, he looks sad and expressionless and has a stooped posture. He infrequently blinks both eyes and his speech is dysarthric. His vital signs are summarized in Table 13.3.

Table 13.3 Vital signs for Case 13.3

Vital signs	Stewart's results	Normal range
Blood pressure (mmHg)	125/70	100/60–135/85
Pulse rate (/min)	90	60–100
Respiratory rate (/min)	18	12–16
Temperature (°C)	36.8	36.6–37.2

- Muscle tone increased in upper limbs; no tremors

- Power normal in all four limbs
- Tender reflexes: slightly brisk in all reflexes
- Both plantar reflexes are flexor
- Sensations normal
- Gait: his walk is stiff, short steps and no swinging of arms during walking.

Integrated medical sciences questions

○ **CASE 13.1 –** Discuss the physiology of the language areas and their role in a normal conversation. Briefly discuss the effects of neurological damage to each area and how a patient might present in each case.

○ **CASE 13.2 –** Briefly discuss the anatomy and function of the cerebrospinal circulation. Discuss the pathogenesis of meningococcal meningitis and the role of cerebrospinal fluid (CSF) examination in detecting the causative micro-organism.

○ **CASE 13.3 –** Briefly discuss the anatomy of the basal ganglia and its function. Discuss the pathophysiological mechanisms by which Parkinson's disease occurs.

🔑 Key concepts

In order to work through the core clinical cases in this chapter, you will need to understand the following key concepts.

The main differences between an upper and a lower motor neuron lesion

Table 13.4 Differences between an upper (UMNL) and lower motor neuron lesion (LMNL)

	UMNL	LMNL
Lesion	Above the anterior horn cell in the spinal cord or above the nuclei of the cranial nerves	Anterior horn cell, motor nerve fibre or neuromuscular junction
Tone	Increased (spasticity) ± clonus	Reduced
Muscle weakness	All muscle groups of the lower limb – more marked in the flexor muscles. In the upper limb weakness is more marked in the extensors	More distally than proximally. Both flexors and extensors affected
Deep tendon reflexes	Increased (but superficial reflexes such as abdominal reflexes are usually absent)	Reduced or absent
Plantar response	Extensor (upgoing toe)	Normal or absent
Fasciculation	Absent	May be present in anterior horn cell lesions
Wasting	Late; mainly because of disuse	Usually present

Power is graded as follows:

0   Complete paralysis.

1   A flicker of contraction

2   Movement possible where gravity is excluded

3   Movement possible against gravity but not if any resistance is added

4   Movement possible against gravity and some resistance is present

5   Normal power.

What is a transient ischaemic attack?

A transient ischaemic attack (TIA) is a focal deficit lasting from a few seconds to 24 hours. It is usually followed by complete recovery, and usually heralds a thromboembolic stroke.

The risk factors for TIAs and stroke

Systemic disorders

- Hypertension
- Hyperlipidaemia
- Diabetes mellitus
- Smoking
- Alcohol-related disorders
- Use of contraceptive pill + smoking.

Arterial disorders

- Carotid artery narrowing/atherosclerosis
- Connective tissue disorders.

Cardiac disorders

- Rheumatic heart disease
- Endocarditis
- Left atrial thrombosis + atrial fibrosis
- Cardiac surgery
- Myxoma.

Blood disorders

- Polycythaemia
- Hyperviscosity
- Thrombocytopenia
- Coagulation disorders
- Sickle-cell disease.

The blood supply to the brain

The brain is supplied by:

1. Two internal carotid arteries
2. Two vertebral arteries.

These four arteries lie in the subarachnoid space and they anastomose on the inferior surface of the brain.

The internal carotid artery

The branches of the cranial portion of this artery are:

● The ophthalmic artery: supplies the eye, other orbital structures and the frontal area of the scalp.

● The posterior communicating artery: runs above the oculomotor nerve. It joins the posterior cerebral artery.

● The choroidal artery: ends in the choroid plexus and gives a number of small branches.

● The anterior cerebral artery: supplies the 'leg area' of the precentral gyrus; also gives branches to the lentiform and caudate nuclei (basal ganglia) and the internal capsule.

● The middle cerebral artery: the largest branch of the internal carotid artery. Supplies the entire lateral surface of the hemisphere, except for a narrow strip supplied by the anterior cerebral artery. In addition, the occipital pole and the inferolateral surface of the cerebral hemisphere are supplied by the posterior cerebral artery.

The vertebral artery

The branches of the cranial portion of this artery are:

● The meningeal branches

● The posterior spinal artery

● The anterior spinal artery

● The posterior inferior cerebellar artery: this is the largest branch of the vertebral artery. It supplies the cerebellum, the undersurface of the cerebellar hemisphere, the medulla oblongata and the choroid plexus of the fourth ventricle.

The main differences between carotid territory and vertebrobasilar TIAs

Table 13.5 Differences between different transient ischaemic attacks (TIAs)

	Carotid territory TIA	Vertebrobasilar TIA
The lesion	Ischaemia of carotid artery or any of its branches (anterior, middle, posterior cerebral arteries)	Ischaemia of vertebrobasilar artery.
Clinical presentation	Contralateral hemiparesis ± hemisensory loss Aphasia, if the dominant hemisphere affected	Vertigo, diplopia, binocular visual blurring, facial weakness, dysarthria, dysphagia, dysphonia, nausea, vomiting, ataxia, hemiparesis

The main differences between Parkinson's disease and Huntington's disease

Table 13.6 Differences between Parkinson's disease and Huntington's disease

Item	Parkinson's disease	Huntington's disease (HD)
Aetiology	Not known but familial forms exist (may be inherited as autosomal dominant or autosomal recessive). In familial types two genes have been identified: α-synuclein (found in the autosomal dominant form) and the protein parkin (found in the autosomal recessive form)	Inherited as autosomal dominant disease. *HD* gene is located on 4p16.3 and it encodes a protein known as 'huntingtin'. Normally *HD* gene contains 5–35 copies of repeat. In this disorder, the number of repeats is increased (trinucleotide repeat disorder)
Main neuronal loss	Pigmented nuclei (substantia nigra and locus ceruleus)	Degeneration of striatal neurons: caudate nucleus, frontal lobes and putamen
Pathological changes	Pallor of the substantia nigra, and locus ceruleus. Loss of catecholaminergic neurons in these regions. Lewy bodies may be present in the remaining neurons	The brain is small and shows atrophy of caudate nucleus and the putamen

The lateral and third ventricles are dilated

Atrophy of frontal lobe |
Neurotransmitter loss	Dopamine (decreased 90 per cent), noradrenaline (decreased 60 per cent), serotonin or 5-hydroxytryptamine (decreased 60 per cent)	Acetylcholine and γ-aminobutyric acid (GABA) (decreased by about 70-80 per cent)
Pathophysiology	Relative excess of acetylcholine	Increased inhibitory input to the subthalamic nucleus (relative excess of dopamine) → subthalamic nuclei failing to regulate the motor activity → involuntary movements
Effect of dopamine receptor agonists	Improvement of symptoms when patients treated with L-dopa (the precursor of dopamine)	Exacerbation of involuntary movement
Effect of dopamine receptor antagonists	Exacerbation of Parkinson's disease	Improvement of involuntary movement
Clinical features	Diminished facial expression, stooped posture, and slowness of voluntary movement, festinating gait, rigidity and tremors, 'pill-rolling'	Progressive movement disorder (jerky, hyperkinetic and dystonic movements) + dementia

Answers

CASE 13.1 – It happened all of a sudden.

Q1: What are the possible causes for the presenting problem?

As discussed earlier neurological examination shows the following:

- Mild hemiparesis of his right face and saliva is dripping from the right angle of his mouth (the facial nerve normally supplies motor fibres to the muscles of the scalp, face, auricular muscles, buccinator, platysma, stapedius, stylohyoid muscles and posterior belly of the digastric muscle. The changes in Jonathan's case are mainly in the lower part of his face and are consistent with an upper motor neuron lesion (UMNL), i.e. supranuclear lesion of cranial nerve VII. As the upper part of the face is normally bilaterally innervated, a unilateral lesion, as in Jonathan's case, will result in partial paralysis of the upper part of the face but the movements of the lower part of the face on the affected side will appear much more affected).

- Weakness of his right arm and normal power of the left side. Able to flex his right hip and knee but cannot raise his right leg straight from bed. Reflexes on the right side – biceps (C5, C6), triceps (C7, C8) and brachioradialis (C5, C6) – are moderately brisk compared with those on the left side. The right knee (L2, L3, L4) and ankle reflexes (S1) are also brisk. Babinski's reflex is present on the right and the plantar response is flexor on the left side. This suggests a UMNL affecting the upper and lower limbs on the right side. The level of the lesion is above the brain stem (i.e. at the internal capsule or the cerebral peduncle in the left cerebral hemisphere).

- He is unable to speak but appears to understand. This suggests that the association cortex at the left angular cortex and 'Wernicke's area' (both areas are responsible for comprehension) have not been affected whereas the motor speech area, 'Broca's area' on the left cerebral hemisphere, has been damaged in the lesion. Broca's area is supplied by the middle cerebral artery.

A1

The following are the most likely hypotheses (causes) for the patient's presentation:

- Right UMNL affecting the lower part of his face and the right upper and lower limbs. He has aphasia and no cognitive impairment or loss of consciousness. The presence of a number of cerebrovascular risk factors (high blood pressure, high blood cholesterol, diabetes mellitus, long history of smoking and a recent history of TIAs), together with the clinical presentation, suggests that Jonathan has developed thrombosis of the left middle cerebral artery.

- Other possible causes are: left-sided cerebral haemorrhage, left-sided cerebral tumour and vasculitis of the middle cerebral artery.

Q2: What further questions would you like to ask to help you differentiate between your hypotheses?

A2

Table 13.7 Further history questions for Case 13.1

History questions	In what way answers can help
Details about the previous attacks of weakness and whether he was admitted to hospital and underwent any investigations	Help to confirm TIAs, if he has had carotid artery stenosis, severity of stenosis and whether he is on antiplatelet therapy or advised to undergo carotid endarterectomy to reduce the risk of stroke
Any history of migraine, dizziness, heart disorders or lung problems?	Atrial fibrillation (AF) in the presence of a valvular disease increases the risk of stroke by approximately 18-fold. Assess whether he was on warfarin therapy and the results of his last international normalized ratio (INR). Chronic lung problems such as lung abscess or bronchiectasis increase the risk of cerebral abscess
Any history of blood disease, e.g. polycythaemia, haemolysis, thrombocytopenia or coagulation disorders?	Blood disorders such as polycythaemia, deficiency of anti-thrombin III, protein C and protein S, thrombocytopenia and coagulation disorders, increase the risk of stroke
Medications, e.g. warfarin, antiplatelet therapy, etc.	To assess the possibility that his problem could be related to the medications that he is receiving (e.g. bleeding related to high dose of warfarin)
Whether he is right or left handed	Handedness indicates the hemisphere that a person prefers for writing. In 90 per cent of individuals, the left hemisphere is dominant for language. In 7.5 per cent, the right hemisphere is dominant in both sexes. In 2.5 per cent, the two hemispheres have an equal share in motor control and language
Family history of cerebrovascular disorders or myocardial infarction at young age	Might be useful in assessment of his risk for cerebrovascular disorder

Q3: What investigations would be most helpful to you and why?

A3

Further investigations

- Full blood examination

- Blood urea and creatinine, sodium and potassium

- ECG/echocardiography

- Computed tomography (CT) or magnetic resonance imaging (MRI) of the brain
- Carotid duplex Doppler.

CASE 13.2 – Her conscious state deteriorated rapidly on the way to hospital.

Q1: What are the possible causes for the presenting problem?

A1

The following are the most likely hypotheses (causes) for the patient's presentation:

- Acute septic (purulent) meningitis, e.g. meningococcal meningitis
- Acute aseptic meningitis, e.g. viral meningitis
- Subarachnoid haemorrhage (signs of subarachnoid haemorrhage are: sudden onset of severe headache, nausea, vomiting and possibly loss of consciousness; meningeal irritation, e.g. neck stiffness and a positive Kernig's sign; and focal neurological signs)
- Cerebral malaria
- Viral encephalitis (less likely)
- Intracerebral haemorrhage (ruptured aneurysm)
- Brain abscess (less likely).

Q2: What further questions would you like to ask to help you differentiate between your hypotheses?

A2

Table 13.8 Further history questions for Case 13.2

History questions	In what way answers can help
Details about her upper respiratory infection, sinusitis or middle-ear infection	Meningitis may complicate middle-ear infection, sinusitis or cavernous sinus infection. History will help in identifying the source of infection and guide antibiotic therapy
Any history of recurrent headache, migraine, cough and expectoration?	Chronic chest problems such as lung abscess, bronchiectasis and tuberculosis (TB) may be complicated by cerebral infections, e.g. cerebral abscess, meningitis
Any history of fall, head trauma or loss of consciousness after a recent head trauma?	Meningitis or cerebral haemorrhage may follow head trauma and skull fracture

Any history of recent travel overseas? History of immune/complement deficiency	A number of disorders such as cerebral malaria and parasitic infections of the central nervous system (CNS) will be missed if history of travelling overseas is missed. Patients with C5–C9 complement deficiencies show increased susceptibility to bacteraemia (invasion of blood and meninges)
Past history of congenital meningeal defects, head injuries, head/neck operations	Patients with a past history of head operations or cranial injury are at a higher risk of developing meningitis
Medications and allergens	To assess whether she was partially treated with antibiotics before hospital admission and whether she has a history of allergy to antibiotics, e.g. penicillin and cephalosporins. Patients on cytotoxic drugs are at higher risk of developing meningeal infection by unusual organisms

 Q3: What investigations would be most helpful to you and why?

A3

Further investigations

- Full blood examination

- Blood urea, creatinine, sodium and potassium

- Chest radiograph

- Brain CT

- Lumbar puncture (Gram stain, special stains and culture)

- Blood culture

- Polymerase chain reaction (PCR) (on cerebrospinal fluid [CSF]).

 CASE 13.3 – My congregation wants a new minister – should I resign?

 Q1: What are the possible causes for the presenting problem?

A1

The following are the most likely hypotheses (causes) for his presentation:

- Parkinson's disease (basal ganglia problem)

- Parkinsonism caused by exposure to toxins or intake of medications

- Involuntary movements, e.g. Wilson's disease.

Q2: What further questions would you like to ask to help you differentiate between your hypotheses?

A2

Table 13.9 Further history questions for Case 13.3

History questions	In what way answers can help
Medications (such as phenothiazine and butyrophenones)	These drugs may induce a parkinsonian syndrome, with slowness, and rigidity but usually little or no tremor. Drug-induced parkinsonism usually subsides on discontinuation of the drug therapy or decreasing the dose
Exposure to chemicals/toxins such manganese	Toxins/metals such as manganese can cause parkinsonism
History of neuropsychiatric changes, or liver disorders, e.g. Wilson's disease	Wilson's disease is inherited as an autosomal recessive disorder. It is characterized by deposition of copper in the basal ganglia, cornea and liver. It may present in young patients with psychiatric changes, involuntary movements and muscle rigidity. The deposition of copper in the liver causes cirrhosis whereas its deposition in the basal ganglia is responsible for the neuropsychiatric changes
Past history of encephalitis or head trauma	Parkinsonism may be the result of postencephalitis parkinsonism

Q3: What investigations would be most helpful to you and why?

A3

Further investigations

- CT or MRI of the brain
- Liver function tests
- Serum copper, urinary copper and serum ceruloplasmin.

Further progress

 CASE 13.1 – **It happened all of a sudden.**

The treating doctor arranges some tests for Jonathan. The results are in Table 13.10.

Table 13.10 Test results for Case 13.1

Test	Jonathan's results	Normal range
Haemoglobin (Hb) (g/L)	125	115–160
Packed cell volume (PCV)	0.42	0.37–0.47
White cell count (WCC) ($\times 10^9$/L)	5.5	4.0–11.0
Platelet count ($\times 10^9$/L)	260	150–400
Sodium (mmol/L)	142	135–145
Potassium (mmol/L)	3.9	3.5–5.0
Blood urea (mmol/L)	3.6	2.5–8.3
Creatinine (mmol/L)	0.08	0.05–0.11
Fasting blood sugar (mmol/L)	7.1	3.6–5.3

ECG: no arrhythmia; left ventricular (LV) hypertrophy.

Echocardiography: normal valves, left LV hypertrophy, no mural thrombi.

MRI: changes in the left middle cerebral artery territory – concurrent MR perfusion-weighted image (PWI) shows reduced cerebral flow in the entire left middle cerebral artery territory.

Carotid duplex Doppler: left internal carotid artery occlusion.

CASE 13.2 – **Her conscious state deteriorated rapidly on the way to hospital.**

The treating doctor arranges some tests for Rebecca. The results are shown in Table 13.11

Table 13.11 Test results for Case 13.2

Test	Rebecca's results	Normal range
Hb (g/L)	121	115–160
PCV	0.43	0.37–0.47
WCC ($\times 10^9$/L)	17.6 (85 per cent neutrophils)	4.0–11.0
Platelet count ($\times 10^9$/L)	290	150–400
Sodium (mmol/L)	141	135–145
Potassium (mmol/L)	3.5	3.5–5.0
Blood urea (mmol/L)	3.0	2.5–8.3
Creatinine (mmol/L)	0.06	0.05–0.11
Fasting blood sugar (mmol/L)	5.5	3.6–5.3

Chest radiograph: Normal.

Urinalysis: Normal.

CT: normal; no evidence of structural damage.

Lumbar puncture: for CSF examination, see Table 13.12.

Table 13.12 Results of lumbar puncture for Case 13.2

CSF fluid	Rebecca's results	Normal range
Appearance	Turbid	Clear
Cells (cells/mm³)	980 (predominantly neutrophils)	0–5
Protein (g/L)	1.7	0.15–0.35
Glucose (mmol/L)	1.6	2.8–4.4 mmol/L
Pressure (cmH₂O)	30	10–18 (patient lying on her side)
Gram stain	Gram-negative bean-shaped diplococci	Nil

Blood culture: meningococci were eventually cultured from the blood.

PCR: supports the diagnosis of *Neisseria meningitidis*.

○ CASE 13.3 – My congregation wants a new minister – should I resign?

The treating doctor arranges some tests for Stewart, and the results are:

● CT scan: no space-occupying lesion

● Liver function tests: normal

● Serum copper, urinary copper and serum ceruloplasmin: all normal,

Further questions

● CASE 13.1 – **It happened all of a sudden.**

Q4: In the light of the clinical presentation, how would you interpret the laboratory test results?

A4

Table 13.13 Interpretation of lab test results for Case 13.1

Test	Change	Interpretation
Full blood examination, urea, creatinine, sodium and potassium	Normal	No evidence of polycythaemia or low platelets. Both are risk factors for stroke
Fasting blood sugar	Raised	Diabetes mellitus is a risk factor. He has had diabetes for a few years
ECG	No arrhythmia; LV hypertrophy	His LV hypertrophy is secondary to high blood pressure
MRI	Changes in the left middle cerebral artery territory. A concurrent MR perfusion-weighted image (PWI) shows reduced cerebral flow in the entire left middle cerebral artery territory	This is consistent with the clinical presentation. Lesions affecting the left middle cerebral artery are expected to cause: – weakness of the right lower part of the face (UMNL) – paralysis of the right arm – reflexes on the right side (triceps, biceps, brachioradialis, knee and ankle) are moderately brisk compared with those on the left side – right plantar reflex is dorsiflexion and flexor on left side – he is unable to speak but appears to understand (aphasia, mainly Broca's area affected)
Echocardiography	Normal valves; LV hypertrophy, no mural thrombi	Again LV hypertrophy secondary to high blood pressure. The source of thrombosis/emboli is not the heart (no mural thrombi and normal heart rhythm)
Carotid duplex Doppler	Left internal carotid artery occlusion	The occlusion of the left carotid artery could be the source of emboli to the middle cerebral artery territory

Q5: What is your final hypothesis?

A5

The clinical picture and the laboratory results are suggestive of stroke (acute UMNL affecting the right lower part of the face and the right upper and lower limbs plus aphasia). The cause is reduction of blood supply in the left middle cerebral artery territory.

Q6: What issues in the given history, examination and laboratory tests support your final hypothesis?

A6

Supportive evidence

History

- Acute-onset right-sided weakness and inability to speak (aphasia)

- Past history of TIAs (visual disturbances, tingling, mild weakness on two occasions)

- Has a number of cerebrovascular risk factors (high blood pressure, high blood cholesterol, diabetes and smoking).

Examination

- Weakness of the right lower part of the face (UMNL)

- Paralysis of his right arm

- Reflexes on right side (triceps, biceps, brachioradialis, knee and ankle) moderately brisk compared with those on left side

- Plantar reflex: dorsiflexion on the right side and flexor on the left

- He is unable to speak but appears to understand (aphasia, mainly Broca's area affected).

Investigations

- No polycythaemia or thrombocytopenia

- ECG: LV hypertrophy

- Echocardiography: normal valves; LV hypertrophy, no mural thrombi

- MRI: changes in the left middle cerebral artery territory; a concurrent MR PWI shows reduced cerebral flow in the entire left middle cerebral artery territory

- Carotid duplex Doppler: left internal carotid artery occlusion.

CASE 13.2 – Her conscious state deteriorated rapidly on the way to hospital.

 Q4: In the light of the clinical presentation, how would you interpret the laboratory test results?

A4

Table 13.14 Interpretation of lab test results for Case 13.2

Test	Change	Interpretation
WCC	Raised (85 per cent neutrophils)	The preliminary results of CSF examination are usually available within 1 h of receipt of CSF sample in the laboratory. Increased neutrophils (85 per cent) indicate acute bacterial (septic) meningitis. Antibiotic therapy (penicillin or ampicillin) should be started immediately if bacterial meningitis is suspected
Blood urea, creatinine, sodium and potassium	Normal	About 40 per cent of patients with meningococcal septicaemia develop a fulminating disease with complications caused by DIC, endotoxaemia, shock and renal failure. Addisonian crisis (acute adrenal failure resulting from bleeding into the adrenal gland and the brain is known as the Waterhouse–Friderichsen syndrome) may occur and result in low blood pressure, electrolyte disturbance and decreased urine production
Chest radiograph	Normal	It is less likely that his meningeal/cerebral infection is secondary to a lung problem such as lung abscess, bronchiectasis or TB
Urinalysis	Normal	The source of her CSF infection is less likely to be the urinary system
CT	Normal	The possibility of cerebral haemorrhage can be excluded. Brain haemorrhage may occur in fulminating meningococcal disease
CSF	Turbid, increased pressure, increased WBCs (mainly neutrophils), increased protein, low glucose, Gram-negative bean-shaped diplococci	These changes suggest acute septic meningitis, most probably caused by Gram-negative diplococci (e.g. *Neisseria meningitidis*). *Haemophilis influenzae* type b (Hib) used to be responsible for most cases of bacterial meningitis. However, with the introduction of new vaccines into childhood immunization regimens, the overall incidence of Hib infection has been lowered and both *N. meningitidis* and *Streptococcus pneumoniae* have become responsible for most cases of bacterial meningitis

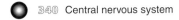
| Blood culture | Meningococci were eventually cultured from the blood | The preliminary results of blood and CSF cultures are usually available within 24 h of receipt of samples in the laboratory. Blood culture is the gold standard and is very useful in identifying the causative bacteria, particularly in patients with a contraindication to performing a lumbar puncture. Blood cultures are positive in 60–80 per cent of untreated patients |
| PCR | *N. meningitidis* | PCR is a rapid method for making the diagnosis of CSF infection. It is able to detect meningococcal meningitis even if the patient has been treated with antibiotics before hospital admission |

DIC, disseminated intravascular coagulation; PCR, polymerase chain reaction.

 Q5: What is your final hypothesis?

A5

The clinical picture and laboratory results are suggestive of acute bacterial (septic) meningitis caused by *N. meningitidis*. No complications such as shock, renal failure or adrenal haemorrhage.

 Q6: What issues in the given history, examination and laboratory tests support your final hypothesis?

A6

Supportive evidence

History

- Headache, fever, rigor, malaise
- Recent history of upper respiratory tract infection
- Looks confused
- Rapid deterioration of her conscious state.

Examination

- Looks drowsy and irritable
- Feverish (39°C)
- Neck stiffness
- Few red blotches on her arms and legs
- Pharynx congested
- Ears normal
- No cranial nerve involvement or focal neurological signs.

Investigations

- Increased WCC (85 per cent neutrophils)

- CSF fluid: turbid, under pressure, increased number of cells (mainly neutrophils), increased proteins and decreased glucose level

- Gram stain: Gram-negative diplococci

- Blood culture: meningococci cultured.

● CASE 13.3 – My congregation wants a new minister – should I resign?

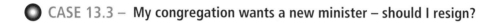

Q4: In the light of the clinical presentation, how would you interpret the laboratory test results?

A4

Table 13.15 Interpretation of lab test results for Case 13.3

Test	Change	Interpretation
Brain CT	No space-occupying lesion	CT may not be able to demonstrate the damage caused by Parkinson's disease. This will not exclude the diagnosis
Liver function tests (AST, ALT, ALP and serum bilirubin)	Normal	Wilson's disease (hepatolenticular degeneration) results from defective excretion of copper. Accumulation of copper causes damage of the liver and brain (basal ganglia). There is no evidence of liver damage
Serum copper, urinary copper and serum ceruloplasmin	Normal	In Wilson's disease, the copper transporter 'ceruloplasmin' is defective and low. As a result, serum copper is low whereas urinary copper is high (excessive excretion of copper via urine). Copper also accumulates in the liver and basal ganglia causing their damage. The patient's results exclude Wilson's disease

ALP, alkaline phosphatase; ALT, alanine aminotransferase; AST, aspartate aminotransferase.

Q5: What is your final hypothesis?

A5

The clinical picture and laboratory results are suggestive of Parkinson's disease.

Q6: What issues in the given history, examination and laboratory tests support your final hypothesis?

A6

Supportive evidence

History

- Clumsiness and stiffness in both arms, more on the right side
- Tremors in hand/fingers
- Handwriting has worsened a lot

Examination

- Looks sad and expressionless
- Infrequently blinks both eyes
- Muscle tone increased in upper limbs
- Power is normal in all limbs
- Reflexes are slightly brisk bilaterally
- Both plantar reflexes are flexor
- Sensations normal
- Gait: stiff, short steps, no swinging of arms during walking.

Investigations

- Brain CT: no space-occupying lesions
- Liver function tests and serum copper are normal.

Integrated medical sciences questions

CASE 13.1 – Discuss the physiology of the language areas and their role in a normal conversation. Briefly discuss the effects of neurological damage to each area and how a patient might present in each case.

The language network is located in the left cerebral hemisphere in 90 per cent of right-handed individuals. This network includes the peri-sylvian portions of the inferior frontal region, known as 'Broca's area', and the temporoparietal region, known as 'Wernicke's area'. In addition to these two areas, other portions of the network are located in the frontal, parietal and temporal cortex.

Handedness indicates the hemisphere preferred for writing or the hemisphere that is dominant for motor control. In most right-handed individuals, the language centres are found in the left hemisphere. Most left-handed people also have language centres in the left hemisphere. The dominance of cerebral hemispheres can be summarized as follows:

- In 90 per cent of individuals, the left hemisphere is dominant for language.

- In 7.5 per cent, the right hemisphere is dominant in both sexes.

- In 2.5 per cent, the two hemispheres have an equal share in motor control and language.

The language areas, their functions and the effect of a lesion are summarized in Table 13.16.

Table 13.16 Language areas, function and effect of lesion

Area	Anatomical location	Connections	Function	Effects of a lesion
Broca's area	Triangular parts of the inferior frontal gyrus of the left cerebral hemisphere, corresponding to areas 44 and 45 of Brodmann's area	Outputs to the face and tongue areas of the adjacent motor area	Motor speech area	Expression aphasia (understands a conversation but unable to speak)
Wernicke's area	The posterior part of the superior temporal gyrus of the left cerebral hemisphere (area 22)	Outputs to nearby areas that aid in comprehension	Sensory speech area (understanding of spoken word)	Receptive aphasia (able to talk fluently but no comprehension)
Arcuate fasciculus	Around the posterior end of the lateral fissure within the underlying white matter – left cerebral hemisphere	Arcuate fibres connect Wernicke's area with Broca's area	Transfer sensory information to Broca's area	Receptive aphasia (able to talk fluently but no comprehension)
Angular gyrus	Area 39 (inferior parietal lobe – left cerebral hemisphere)	Receives a projection from the inferior part of area 19 and the area itself projects to Wernicke's area	Commonly included as part of Wernicke's area. It is believed that the neurons of this area are the lexicon (dictionary) of words, syllables, numerical and written syllables	Receptive aphasia (able to talk fluently but no comprehension)

CASE 13.2 – Briefly discuss the anatomy and function of the cerebrospinal circulation. Discuss the pathogenesis of meningococcal meningitis and the role of CSF examination in detecting the causative micro-organism.

Cerebrospinal fluid is a clear, colourless fluid that fills the ventricles and canals of the CNS and bathes its surfaces. It is produced by the brain (about 500 mL/day). It is constantly absorbed and only 150 mL is present at one time.

The formation of CSF may be summarized as follows:

- CSF is generated by the choroidal plexus in the lateral ventricles → CSF moving to the interventricular foramina → entering the third ventricle → more CSF being secreted in the third ventricle → CSF moving to the cerebral aqueduct → CSF reaching the fourth ventricle → more CSF secreted in the fourth ventricle → CSF moving out of the lateral apertures and a median aperture → CSF bathing the surfaces of the brain and spinal cord → finally, at the arachnoid villi, CSF being absorbed into venous blood of dural venous sinuses. The circulation is repeated.

- The main functions of CSF are: protection of the brain and spinal cord; rinsing and secretion of wastes formed in the CNS; and provision of a physiological environment for the neurons to function.

The pathogenesis of meningococcal meningitis

Neisseria meningitidis is a Gram-negative diplococcus. This bacterium is characterized by the presence of a number of virulence factors that enable it to produce meningitis. These virulence factors are: the wall of the bacteria containing lipopolysaccharide or endotoxin; meningococci expressing pili (attachment organelles); meningococci expressing polysaccharide capsule (important virulent factor); and 13 serologically distinct encapsulated forms that have been responsible for the production of infection.

Attachment of *N. meningitidis* by their pili to the epithelial cells (non-ciliated cells) of nasopharynx → engulfment process → organism transmigration → submucosa → into capillaries → into arteries → invasion of the vascular system → rapid doubling of meningococci (produce large amounts of endotoxin) → septic state + shock → endotoxins of meningococci interacting with macrophages → release of cytokines, free radicals → damage of vascular system + platelet deposition + vasculitis → vascular disruption (development of petechiae and ecchymoses). The changes in blood coagulability → intravascular clotting and occlusion of blood vessels of limbs (ischaemia).

Meningococci invade the blood–CSF barrier which consists of: fenestrated endothelium cells of blood vessels at the choroids plexus; and tightly joined choroid plexus epithelial cells. Invasion of this barrier by micro-organisms results in meningitis. The organisms may traverse these barriers by one or more of the following mechanisms:

- Infection of the cells forming the barrier
- Passive transport of microbes across the intracellular vacuoles.

Organisms gain entry through the arachnoid villi → release of endotoxin in the CSF → meningeal inflammation → increased cerebrovascular permeability and brain oedema → more organisms gaining entry into the CSF.

Table 13.17 summarizes the normal composition of the CSF and changes expected to occur in CSF composition in acute septic (purulent) meningitis, viral meningitis and tuberculous meningitis.

Table 13.17 Normal composition of CSF and changes in different forms of meningitis

Characteristic	Normal values	Acute septic (purulent) meningitis	Aseptic meningitis	Tuberculous meningitis
Appearance	Clear	Cloudy	Usually clear	Turbid/opalescent
Cells (/mm³)	0–5	200–100 000 (mainly neutrophils)	100–1000 (mainly monocytes/ lymphocytes)	250–500 (mainly lymphocytes)
Protein (g/L)	0.15–0.35	0.5–5.0	0.2–1.25	0.45–5.00
Glucose (mmol/L)	2.8–4.4 (about 60–70 per cent of plasma level)	Low	Normal	Very low
Pressure (cmH₂O)	10–18 (lying on side) and bout 30 (sitting)	Raised	Raised	Raised

CASE 13.3 – Briefly discuss the anatomy of the basal ganglia and its function. Discuss the pathophysiological mechanisms by which Parkinson's disease occurs.

The major components of the basal ganglia are:

- Striatum (caudate and the putamen)

- Globus pallidus (pars medialis, pars lateralis)

- Substantia nigra (pars reticulate and pars compacta)

- Subthalamic nuclei

- Thalamus (ventroanterior and ventrolateral).

The basal ganglia are connected with several subthalamic nuclei and also with cerebral cortex, and specific brain-stem nuclei.

A number of neurotransmitters are found in the basal ganglia and are important for their normal function. The main transmitters produced in basal ganglia are summarized in Table 13.18.

Table 13.18 Main transmitters of basal ganglia

Chemical transmitter	Source	Function	Effects of its loss and clinical significance
Acetylcholine	Corpus striatum	Excitatory (e.g. at medium-sized striatal neurons)	Development of dementia that eventually affects one-third of patients with Parkinson's disease
Glutamate	Thalamocortical connections and corticostriate fibres	Excitatory	
γ-Aminobutyric acid (GABA)	Striopallidal fibres and pallidothalamic fibres	Inhibitory	In Huntington's disease loss of the GABAergic neurons in the corpus striatum is responsible for the clinical changes of the disease. Both acetylcholine and GABA are decreased (about 70–80 per cent)
Dopamine	Nigroreticular fibres	D_1 = excitatory D_2 = inhibitory	In Parkinson's disease: dopamine (decreased 90 per cent), noradrenaline (decreased 60 per cent), serotonin (decreased 60 per cent) Parkinson's disease is treated with levodopa (taken up by dopaminergic neurons and converted to dopamine by decarboxylation). Usually combined with peripheral decarboxylase inhibitor (carbidopa). It is also treated with specific dopamine receptor agonist (bromocriptine)
Noradrenaline	Locus ceruleus	Excitatory	Development of autonomic changes and depression in patients with Parkinson's disease

The main function of the basal ganglia is coordination of cortical motor commands. The direct (excitatory and the indirect (inhibitory) pathways of the basal ganglia provide a counter and balanced control on activities of the motor cortex.

The mechanism underlying the pathogenesis of Parkinson's disease may be summarized as:

Degeneration of the substantia nigra → degeneration of the pathway from the substantia nigra to the striatum → loss of tonic facilitation of spiny striatal neurons bearing D_1 receptors → the 'direct pathway' not functioning and the 'indirect pathway' being activated → activation of GABAergic neurons in the striatum → disinhibition of the subthalamic nuclei → subthalamic nuclei being discharged (activated) into the medial pallidal segment → increased inhibitory control of the thalamus → loss of the excitatory drives to the motor cortex → clinical signs such as tremors and rigidity in Parkinson's disease.

Further reading

Clarke C, Moore AP. Parkinson's disease. *Clinical Evidence* 2003;**10**:1582–1598.

Correia JB, Hart CA. Meningococcal disease. *Clinical Evidence* 2003;**10**:931–941.

Dewey RB Jr. Autonomic dysfunction in Parkinson's disease. *Neurologic Clinics* 2004;**22**(suppl 3):S127–139.

Eriksen JL, Wszolek Z, Petrucelli L. Molecular pathogenesis of Parkinson disease. *Archives of Neurology* 2005;**62**:353–357.

Gendelman HE, Persidsky Y. Infections of the nervous system. *Lancet Neurology* 2005;**4**:12–13.

Martin RC. Language processing: functional organization and neuroanatomical basis. *Annual Review of Psychology* 2003;**54**:55–89.

Mastronardi L, Ruggeri A. Cervical disc herniation producing Brown–Séquard syndrome: case report. *Spine* 2004;**29**:E28–31.

Nishitani N, Schurmann M, Amunts K, Hari R. Broca's region: from action to language. *Physiology (Bethesda)* 2005;**20**:60–69.

Sinner SW, Tunkel AR. Antimicrobial agents in the treatment of bacterial meningitis. *Infectious Disease Clinics of North America* 2004;**18**:581–602.

Takakusaki K, Saitoh K, Harada H, Kashiwayanagi M. Role of basal ganglia-brainstem pathways in the control of motor behaviour. *Neuroscience Research* 2004;**50**:137–151.

Trisch S, Silberstein P, Limousin-Dowsey P, Jahanshahi M. The basal ganglia: anatomy, physiology and pharmacology. *Psychiatric Clinics of North America* 2004;**27**:757–799.

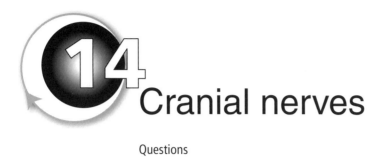

Cranial nerves

Questions

Clinical cases

Key concepts

Answers

Clinical cases

CASE 14.1 – I feel like my surroundings are spinning.

Melinda Shaun, a 25-year-old librarian, comes in with her boyfriend to see her GP, Dr Jessica Brooks. Over the last 2 days Melinda has had an intense sense of rotation of her surroundings which is aggravated by moving her head, rolling over in bed or moving from an upright to a recumbent posture. As a result of this problem she has had difficulty standing or walking and she needs her boyfriend to help her. Melinda has a history of upper respiratory tract infection about 4–5 days earlier. Today she has felt nauseous and vomited once on her way to the clinic. On examination, Melinda looks pale and is unable to stand on her own. Her vital signs are summarized in Table 14.1.

Table 14.1 Vital signs for Case 14.1

Vital signs	Melinda's results	Normal range
Blood pressure (mmHg)	110/70 (sitting)	100/60–135/85
	105/60 (lying)	
Pulse rate (/min)	90 (sitting)	60–100
	86 (lying)	
Respiratory rate (/min)	18	12–16
Temperature (°C)	37.5	36.6–37.2

- Ear, throat and nose examination: both drums are intact; no discharge. Some wax present in both ears. Running nose, congested mucous membrane with a clear watery secretion in both nostrils. Pharynx is slightly congested. Some postnasal discharge is noted.

- Neurological examination: conscious and oriented, no neck stiffness, and cranial nerves are normal. Moving all limbs and reflexes are bilaterally normal. No sensory loss.

- Eye examination: horizontal nystagmus with rotational component. The fast phase is directed to the left.

- Cardiovascular and respiratory examinations: heart is regular and chest is clear to auscultation.

- Abdominal examination: normal.

● CASE 14.2 – I am unable to close my right eye.

Mr Adam Wesley, a 69-year-old senior citizen, comes in with his wife to see his GP, Dr Alan Ramsis, because of right-sided facial weakness. Two days ago Adam and his wife returned to their house after visiting their eldest son in a nearby city. A few hours after their arrival home Adam's wife noticed that her husband's mouth was drooping on the right side and he could not close his right eye. Adam mentions that he has had mild aching pain behind his right ear for the last 2 weeks and took paracetamol on several occasions. About 10 years ago, Adam underwent a surgical operation to remove a right parotid tumour. The operation was successful and no neurological deficit occurred after the operation. He does not drink or smoke and he is not on any medications. On examination, Adam's face is asymmetrical and the right angle of his mouth is drooped. His vital signs are summarized in Table 14.2.

Table 14.2 Vital signs for Case 14.2

Vital signs	Adam's results	Normal range
Blood pressure (mmHg)	110/70	100/60–135/85
Pulse rate (/min)	90	60–100
Respiratory rate (/min)	18	12–16
Temperature (°C)	37.4	36.6–37.2

- Neurological examination: Adam is unable to move his forehead on the right side or close his right eye. He has lost the right nasolabial fold and sensation in the anterior two-thirds of his tongue, the right angle of his mouth is drooping and he has lost taste sensation in the anterior two-thirds of the tongue.

- A few vesicles are noticed on the right auditory canal and the right auricle.

- Cardiovascular and respiratory examinations are normal. Abdominal examination is normal.

● CASE 14.3 – It feels like electricity is radiating through my jaw.

Mrs Anne Schaeffer, a 70-year-old retired primary school principal, comes in to see her GP, Dr Mark Eugene, because of excruciating facial pain. Anne has had dull aching pain in her left face for the last 3 weeks. At first she thought it was related to her teeth and went to see her dentist. As the pain continued and her dentist suggested that she needed to see a doctor, Anne came in to see Dr Eugene. Her pain feels like electricity, radiating in her jaw. It usually starts on the left side of her lower jaw, and then spreads upwards to the upper jaw and ends around her left eye region. It lasts for a few seconds and reappears several times a day. She noticed that the pain reappears when she chews, talks or is exposed to cold wind. It is also produced by the lightest touch to her lips and gums. The pain does not occur at night. She used to have tension headache when she was working as a principal but it ceased after her retirement. About 10 years ago she experienced whiplash to her neck after a motor collision with no complications.

On examination, her face is screwed up in agony. Her vital signs are normal.

Neurological examination:

- Pain triggered by the lightest touch to the right angle of her mouth

- Corneal reflex present bilaterally

- All cranial nerves normal

- No power loss or sensory loss bilaterally

- Deep tendon reflexes normal bilaterally.

Cardiovascular and respiratory examinations are normal.

Integrated medical sciences questions

CASE 14.1 – Maintaining an upright posture and balance (feeling of equilibrium) when we stand is dependent on a number of anatomical structures and physiological mechanisms. Briefly list these structures and explain their physiological role in maintaining the normal feeling of equilibrium.

CASE14.2 – What are the main causes of facial (cranial nerve VII) palsy? List the clinical characteristics of each cause.

CASE 14.3 – What are the cranial nerves that may be compressed/affected by a cerebellopontine angle tumour (acoustic neuroma)? Briefly discuss the clinical consequences of a left cerebellopontine angle tumour.

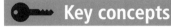

Key concepts

In order to work through the core clinical cases in this chapter, you will need to understand the following key concepts.

Important terms

- Dizziness: a non-specific term that may mean vertigo, presyncope or disequilibrium.

- Vertigo: definite rotational sensation. With the eyes open, the patient sees the environment move and with the eyes closed he or she feels a sense of rotation in the space.

- Presyncope: light-headedness, impending fainting, visual disturbances. Presyncope is usually a result of decreased blood flow in the cerebral circulation (e.g. acute myocardial infarction, cardiac arrhythmias).

- Instability and disequilibrium: impaired balance or loss of balance on walking.

- Nystagmus: a rapid involuntary oscillation of the eyeballs, occurring normally during or after bodily rotation. Nystagmus may be physiological or pathological.

- Cranial nerves: any nerve that exits the brain within the skull (above the foramen magnum).

Table 14.3 The main differences between peripheral and central vertigo

Item	Peripheral vertigo	Central vertigo
Causes	Vestibular neuronitis, labyrinthitis, Menière's disease, acoustic neuroma	Vertebral basilar insufficiency Infarction of the lateral brain stem
Severity	++++	+ to +++
Onset	Sudden	Non-paroxysmal
Nausea and vomiting	+++	±
Nystagmus	Always present, usually horizontal + rotatory component	May be absent. May occur in more than one direction of gaze Nystagmus is usually vertical Eye movements are dysconjugate
Tinnitus and hearing loss	Often present	±

The cranial nerves and the major functions of each nerve

I The olfactory nerve: smell

II The optic nerve: vision

III The oculomotor nerve: eye movement, pupillary constriction (the oculomotor nerve supplies the levator palpebrae superioris and all the internal and external muscles of the ipsilateral eye except the superior oblique, lateral rectus and papillary dilator)

IV   The trochlear nerve: eye movement (the trochlear nerve supplies the superior oblique, the muscle that is purely a depressor when the eye is adducted)

V   The trigeminal nerve: facial sensation, mastication

VI   The abducens nerve: eye movement (the abducens nerve supplies the lateral rectus muscle which moves the eye laterally)

VII   The facial nerve: facial expression, taste sensation from the anterior two-thirds of the tongue, lacrimation, salivation

VIII The vestibulocochlear (acoustic) nerve: hearing, balance

IX   The glossopharyngeal nerve: taste sensation from the posterior third of the tongue, salivation, swallowing, visceral sensation from the posterior third of tongue and pharynx

X   The vagus nerve: swallowing, autonomic, visceral sensation

XI   The accessory nerve: neck and shoulder movement (supplies the sternomastoid and trapezius muscles)

XII   The hypoglossal nerve: tongue movement.

Answers

 CASE 14.1 – I feel like my surroundings are spinning.

 Q1: What are the possible causes for the presenting problem?

A1

The following are possible causes (hypotheses) for Melinda's presentation.

The most likely causes are:

- vestibular neuronitis

- labyrinthitis

- benign positional vertigo.

The following are less likely causes:

- Menière's disease: characterized by vertigo, unilateral hearing loss and tinnitus. Absence of hearing loss and tinnitus will make this hypothesis less likely. These two symptoms should be part of our history taking.

- Acoustic neuroma: patients with acoustic neuroma usually present with hearing loss, tinnitus and unsteadiness, and in advanced cases cranial nerve V lesion. Absence of hearing loss and tinnitus will make this hypothesis less likely. These two symptoms should be part of our history taking.

- Vertebrobasilar ischaemia: patients with vertebrobasilar ischaemia manifest with vertigo, diplopia, ataxia, bilateral sensory or motor symptoms, and fluctuating episodes of drowsiness. Distinguishing the vertigo of vertebrobasilar ischaemia from labyrinthine vertigo may be difficult in elderly patients. However, in Melinda's case there is enough evidence to support her vertigo most probably being caused by labyrinthine pathology.

- Infarction of the lateral brain stem supplied by the posterior inferior cerebellar artery, known as Wallenberg's syndrome: this syndrome involves cranial nerves IX and X, Horner's syndrome, cerebellar ataxia and crossed hemibody pain, and temperature loss.

- Postural hypotension: no significant changes in her blood pressure readings with changes of body position, sitting versus lying.

- Central vertigo caused by meningitis: apart from fever and vertigo, there are no signs and symptoms to support this hypothesis. However, this should be part of our differential diagnosis.

Q2: What further questions would you like to ask to help you differentiate between your hypotheses?

A2

Table 14.4 Further history questions for Case 14.1

History questions	In what way answers can help
Has she noticed global weakness, sweating, dimming of vision on changing her position?	Very early in your assessment, it is important to differentiate between vertigo (definite rotational sensation) and presyncope (light-headedness, impending fainting, with visual disturbances). Presyncope is usually the result of postural hypotension or cardiac arrhythmias whereas vertigo may be peripheral or central in its origin. Peripheral vertigo is caused by: vestibular neuronitis; labyrinthitis; benign positioning vertigo; Menière's disease; and acoustic neuroma. Central vertigo is caused by: vertebrobasilar ischaemia; infarction of the lateral brain stem; cerebral haemorrhage; and meningitis. Presyncope is usually associated with global weakness, dimming of vision and sympathetic stimulation (sweating and increased heart rate)
More information about her upper respiratory tract infection and her vertigo (sense of rotation)	Some medications used in treatment of upper respiratory tract may produce dizziness and a sense of rotation. You will also need to assess whether she has developed any complications such as sinusitis, otitis media, meningitis, etc.
Any history of severe headaches, fever, rigors, neurological deficit or changes in her conscious state	Central vertigo may be caused by cerebral haemorrhage, cerebral infarction or meningitis. You need to exclude these conditions first. History and clinical examination are usually helpful in this process
If she has noticed any neurological changes such as diplopia, facial pain, disequilibrium, dysphagia, dysphonia, or sensory or motor loss	Central vertigo is usually associated with neurological deficit. Absence of these symptoms will make central vertigo less likely and favours peripheral vertigo
If she has trouble with her ears, tinnitus or decreased hearing in one of her ears	You need to exclude or confirm conditions such as acoustic neuroma and Menière's disease in your differential diagnosis
Past history of ear infection, sinusitis, recurrent pharyngitis and similar illnesses	To assess whether she has had chronic ear problems
History of diabetes mellitus, low blood pressure, heart problems, or low blood sugar	Patients with diabetes mellitus may develop autonomic dysfunction and postural hypotension. Hypoglycaemia may cause presyncope-like symptoms
Medications and allergies	Many drugs are potentially ototoxic and may damage the vestibular system (e.g. gentamicin)

Q3: What investigations would be most helpful to you and why?

A3

Further investigations

- Computed tomography (CT)/magnetic resonance imaging (MRI) of the brain

- Audiometry

 CASE 14.2 – I am unable to close my right eye.

 Q1: What are the possible causes for the presenting problem?

A1

The following are possible causes (hypotheses) for Adam's presentation.

Most likely causes

With an upper motor neuron lesion (UMNL) of the facial (VII) cranial nerve, the lower part of the face is much weaker than the upper part. This is because there is bilateral corticobulbar projection to the nucleus of the cranial nerve VII nucleus supplying the upper facial nucleus, whereas the nucleus supplying the lower part of nerve VII is unilateral.

In a lower motor neuron lesion (LMNL) of nerve VII, both upper and lower muscles of the face are equally affected.

Right lower motor neuron lesion (RMNL) of the facial nerve can be caused by one of the following:

- A lesion affecting cranial nerve VII as it crosses the petrous temporal bone (the supportive evidence for this hypothesis is loss of taste sensation in the first two-thirds of the tongue and the presence of facial weakness involving the right upper and lower parts of the face equally, i.e. LMNL signs; we might need to ask him about hyperacusis (hearing loud sounds in the affected ear) which may also present in lesions at this level). The causes of cranial nerve VII palsy at this level are:

  - Bell's palsy

  - trauma

  - middle-ear infection

  - herpes zoster infection of the geniculate ganglion of cranial nerve VII (Ramsay Hunt syndrome).

  There is no history of middle-ear infection or trauma. The presence of vesicles in his right auditory canal and the right auricle supports herpes zoster infection.

- A lesion involving the base of the skull, or parotid gland, e.g. Paget's disease of bone causing cranial nerve VII compression at the stylomastoid foramen; recurrence of the parotid tumour and involvement of the cranial nerve VII branches; mumps; trauma; and sarcoidosis. Paget's disease of bone, mumps and trauma are less likely. If his symptoms are caused by recurrence of the parotid tumour, he will have LMNL without loss of taste sensation. This is because the chorda tympani nerve that carries taste sensation from the anterior two-thirds of the tongue joins the facial nerve at the petrous temporal bone (i.e. at a higher level). However, MR images of the brain, brain stem and parotid region are required to rule out this hypothesis.

Less likely causes

● Neuromuscular junction disease, e.g. myasthenia gravis

● Muscle disease, e.g. dystrophia myotonica

● A cerebellopontine angle tumour involving cranial nerve VII (in cerebellopontine angle tumour, cranial nerves V, VI, VII and VIII are involved)

● A lesion at the pons (this is characterized by convergent squint as a result of lateral rectus palsy, unilateral facial weakness and contralateral hemiparesis)

● A lesion above the seventh nucleus (usually produced by cerebral infarction and results in UMNL of the facial nerve).

Q2: What further questions would you like to ask to help you differentiate between your hypotheses?

A2

Table 14.5 Further history questions for Case 14.2

History questions	In what way answers can help
Does he hear loud sounds in the affected side (hyperacusis)?	The motor nucleus of the facial nerve supplies the facial muscles, the stapedius muscle, the posterior belly of the digastric and the stylohyoid muscle. Involvement of the nerve to stapedius results in hyperacusis (patient hears sounds louder in the affected side). This change is usually present in cranial nerve VII lesions at the petrous temporal bone level
Any associated neurological changes, e.g. weakness of arm/leg on opposite side, sensory changes, involvement of other cranial nerves?	Cerebellopontine angle tumours may be associated with cranial nerve V, VI, VII and VIII lesions
History of recent head trauma	Trauma to the base of the skull and the parotid region may result in cranial nerve VII lesion
The pathology results of his parotid tumour, any other therapy after the surgery and follow-up by the surgeon	To assess whether the parotid tumour was benign or malignant and the nature of his tumour (e.g. possibility of recurrence)

Q3: What investigations would be most helpful to you and why?

A3

Further investigations

● MRI of the brain, brain stem and parotid region

● Chest and skull radiographs.

CASE 14.3 – It feels like electricity is radiating through my jaw.

 Q1: What are the possible causes for the presenting problem?

A1

The following are possible causes (hypotheses) for Anne's presentation.

Most likely causes

Trigeminal neuralgia caused by: idiopathic causes; secondary causes, e.g. multiple sclerosis, trauma of the cranial nerve V; and lesions of the cerebrospinal angle regions. Secondary causes of trigeminal neuralgia are less likely.

Less likely causes

- Brain-stem lesions involving cranial V nuclei, e.g. glioma, infarction, syringobulbia

- Cerebellopontine angle tumours, e.g. acoustic neuroma, meningioma, neoplasms

- Lesions at the apex of the petrous temporal bone: in Gradenigo's syndrome, cranial nerves V and VI are affected

- Cavernous sinus problems, e.g. aneurysm, lateral extension of pituitary tumour

- Neoplasms infiltrating the base of the skull and involving the peripheral branches of cranial nerve V on the left side

- Related to the patient's old neck trauma.

Q2: What further questions would you like to ask to help you differentiate between your hypotheses?

A2

Table 14.6 Further history questions for Case 14.3

History questions	In what way answers can help
Duration of the pain: How long does it last? How many times on average does it occur? Distribution of pain and any other characteristics, e.g. what relieves and precipitates her pain?	The pain in trigeminal neuralgia is electric shock-like, lasting for seconds, but it occurs many times a day for weeks. It commences in the mandibular division of the fifth division (V3), spreads upwards to the maxillary division (V2) and then ends at the ophthalmic division (V1)
Any neurological deficit, e.g. facial weakness, vertigo, unsteadiness, sensory loss, eye changes, hemiplegia, hemiparesis?	In cerebellopontine angle tumour, cranial nerves V, VI, VII and VIII are involved. Lesions at the apex of the petrous temporal bone may result in cranial nerve V and VI lesions (Gradenigo's syndrome)

Past history of multiple sclerosis, cancer therapy, meningiomas, neck pain, tension headache, migraine

Secondary causes of trigeminal neuralgia are: multiple sclerosis; trauma to cranial nerve V; and lesions of the cerebellopontine angle. These causes need to be excluded or confirmed

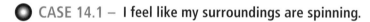
Q3: What investigations would be most helpful to you and why?

A3

Further investigations

MRI of the brain, brain stem and cerebellopontine angle region.

Further progress

● CASE 14.1 – I feel like my surroundings are spinning.

Dr Brooks arranges some tests for Melinda. The results are shown in Table 14.7.

Table 14.7 Test results for Case 14.1

Test	Melinda's results
CT of the brain stem	MRI is recommended
MRI of the brain	No ischaemic injuries in the brain, cerebellum or brain stem. No evidence of vertebral basilar ischaemia
Audiometry	Normal study

● CASE 14.2 – I am unable to close my right eye.

Dr Ramsis arranges some tests for Adam. The results are shown in Table 14.8

Table 14.8 Test results for Case 14.2

Test	Adam's results
MRI of the brain, brain stem and parotid region	Normal study. No evidence of infarction, cerebellopontine angle tumours or metastasis. Compared with previous postoperative studies there are no changes in the parotid region
Chest and skull radiographs	Chest radiograph normal
	Skull radiograph: no fractures, no evidence of Paget's disease

● CASE 14.3 – It feels like electricity is radiating through my jaw.

Dr Eugene arranges some tests for Anne. The results are shown in Table 14.9

Table 14.9 Test results for Case 14.3

Test	Anne's results
MRI of the brain, brain stem and cerebellopontine angle region	Normal study. No evidence of multiple sclerosis or cerebellopontine angle tumours

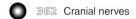

Further questions

 CASE 14.1 – I feel like my surroundings are spinning.

 Q4: In the light of the clinical presentation, how would you interpret the laboratory test results?

A4

Table 14.10 Interpretation of lab test results for Case 14.1

Test	Change	Interpretation
CT of the brain stem	MRI recommended	CT is rarely helpful because the brain stem is poorly seen with this technique
MRI of the brain	No ischaemic injuries in the brain, cerebellum or brain stem. No evidence of vertebral basilar ischaemia	These results exclude central causes of vertigo, e.g. vertebrobasilar ischaemia (characterized by vertigo, diplopia, ataxia, bilateral sensory or motor symptoms, fluctuating episodes of drowsiness); and infarction of the lateral brain stem supplied by the posteroinferior cerebellar artery (Wallenberg's syndrome)
Audiometry	Normal study	This helps in excluding causes such as Menière's disease (characterized by vertigo, unilateral hearing loss and tinnitus) and acoustic neuroma (characterized by hearing loss, tinnitus, unsteadiness and, in advanced cases, cranial nerve V lesion). Absence of hearing loss and tinnitus will exclude these hypotheses

 Q5: What is your final hypothesis?

A5

The clinical picture and the laboratory results are suggestive of vestibular neuronitis, most probably caused by viral infection.

 Q6: What issues in the given history, examination and laboratory tests support your final hypothesis?

A6

Supportive evidence

History

- Intense sense of rotation of the surroundings – last 2 days
- Sense of rotation is aggravated by changes of position

- Recent history of upper respiratory tract infection

- Nausea and vomiting (resulting from associated autonomic changes).

Examination

- Looks pale (caused by associated autonomic changes)

- No postural hypotension

- Temperature 37.5°C

- Running, congested nose and congested pharynx

- Conscious; no neck stiffness

- No sensory or motor loss

- Horizontal nystagmus with rotating component

- Normal cardiovascular and respiratory examinations

- Normal abdominal examination.

Investigations

- MRI of brain: no ischaemic injuries in the brain, cerebellum or brain stem; no evidence of vertebral basilar ischaemia

- Audiometry: normal study.

CASE 14.2 – I am unable to close my right eye.

Q4: In the light of the clinical presentation, how would you interpret the laboratory test results?

A4

Table 14.11 Interpretation of lab test results for Case 14.2

Test	Change	Interpretation
MRI of the brain, brain stem and parotid region	Normal study. No evidence of infarction, cerebellopontine angle tumours or metastasis. Compared with previous postoperative studies there are no changes in the parotid region	This might help in excluding recurrence of the parotid tumour
Chest and skull radiographs	Chest radiograph normal Skull radiograph: no fractures, no evidence of Paget's disease	A normal chest radiograph will make sarcoidosis less likely. A normal skull radiograph and a normal ALP will exclude Paget's disease

ALP, alkaline phosphatase.

Q5: What is your final hypothesis?

A5

The clinical picture and the laboratory results are suggestive of right-sided LMNL of cranial nerve VII (facial nerve), most probably caused by herpes zoster infection of the geniculate ganglion (Ramsay Hunt syndrome).

Q6: What issues in the given history, examination and laboratory tests support your final hypothesis?

A6

Supportive evidence

History

- Right-sided facial weakness
- Mouth drooped on the right side
- Cannot close his right eye
- Aching pain behind his right ear – last 2 weeks
- Underwent a surgical operation – removal of a right parotid tumour, 10 years ago
- No complications after surgery
- Not on medications/no allergy.

Examination

- Face asymmetrical
- Right angle of mouth drooped
- Unable to move his forehead, right side
- Unable to close right eye
- Loss of right nasolabial fold
- Loss of taste sensations – anterior two-thirds of tongue
- No lymphadenopathy
- A few vesicles on the right auditory canal and right auricle
- Cardiovascular and respiratory examinations normal.

Investigations

- MRI (brain and brain stem): normal
- Chest and skull radiographs: normal.

CASE 14.3 – It feels like electricity is radiating through my jaw.

 Q4: In the light of the clinical presentation, how would you interpret the laboratory test results?

A4

Table 14.12 Interpretation of lab test results for Case 14.3

Test	Change	Interpretation
MRI of the brain, brain stem and cerebellopontine angle region	Normal study. No evidence of multiple sclerosis or cerebellopontine angle tumours	The normal studies help to exclude secondary causes of trigeminal neuralgia, such as multiple sclerosis, infarction and cerebellopontine angle tumours

 Q5: What is your final hypothesis?

A5

The clinical picture and the laboratory results are suggestive of trigeminal neuralgia.

 Q6: What issues in the given history, examination and laboratory tests support your final hypothesis?

A6

Supportive evidence

History

- Excruciating left-sided facial pain – 3 weeks
- Pain not related to her teeth (consulted with her dentist)
- Pain feels like electricity radiating in her left jaw
- Pain commences in her lower jaw, progresses to the upper jaw and ends around left eye
- Pain lasts a few seconds and repeats several times a day
- Pain appears when she chews, talks and touches her lip or gums
- No pain at night.

Examination

- Corneal reflex bilaterally present
- Other cranial nerves normal

- No sensory or motor loss
- Deep tendon reflexes bilaterally normal
- Cardiovascular and respiratory examinations are normal.

Investigations

- MRI (brain, brain stem, cerebellopontine angle): normal

ᐦᐦ Integrated medical sciences questions

● CASE 14.1 – Maintaining an upright posture and balance (feeling of equilibrium) when we stand is dependent on a number of anatomical structures and physiological mechanisms. Briefly list these structures and explain their physiological role in maintaining the normal feeling of equilibrium.

Normal feeling of equilibrium depends on the following structures and functions:

● Receiving appropriate information from the eyes, vestibular system, peripheral sensory receptors in the feet, and the presence of a normal sensory pathway in the dorsal column of the spinal cord.

● Coordinating nuclei in the brain stem, basal ganglia, cerebellum, reticular information and cerebral cortex.

● Vestibular system, semicircular canals, ampullae, utricle and saccule: the vestibular input is composed of information from utricular maculae and the cristae of the semicircular canals. The utricular maculae respond to changes in gravity and linear acceleration, whereas the semicircular canals are responsive to angular acceleration. The body, via the vestibulo-ocular reflex, vestibulo-cerebellocortical connections and vestibular nuclei in the pons and upper medulla, is able to make adjustment and compensatory movements to maintain balance.

● Cranial nerve VIII: balance is dependent on sensory input from the vestibular system.

● Vestibular nuclei in the pons and upper medulla.

● Cerebellum: the cerebellum receives afferent fibres from the spinal cord, vestibular system, basal ganglia and cerebral cortex. Lesions of the cerebellum could result in incoordination (ataxia) and reduced muscle tone.

● CASE 14.2 – What are the main causes of facial (cranial nerve VII) palsy? List the clinical characteristics of each cause.

Table 14.13 Main characteristics of facial palsy

Level of the lesion	Pathological causes	Clinical presentation
Supranuclear lesion	Cerebral infarction	UMNL of cranial nerve VII on the side opposite the lesion (facial weakness of the lower part of the face and hemiparesis)
		Frontalis muscle is spared, eye closure and blinking not affected
Pons: usually cranial nerve VI (abducens) and VII (facial) involved together	Pontine lesion is usually caused by infarction or a tumour (glioma) in the brain stem. The facial nucleus may be affected in motor neuron disease and poliomyelitis	Cranial nerves VI and VII are usually involved (LMNL). LMNL and convergent squint (lateral rectus muscle palsy + unilateral facial weakness + contralateral hemiparesis)
Cerebellopontine angle tumour	Acoustic neuroma, meningioma, metastasis (secondary tumour mass)	Usually cranial nerves V, VI and VIII together with VII are involved

Petrous temporal bone	Idiopathic (Bell's palsy), trauma, middle-ear disease, herpes zoster, tumour	Loss of taste sensation on the anterior two-thirds of the tongue + hyperacusis (loss of nerve supply to stapedius muscle) + LMNL of cranial nerve VII on the same side of the lesion (weakness of both upper and lower muscles of the face)
Base of the skull, parotid gland and peripheral distribution of cranial nerve VII	Paget's disease of bone, tumours of the base of the skull, tumours of the parotid gland, mumps, sarcoidosis, trauma, polyneuritis	LMNL of cranial nerve VII on the same side of the lesion (weakness of both upper and lower muscles of the face)
Neuromuscular junction	Myasthenia gravis	Bilateral LMNL
Muscle disease	Dystrophia myotonica	Bilateral LMNL

● CASE 14.3 – What are the cranial nerves that may be compressed/affected by a cerebellopontine angle tumour (acoustic neuroma)? Briefly discuss the clinical consequences of a left cerebellopontine angle tumour.

The cranial nerves that may be compressed/affected by a cerebellopontine angle tumour (acoustic neuroma) are shown in Table 14.14.

Table 14.14 Cranial nerves affected by cerebellopontine angle tumour

Cranial nerve	Function	Effects of a left cerebellopontine angle tumour
The trigeminal (cranial V) nerve	Sensory function: light touch and pain sensations in the territory of the three sensory divisions of the trigeminal nerve, ophthalmic, maxillary and mandibular divisions, supplying the forehead, cheeks and jaw Motor function: the muscles of mastication mainly the pterygoid and masseter muscles Reflexes: the corneal reflex (a brisk closure of the eye evoked by touching the cornea gently with a wisp of cotton wool) and the jaw reflex (the afferent and the efferent pathways are provided by cranial nerve V)	Loss of light touch and pain sensations on the left side of the face (forehead, cheeks and jaw) Weakness of the muscles of mastication Loss of corneal reflex (left side) and the jaw reflex
The abducens (cranial VI) nerve	The abducens nerve supplies the lateral rectus which moves the eyeball laterally	Loss of the ability to move the left eye laterally

The facial (cranial VII) nerve	Motor function: it supplies all the muscles of the face and scalp, except the levator palpebrae superiors. It also supplies the platysma Sensory function: taste sensation from the anterior two-thirds of the tongue is transmitted by the facial nerve via the chorda tympani nerve	Left-sided facial muscle weakness Loss of taste sensations from the anterior two-third of the tongue
The vestibulocochlear (cranial VIII) nerve	This nerve comprises two components: the vestibular and the auditory	Decreased hearing on the left side and incoordination (a sense of rotation of the surroundings)

Further reading

Dieterich M. Dizziness. *Neurologist* 2004;**3**:154–164.

Gilden DH. Clinical practice. Bell's palsy. *New England Journal of Medicine* 2004;**351**:1323–1331.

Minor LB, Schessel DA, Carey JP. Meniere's disease. *Current Opinion in Neurology* 2004;**17**:9–16.

Pames LS, Agrawal SK, Atlas J. Diagnosis and management of benign paroxysmal positioning vertigo (BPPV). *Canadian Medical Association Journal* 2003;**169**:681–693.

Salinas R. Bell's palsy. *Clinical Evidence* 2003;**10**:1504–1507.

Ward BA, Gutmann DH. Neurofibromatosis 1: From lab bench to clinic. *Pediatric Neurology* 2005;**32**:221–228.

Zakizewska JM, Lopez BC. Trigeminal neuralgia. *Clinical Evidence* 2003;**10**:1599–1609.

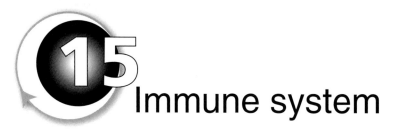

Immune system

Clinical cases

● CASE 15.1 – I came because of my joint pains.

Lillian Lucado, a 21-year-old university student, comes in to see her GP, Dr Edward Nelson, because of joint pains in both hands. Over the last few months, Lillian has noticed a gradual deterioration in her health and she always feels tired after minor exercise. She also gives a history of skin rash over her cheeks, particularly after exposure to the sun. She is not on any medications. She has had no past history of loose bowel motions, urinary tract infection, allergy or recent upper respiratory tract infection. She has no family history of arthritis. On examination, she looks ill and has an erythematous rash over the nose spreading to her checks. No lymphadenopathy. Her vital signs are summarized in Table 15.1.

Table 15.1 Vital signs for Case 15.1

Vital signs	Lilllan's results	Normal range
Blood pressure (mmHg)	120/70	100/60–135/85
Pulse rate (/min)	80	60–100
Respiratory rate (/min)	16	12–16
Temperature (°C)	37	36.6–37.2

- Scalp: patches of permanent alopecia

- Buccal cavity: multiple ulcers noticed

- Hands: tenderness in the proximal interphalangeal and metacarpophalangeal joints of both hands; no psoriatic changes

- No subcutaneous nodules

- Cardiovascular and respiratory examinations normal

- Abdominal examination normal

- Urinalysis normal.

● CASE 15.2 – It all happened in seconds.

Ms Patricia Stephen, a 41-year-old manager, is admitted to hospital on New Year's Eve because of a motor-car accident. Assessment of her condition by the trauma registrar reveals that she has a compound fracture her right tibia and fibula that requires surgical management. She develops wound infection and the registrar decides to start her on cephalothin. Within 20 min, her face begins to swell and she is wheezing. On examination, she looks anxious, flushed and short of breath. Her vital signs are shown in Table 15.2.

Table 15.2 Vital signs for Case 5.2

Vital signs	Patricia's results	Normal range
Blood pressure (mmHg)	80/50	100/60–135/85
Pulse rate (/min)	120	60–100
Respiratory rate (/min)	30	12–16
Temperature (°C)	37	36.6–37.2

- Her face and lips are oedematous.

- Her tongue and uvula are swollen and she is unable to open her eyes because of swelling of her eyelids and face.

- Auscultation of her chest: wheezing all over her lungs.

- Multiple urticarial lesions of her trunk and limbs.

CASE 15.3 – I was diagnosed with HIV infection about 3 years ago.

Michael Johnson, a 37-year-old engineer who was diagnosed with HIV infection about 4 years ago, comes in to see his GP because of fever, cough and shortness of breath. Michael was treated with combination antiretroviral therapy (HAART) and stayed on this regimen until 9 months ago. At that time he had a number of challenges at work and felt down, so he decided to discontinue his treatment and stop visiting his physician. Over the last couple of weeks, he has developed a productive cough, fever and shortness of breath. He has no chest pain but his breathing is noisy and musical. On examination, he looks ill and depressed. There are multiple white patches overlying his buccal mucosa. His vital signs are summarized in Table 15.3.

Table 15.3 Vital signs for Case 15.3

Vital signs	Michael's results	Normal range
Blood pressure (mmHg)	110/70	100/60–135/85
Pulse rate (/min)	110	60–100
Respiratory rate (/min)	30	12–16
Temperature (°C)	38.5	36.6–37.2

- Respiratory examination: crackles heard on auscultation of both lungs

- Central nervous system (CNS) examination normal

- Abdominal and cardiovascular examinations normal.

👥 Integrated medical sciences questions

CASE 15.1 – Briefly discuss the mechanisms underlying the pathogenesis of systemic lupus erythematosus (SLE).

CASE15.2 – Briefly compare the characteristics of different types of hypersensitivity. Briefly discuss the mechanisms responsible for the development of bronchial asthma.

CASE 15.3 – Discuss the pathogenesis of HIV infection and the mechanisms by which HIV infection produces immune deficiency.

🗝 Key concepts

In order to work through the core clinical cases in this chapter, you will need to understand the following key concepts.

New terms

- Antigen: any substance that may be specifically bound by an antibody molecule or T-cell receptor.

- Antibody: any of a large number of proteins of high molecular weight that are normally produced by specialized B cells after stimulation by an antigen. These antibodies act specifically against the antigen.

- Epitope: any antibody that binds to only a portion of the macromolecule, which is known as an epitope or a determinant.

- Hapten: a small separable part of an antigen that reacts specifically with an antibody but is incapable of stimulating antibody production except in combination with an associated protein molecule.

- Opsonization: the process of modifying antigen (usually a bacteria) by the action of opsonins.

Table 15.4 The main differences between innate and adaptive immune systems

Innate immunity	Adaptive immunity
This is the non-specific host defence mechanism. It does not need a 'memory' to function	This is the specific immune system. It requires a 'memory' to function
It comprises: the physical barriers such as skin and mucous membranes; the chemical barriers such as lysozyme in tears and gastric acid; interferons and cytokines; phagocytes; and the complement system	It comprises antibodies and lymphocytes (B and T cells)

Table 15.5 The main differences between B and T lymphocytes

B lymphocytes	T lymphocytes
Originate from stem cells in the bone marrow	Originate from stem cells in the bone marrow
Mature in bone marrow	Mature in thymus gland and become able to identify 'self proteins'
Make up 25 per cent of lymphocytes	Make up 75 per cent of lymphocytes
5–10 per cent are present in peripheral blood	70–90 per cent present in peripheral blood
When activated, become plasma cells which secrete large amounts of immunoglobulins (IgA, IgD, IgM, IgG and IgE). B-memory cells are also present	Two types: T-helper cells (CD4) forming 75 per cent of T cells; and T-cytotoxic killer cells (CD8) forming 25 per cent of T cells
	They are able to eliminate viruses, fungi and protozoa, and kill malignancy-transformed cells and transplanted cells

May require signals from T-helper cells in order to differentiate to plasma cells and secrete antibodies	All T cells bear CD3 antigen on their surface. In addition, T-helper cells bear CD4$^+$ antigen, whereas T-cytotoxic cells bear CD8$^+$

Complement system

The complement system is an important component of the innate immune system. It is made up of many plasma enzymes, and regulatory proteins that react with each other to opsonize pathogens. There are four pathways to activate the complement system:

1. Classic pathway: activated by antigen–antibody immune complex. It is initiated by binding of C1q (the first protein in the complement cascade) to the pathogen surface.

2. The mannose-binding lectin activation pathway (MB-lectin pathway): activated by microbes with terminal mannose groups.

3. The alternative activation pathway: activated by tumour cells or microbes. It is activated by binding of activated C3 in plasma to the surface of a pathogen.

4. The terminal pathway: this pathway is common to the first three pathways, which lead to a membrane attack complex that lyses cells.

The following are the functions of the complement system:

● It is a critical component of the innate immunity.

● It promotes activation of inflammation (anaphylatoxins, C3a, C5a).

● It promotes opsonized cell lysis (membrane attack complex)

● It allows activation of the immune system pathway by 'altered self' cells such as cancer cells.

The different types of immunoglobulins

Table 15.6 Comparison of different immunoglobulins

Characteristic	IgA	IgD	IgE	IgG	IgM
Molecular form	Monomer, dimer	Monomer	Monomer	Monomer	Pentamer, hexamer
Subclass	A1, A2	–	–	G1, G2, G3, G4	–
Molecular mass (kDa)	160, 400	170	190	150	950–1150
Percentage of total serum Ig	7–15	0.3	0.013	75–85	5–10
Antibody valence	2, 4	2	2	2	10, 12
Biological characteristics	Secretory Ig	Marker for mature B cells	Allergic reactions	Can be transferred in the placenta, secondary antibody response	Primary antibody response

The mechanisms by which CD4$^+$ loss/dysfunction occurs in HIV infection

- Direct effects of HIV on CD4$^+$ T cells

- Lysis of infected cells by cytotoxic T cells

- Expression of HIV peptides on infected CD4$^+$ T cells $\rightarrow$ killing of the infected cells by immunosuppressive effects of soluble HIV proteins on unaffected cells.

Answers

CASE 15.1 – I came because of my joint pains.

The findings from history and examinations suggest that the patient has multiple systems affected by the disease process:

- Skin: skin rash over her cheeks particularly after exposure to the sun and alopecia

- Mucous membrane: ulcers

- Joints: pain of interphalangeal and metacarpophalangeal joints of her hands.

Q1: What are the possible causes for the presenting problem?

A1

All these findings suggest a connective tissue disorder. The following are possible causes (hypotheses) for her problems:

- Postviral arthritis, although she has no recent history of viral infection.

- Rheumatoid arthritis: usually there is stiffness of the small joints of the hands (metacarpophalangeal, proximal and distal interphalangeal joints) and feet (metatarsophalangeal joints). The wrist, elbows, shoulders, knees and ankles may also be affected. The pain and stiffness are significantly worse in the morning. Non-articular signs include subcutaneous nodules, serositis and pleural effusion, vasculitis, neuropathies, scleritis and episcleritis. Lymph nodes may be palpable in rheumatoid arthritis. It is obvious that rheumatoid arthritis is less likely as a cause for her presentation.

- Systemic lupus erythematosus (SLE): a multisystem disorder with arthralgia, skin rash, mucus ulcers, cerebral and kidney disease. SLE is the most likely cause for her presentation.

- Systemic sclerosis: this multisystem disorder is characterized by Raynaud's phenomenon, calcinosis, oesophageal involvement (heartburn, reflux, dysphagia), sclerodactyly (diffuse swelling, stiffness and changes of the skin of fingers) and telangiectasia. This cause is less likely to be responsible for her problems.

Q2: What further questions would you like to ask to help you differentiate between your hypotheses?

A2

Table 15.7 Further history questions for Case 15.1

History questions	In what way answers can help
History of malaise, tiredness and fever	Fever is common in disease exacerbation. It may be present in about 50 per cent of patients
Joint swelling, morning stiffness, any deformity	Rheumatoid arthritis is characterized by symmetrical involvement of the small joints of the hands and feet. The wrist, elbows, shoulders, knees and ankles may also be affected. The pain and stiffness are significantly worse in the morning

Shortness of breath, cough or chest pain	SLE may be associated with lung involvement in 60 per cent of patients (recurrent pleurisy, pleural effusions are most common and often bilateral)
Any changes in her mood, feeling 'run down', headaches, psychological changes	The nervous system is involved in about 60 per cent of patients with SLE. There may be mild depression, psychological and mood changes, cerebellar ataxia and cranial nerve lesions
Medications such as hydralazine, isoniazide, D-penicillamine	These drugs are able to induce lupus (not associated with anti-dsDNA)

 Q3: What investigations would be most helpful to you and why?

A3

Further investigations

- Full blood examination
- Erythrocyte sedimentation rate (ESR)
- Antinuclear antibodies (ANAs)
- Anti-double-stranded-DNA (dsDNA) antibodies
- Radiograph of her hands
- Blood urea, creatinine, sodium and potassium
- Urinalysis.

 CASE 15.2 – **It all happened in seconds.**

 Q1: What are the possible causes for the presenting problem?

A1

The likely cause (hypothesis) for Patricia's presentation is drug-induced anaphylaxis (type 1 hypersensitivity). Her anaphylaxis is most probably related to cephalothin treatment. Penicillin and the penicillin group of related antibiotics act as a hapten. The highly reactive β-lactam ring of penicillin is crucial for its antibiotic activity. This ring also reacts with amino groups on the host proteins to form covalent conjugates, resulting in penicillin-modified self-peptides that provoke a T-helper 2 (Th2) response in some individuals. The Th2 cells activate penicillin-binding B cells to produce IgE antibodies against the penicillin hapten.

Q2: What further questions would you like to ask to help you differentiate between your hypotheses?

A2

The patient should be managed immediately without any delay:

1. Lay patient down and raise her feet.

2. Ensure that her airway is free, give O_2 by mask.

3. Monitor her blood pressure, pulse rate and oximetry (determination of the O_2 saturation of blood using finger oximetry).

4. Give her 0.5 ml of 1:1000 adrenaline (epinephrine) intramuscularly (0.5 mg), to be repeated after 5 min if her blood pressure remains low.

5. Give her hydrocortisone 100 mg.

6. Give her antihistamine 10 mg by slow intravenous drip over 48 h.

Further history questions may be taken after full management of her anaphylaxis (Table 15.8).

Table 15.8 Further history questions for Case 15.2

History questions	In what way answers can help
History of anaphylaxis with drugs, food or insect stings	It is important to ask about history of allergy before prescribing medications. People allergic to penicillin should not be treated with penicillin or related chemicals (e.g. cephalosporin antibiotics)
What provokes your allergy, e.g. penicillin antibiotics and related drugs, or peanuts	In people with IgE antibodies against penicillin, giving the drug or closely related structurally antibiotics (e.g. cephalothin) by injection can cause anaphylaxis and even death
Past history of treatment for anaphylaxis or allergy, e.g. urticaria, bronchial asthma	Usually positive

 Q3: What investigations would be most helpful to you and why?

A3

Further investigations

- Full blood examination
- Serum IgE
- Urinary histamine
- Serum β-tryptase.

CASE 15.3 – I was diagnosed with HIV infection about 3 years ago.

Q1: What are the possible causes for the presenting problem?

A1

The following are the most likely causes (hypotheses) for Michael's presentation (productive cough, fever, noisy breathing, wheezing and shortness of breath):

- Pneumonia caused by bacterial infection or *Pneumocystis carinii* infection. Michael discontinued his treatment for HIV infection, combination antiretroviral therapy (HAART), about 9 months ago and we do not know his current CD4⁺ T-cell count. As a result of his low CD4⁺ T-cell count, altered B-cell function and defects in neutrophil function, he is at high risk of developing infection caused by encapsulated organisms such as *Streptococcus pneumoniae* and *Haemophilus influenzae*. HIV-infected individuals have a sixfold increase in the incidence of pneumococcal pneumonia. They are at high risk of pneumococcal disease when the CD4⁺ T-cell count is $< 200/\mu$L. He is also at high risk of *P. carinii* infection (patients with a CD4⁺ T-cell count $< 200/\mu$L should be placed on a regimen for *P. carinii* prophylaxis).

- Pneumonia caused by mycobacterial infection: reactivation of pulmonary tuberculosis (TB) often develops relatively early in the course of HIV infection and may be an early sign of HIV disease.

- Fungal infection of the lung (e.g. cryptococcal infection). In 90 per cent of patients with fungal lung infection, however, there is concomitant CNS infection. Michael has no signs or symptoms suggesting CNS infection.

 Q2: What further questions would you like to ask to help you differentiate between your hypotheses?

A2

Table 15.9 Further history questions for Case 5.3

History questions	In what way answers can help
History of fever, cough, expectoration, oral thrush, unexpected weight loss, night sweats, chest pain	These symptoms are usually associated with pulmonary infections caused by *P. carinii*. Fever and weight loss may be the result of disseminated disease such as mycobacteria or fungi or may indicate non-Hodgkin's lymphoma
Amount and colour of his sputum. Duration of symptoms	Patients with *P. carinii* usually present with a cough that is non-productive, or productive of scant amounts of white sputum. The symptom duration is usually a few weeks (2–4 weeks). In contrast, the presence of cough productive of purulent sputum and symptom duration of a few days favour the diagnosis of bacterial pneumonia
His last CD4⁺ T count results. When did his doctor start him on antiretroviral therapy? What was his CD4⁺ T-cell count then?	HIV-infected individuals with CD4⁺ T-cell counts $< 200/\mu$L are at higher risk of infection with *P. carinii*. Patients with CD4⁺ T-cell counts $< 50/\mu$L are at higher risk of infection with cytomegalovirus and mycobacteria of *Mycobacterium avium* complex (MAC)

History of immunization with pneumococcal polysaccharide	HIV-infected individuals have a sixfold increase in the incidence of pneumococcal pneumonia. Immunization is recommended particularly when the CD4⁺ T-cell count is < 200/µL
Any prior bouts of pneumonia	Patients with HIV infection and low CD4⁺ T-cell count are at higher risk of developing pneumonia possibly because of altered B-cell function or defects in neutrophil functions. Those who give a past history of bouts of pneumonia are at higher risk of recurrence of pneumonia
Details about his combination antiretroviral therapy and when exactly he stopped the treatment. Any prophylactic therapy?	Patients with HIV infection are at higher risk of developing pneumonia when they are not on antiretroviral therapy. Once the CD4⁺ T-cell count is < 200/µL, patients should be placed on a regimen of *P. carinii* prophylaxis

 Q3: What investigations would be most helpful to you and why?

A3

Further investigations

- Full blood examination

- CD4 and CD8 counts

- HIV viral load

- Serum lactate dehydrogenase (LDH)

- Chest radiograph

- Sputum-microbiological studies

- Blood culture

Further progress

CASE 15.1 – I came because of my joint pains.

Dr Nelson arranges some tests for Lilian. The results are shown in Tables 15.10 and 15.11.

Table 15.10 Blood test results for Case 15.1

Test	Lilian's results	Normal range
Haemoglobin (Hb) (g/L)	95	115–160
Packed cell volume (PCV)	0.38	0.37–0.47
White cell count (WCC) ($\times 10^9$/L)	3.3	4.0–11.0
Platelet count ($\times 10^9$/L)	120	150–400

Table 15.11 Other test results for Case 15.1

Test	Lilian's results
ESR (mm/h)	114 (normal range 0–20)
Antinuclear antibodies (ANAs)	Titre of 1:640
dsDNA antibodies.	Elevated
Radiograph of her hands	No articular damage or change

Blood urea, creatinine, sodium and potassium: within normal limits.

Urinalysis: normal.

● CASE 15.2 – It all happened in seconds.

The registrar arranges some tests for Patricia. The results are shown in Table 15.12.

Table 15.12 Test results for Case 15.2

Test	Patricia's results	Normal range
Hb (g/L)	143	115–160
PCV	0.40	0.37–0.47
WCC ($\times 10^9$/L)	8.97	4.0–11.0
Platelet count ($\times 10^9$/L)	310	150–400
Neutrophils ($\times 10^9$/L)	5.10	2.00–7.50
Lymphocytes ($\times 10^9$/L)	2.49	1.50–4.00
Monocytes ($\times 10^9$/L)	0.51	0.20–0.80
Eosinophils ($\times 10^9$/L)	0.83	0.04–0.44
Basophils ($\times 10^9$/L)	0.04	0.00–0.10
Serum IgE level (g/L)	Raised	<0.00025

CASE 15.3 – I was diagnosed with HIV infection about 3 years ago.

The treating doctor arranges some tests for Michael. The results are shown in Tables 15.13 and 15.14.

Table 15.13 Full blood examination, T-cell subtypes and serum LDH: test results for Case 15.3

Test	Michael's results	Normal range
Hb (g/L)	111	115–160
PCV	0.39	0.37–0.47
WCC ($\times 10^9$/L)	2.7	4.0–11.0
Platelet count ($\times 10^9$/L)	122	150–400
CD4 count ($\times 10^9$/L)	0.040	0.55–1.20
CD8 count ($\times 10^9$/L)	1.09	0.40–0.80
CD4/CD8 ratio	0.036	1.3–1.5
Serum LDH (IU/L)	540	208–378

LDH, lactate dehydrogenase.

Table 15.14 Sputum: test results for Case 15.3

Sputum test	Michael's results
Gram stain	Negative
Toluidine blue	Positive for *Pneumocystis carinii*
Ziehl–Neelsen (ZN) stain	No acid-fast bacilli
Culture for TB	Results to be followed
Culture and sensitivity	Negative

Blood culture: no growth.

Chest radiograph: diffuse bilateral pulmonary infiltrate; no cavitations or pleural effusion; no hilar or mediastinal adenopathy.

HIV viral load: 69 000 copies/mL (detected by reverse transcription poylmerase chain reaction or RT-PCR).

Further questions

 CASE 15.1 – I came because of my joint pains.

 Q4: In the light of the clinical presentation, how would you interpret the laboratory test results?

A4

Table 15.15 Interpretation of lab test results for Case 5.1

Test	Change	Interpretation
Hb	Low	Anaemia occurs in about 50 per cent of patients with SLE. Red blood cells are usually normocytic and normochromic. The most likely cause of her anaemia is haemolysis of red blood cells. Other possible causes are: excessive menstrual bleeding); and blood loss from the gastrointestinal tract (this is less likely because she has not been treated with an NSAID)
WCC	Low	Leukopenia occurs in about 50 per cent of patients with SLE. It is usually the result of immune mechanisms (e.g. anti-neutrophil antibodies, immune complexes)
Platelet count	Low	Thrombocytopenia has been reported in about 50 per cent of patients with SLE. The causes of low platelets are: abnormal immune mechanisms; antiplatelet antibodies; DIC; and ITP (possibly the first manifestation of SLE)
ESR	Raised (> 100 mm/h)	ESR is raised in most patients and it has been claimed that it correlates with disease activity
ANAs	Raised (titre of 1:640)	A positive ANA test results has a 25–35 per cent predictive value for SLE. The test has a sensitivity of 99 per cent and specificity of 80 per cent
dsDNA antibodies	Elevated	dsDNA should be ordered if ANA test is positive. The test has 70 per cent sensitivity but 95 per cent specificity. Other tests you may order are Sm, RNP, Ro (SS-A) and La (SS-B) nuclear RNA proteins. Sm test has a sensitivity of about 25 per cent, but a specificity of 99 per cent. Both dsDNA and Sm are useful in confirming the diagnosis
Radiograph of hands	No articular damage or change	Joint erosion is very rare in SLE. This might be useful in differentiating SLE from rheumatoid arthritis (joint erosion, damage of periarticular tissue and deformity usually occur in rheumatoid arthritis)
Blood urea, creatinine, sodium and potassium	Normal	Renal involvement occurs in 50 per cent of patients with SLE (lupus nephritis). Usually serum complement levels are useful. Decreased levels of CH50, C4 and C3 tend to occur with disease activity especially with associated renal disease. Measurement of complement levels may be useful in assessing this issue further

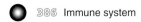

Urinalysis	Normal	Haematuria and proteinuria may be present with renal involvement (lupus nephritis). However, a negative urinalysis does not exclude renal involvement and more tests are needed to assess the kidney function. In SLE the kidney could be affected by the disease process itself or drug-induced renal damage

CH50, total haemolytic complement; DIC, disseminated intravascular coagulation; ITP, idiopathic thrombocytopenic purpura.

 Q5: What is your final hypothesis?

A5

Systemic lupus erythematosus.

 Q6: What issues in the given history, examination and laboratory tests support your final hypothesis?

A6

Supportive evidence

History

- Joint pains in both hands
- Gradual deterioration in her health and always feels tired after minor exercise
- Skin rash over her cheeks, particularly after exposure to the sun
- She is not on any medications
- No past history of urinary tract infection, allergy or recent upper respiratory tract.

Examination

- She looks ill, but vital signs normal
- Erythematous rash over the nose spreading to her cheeks
- No lymphadenopathy
- Areas of permanent alopecia
- Buccal cavity: multiple mucosal ulcers
- Tenderness in the proximal interphalangeal and metacarpophalangeal joints of the hands
- No psoriatic changes.

Investigations

- Hb, WCC and platelets: all low
- ESR: raised > 100 mm/h

- Anti-dsDNA antibodies: elevated

- Radiograph of hands: no articular damage or change

- Blood urea, creatinine, sodium and potassium: normal

- Urinalysis: normal.

⬤ CASE 15.2 – It all happened in seconds.

 Q4: In the light of the clinical presentation, how would you interpret the laboratory test results?

A4

Table 15.16 Interpretation of lab test results for Case 5.2

Test	Change	Interpretation
Eosinophil count	Raised	Eosinophils migrate to the site of allergic reactions and in anaphylaxis large amounts of eosinophils are released and appear in the circulation and organs involved in the inflammatory reaction
Serum IgE level	Raised	This is not a useful test and in clinical practice is not used. It may suggest IgE-dependent hypersensitivity
Serum β-tryptase	Raised	Suggests mast cell activation. This test is rarely used in clinical practice
Urinary histamine	Slightly raised	This is not a practical test in anaphylaxis. Urinary histamine reflects a small portion of histamine released from mast cells and basophils during anaphylaxis. Histamine will be immediately metabolized in the circulation before its renal clearance

 Q5: What is your final hypothesis?

A5

Drug-induced hypersensitivity.

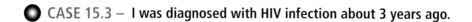

Q6: What issues in the given history, examination and laboratory tests support your final hypothesis?

A6

Supportive evidence

History

- Changes started 20 min after starting her on cephalothin antibiotics
- Her face begins to swell and she is wheezing.

Examination

- She looks anxious, flushed and short of breath.
- Vital signs: low blood pressure, increased pulse rate and respiratory rate.
- Face and lips are oedematous; unable to open her eyes because of swelling of her eyelids and face.
- Tongue and uvula are swollen.
- Wheezing all over her lungs.
- Multiple urticarial lesions of her trunk and limbs.

Investigations

- Raised eosinophils
- Increased serum Ig E levels
- Urinary histamine: slightly elevated.

 CASE 15.3 – I was diagnosed with HIV infection about 3 years ago.

Q4: In the light of the clinical presentation, how would you interpret the laboratory test results?

A4

Table 15.17 Interpretation of lab test results for Case 5.3

Test	Change	Interpretation
Hb	Decreased	In patients with HIV infection, anaemia is usually the result of chronic infection, bone marrow suppression, drug association, haemolytic/immune association or nutrition

WCC	Decreased	WBCs are frequently elevated in the presence of infection. This elevation may be relative to their baseline value. This is particularly important in patients with WCC less than the normal laboratory range. Neutropenia is usually present
Platelet count	Decreased	In patients with HIV infection, platelet count is usually low
CD4 count	Decreased	CD4+ T-cell count remains a good indicator of an HIV-infected patient's risk of developing opportunistic infection. At count of < 200/μL, the risk of infection with *P. carinii* is high
CD4/CD8 ratio	Decreased	A decreased CD4/CD8 ratio indicates increased risk of opportunistic infection
Serum LDH	Raised	Serum LDH is usually raised in patients with PCP. Several other conditions may be associated with elevated LDH such as bacterial pneumonia and tuberculosis. Serum LDH has been shown, however, to correlate with prognosis and response to therapy in patients with *P. carinii*
Sputum: toluidine blue	Positive for *P. carinii*	*P. carinii* is the cause of his presentation (cough, fever, shortness of breath, wheezing)
Sputum: Gram stain and ZN stain	Negative	This will make TB less likely. However, a sputum culture for TB is needed to confirm this
Blood culture	No growth	The possibility that infection caused by *S. pneumonia* and *Haemophilus* species less likely
Chest radiograph	Diffuse bilateral pulmonary infiltrate	This picture is consistent with PCP
HIV viral load	69 000 copies/mL	This test predicts what will happen to the CD4+ T-cell counts in the near future. Effective therapy should bring the level to < 50 copies/mL

PCP, *P. carinii* pneumonia.

 Q5: What is your final hypothesis?

A5

P. carinii pneumonia (PCP) in a patient with AIDS.

Q6: What issues in the given history, examination and laboratory tests support your final hypothesis?

A6

Supportive evidence

History

- Diagnosed with HIV infection 4 years earlier
- Discontinued HAART and stopped visiting his physician about 9 months ago
- Presents with fever, cough and shortness of breath for 2 weeks.

Examination

- Looks ill and depressed
- Multiple white patches overlying his buccal mucosa
- Feverish 38.5°C
- Increased pulse rate and respiratory rate
- Crackles heard on auscultation of both lungs
- Cardiovascular examination and CNS examination both normal
- Abdominal examination normal.

Investigations

- Low Hb, WCC and platelets
- Decreased CD4 count
- Decreased CD4/CD8 ratio
- Increased serum LDH
- Sputum is positive for *P. carinii*
- Sputum negative for Gram stain and ZN stain
- Sputum culture negative
- Blood culture: no growth
- Chest radiograph: diffuse bilateral pulmonary infiltrate; no cavitations or pleural effusion; no
- HIV viral load: 69 000 copies/mL (detected by RT-PCR)

⚇ Integrated medical sciences questions

⚫ CASE 15.1 – Briefly discuss the mechanisms underlying the pathogenesis of SLE.

Predisposing factors

- Genetic risk for SLE (14–48 per cent in monozygotic twins) and increased frequency of SLE in HLA-B8, -DR2, -DR3, - DQA1 and -DQB1

- More common in females in the childbearing years (possibly female sex hormones play a role)

- Common in China and south-east Asia, and in black populations

- Environmental factors: viral infection, exposure to ultraviolet (UV) light

- Immunological factors: abnormalities in immune system regulation and loss of 'self' tolerance (it is not clear whether this is a primary or a secondary problem); and abnormality in the immune system and decreased ability to clear autoantibodies formed.

Immunological changes and its role in pathogenesis

- Decreased suppressor T cells (cause unknown)

- Defects in apoptosis (cells break down abnormally resulting in the release of nuclear antigens → processing by antigen-presenting cells (macrophages, B lymphocytes) → formation of peptides → formation of peptide–major histocompatibility complex → stimulation of Th cells (CD4) → release of cytokines (interleukins IL-6, IL-4 and IL-10) → activation of B cells to produce antibodies to many nuclear antigens (e.g. ANA to DNA, Sm, RNP, Ro, La).

Hormonal role in pathogenesis

- Oestrogen and progesterone promote B-cell hyperactivity whereas male sex hormones suppress B-cell proliferation.

- Males with Klinefelter's syndrome and those with abnormal oestrogen metabolism are at a higher risk of developing SLE.

Consequences of immunological changes

Most of the changes in different body systems are caused by antibodies formed during the disease progress and deposition of immune complex → activation of the complement system (consumption of the complement system during this process) and chemotactic factors → attraction of WBCs which phagocytose the immune complex → release of mediators → further inflammation → chronic inflammation of body organs + fibrosis + necrosis (e.g. development of glomerulonephritis) → progressive loss of function.

Antibodies are formed to cell surface antigens and coats red blood cells, WBCs and platelets → cytotoxicity → haemolytic anaemia, leukopenia and thrombocytopenia.

Antibodies to endothelial cells of blood vessels → arterial and venous thromboses and development of placental infarcts and abortion in pregnant patients with SLE.

Skin changes are mainly caused by: damage of DNA by UV light; antibodies formed by the patient's body forms immune complex and a local inflammatory reaction occurs in the exposed area of the face; increased binding of autoantibodies (anti-Ro) to UV-activated keratinocytes; and increased interleukin release from UV-activated keratinocytes and development of acute inflammatory response (redness, swelling, increased blood supply to the area, itching of the butterfly area).

● **CASE15.2 – Briefly compare the characteristics of different types of hypersensitivity. Briefly discuss the mechanisms responsible for the development of bronchial asthma.**

Table 15.18 The Gel and Coombs' classification of hypersensitivity

	Type I	Type II	Type III	Type IV	Type V
Description	Immediate	Cytotoxic	Immune complex	Delayed	Stimulating/blocking
Mechanism	Formation of IgE antibody specific to inducing antigen. Antibody binds via Fc receptor to mast cells and basophils. Degradation of mast cells and release of mediators	Reaction of antibody with cell surface-bound antigen. Activation of complement system. IgG and IgM involved	Exogenous (viruses, bacteria, fungi, parasites)	Delayed type of hypersensitivity. Activation of macrophages and lymphokines	Interaction of antibodies to cell surface receptors causing malfunction
Pathological features	Oedema, vasodilatation, smooth muscle contraction, cytokine release	Antibody-mediated damage to target cells (e.g. haemolysis)	Acute inflammatory reaction, vasculitis	Granuloma formation, caseation, necrosis, chronic inflammation, fibrosis	Hypertrophy
Clinical examples	Bronchial asthma, anaphylaxis	Haemolytic anaemia, Goodpasture's syndrome, blood transfusion reaction, hyperactive graft rejection	Serum sickness, SLE, rheumatoid arthritis	Pulmonary TB, contact dermatitis, graft-versus-host disease, leprosy	Graves' disease, myasthenia gravis

The following are the mechanisms underlying the development of bronchial asthma.

Predisposing factors

● Genetic factors: two asthma genes have been identified – *ADAM-33* on human chromosome 20 and *PhF11* on human chromosome 13. It is expected that more genes involved in asthma will be identified in the near future.

● Environmental factors: those initiating an immune response.

Pathological changes

● Oedema of the airway-lining mucosa

● Hyperaemia

- Infiltration of the mucosa with inflammatory cells

- Hypertrophy and hyperplasia of the airway glands

- Hyperplasia of the airway smooth muscles

- Production of chemokines

- Production on hyerviscous sputum.

Mediators involved in acute asthma

- Acetylcholine: constriction of airways (stimulates muscarinic receptors)

- Histamine released from esinophils

- Platelet-activating factor (PAF)

- Neuropeptides

- Kinins

- Leukotrienes

- Nitric oxide (NO).

Pathophysiological changes

- Increased resistance to airway flow (because of obstruction)

- Decreased flow rates

- No changes in the pressure–volume curves

- During inspiration, the pleural pressure becomes more negative

- During expiration, high pleural pressure is present

- Thus, wide pressure swings and a much higher resistance

- Increased respiratory rate during acute asthmatic attack.

CASE 15.3 – Discuss the pathogenesis of HIV infection and the mechanisms by which HIV infection produces immune deficiency.

Human immunodeficiency virus

There are at least two types of the human immunodeficiency virus responsible for the development of acquired immune deficiency syndrome (AIDS):

1. HIV-1: the more virulent type, which is responsible for immune deficiency worldwide

2. HIV-2: endemic in West Africa and India.

HIV-1 shows marked genetic variability and is classified into three major groups:

1. M (main)

2. O (outlier)

3. N (non-M, non-O).

The M group of HIV-1 is the major cause of immune deficiency worldwide.

The characteristics of the HIV-1 virus may be summarized as follows:

- HIV is an enveloped retrovirus.

- It belongs to the lentiviruses (slowly producing a disease).

- It contains two copies of an RNA genome.

- It contains reverse transcriptase, integrase and protease enzymes.

- It has an outer viral glycoprotein, gp 120, and gp 41 in the viral envelope.

The HIV has several genes, including:

- *gag* gene (group-specific antigen): encodes the structural proteins of viral core

- *pol* gene (polymerase): encodes the enzymes involved in viral replication and integration

- *env* gene (envelope): encodes the viral envelope glycoprotein.

The different modes of infection with HIV

Infection occurs via the transfer of body fluids from an infected person to an uninfected one, and fluids are:

- vaginal fluid (during sexual intercourse)

- semen (during sexual intercourse)

- mother's milk (lactation of a newborn)

- blood (contaminated needles used for intravenous use, during delivery, use of infected blood products). The virus may be free in these body fluids or carried in infected CD4 T cells, macrophages and dendritic cells.

The changes that may follow an infection with HIV

Infection with HIV → acute viraemia → influenza-like symptoms (80 per cent of patients) + activation of CD8 T cells to kill infected cells + marked decrease in CD4 T cells, although the diagnosis is usually missed at this stage → recovery from the influenza-like symptoms in a few days + gradual decline in the number of CD4 T cells over the next 2–12 years or more → development of AIDS (in most patients) + opportunistic infections and increased tendency to develop cancer.

How the virus is attached to the host cells

There are a number of receptors that can facilitate the process by which the HIV is attached to CD4 T cells, macrophages or other cells. These receptors are:

- CD4 receptors: present in CD4 T cells, dendritic cells and macrophages

- Co-receptors (chemokine receptors): mainly CCR5 (expressed on dendritic cells, macrophages and CD4 T cells)

- CXCR4: expressed on the activated T cells.

How does binding of the virus occur?

- Binding of gp 120 to the CD4 receptor or co-receptors (CCR5 or CXCR4).

- The gp 41 is responsible for the fusion of the viral envelope with the plasma membrane of the host cells.

The changes that might occur next in the host cell

The viral genome and the viral reverse transcriptase → transcription of the viral RNA into a complementary DNA (cDNA) → integration into the cell host genome by viral integrase (integrated cDNA copy is known as provirus) → viral replication is initiated by transcription of the provirus when a T-helper cell is activated (some cells may remain in a latent state for years after integration).

The viral genes (*gag, pol* and *env*) are essential for the viral replication in activated T cells, e.g. the *gag* and *pol* mRNAs → giving the individual functional proteins of HIV and the *env* mRNA → giving gp 160 which cleaves by cell proteases into gp 120 and gp 41 required for the virus envelope glycoprotein.

Immunological changes in HIV-infected patients

Loss of CD4 T cells: might occur by these mechanisms:

- Direct viral killing of infected cells

- Induction of apoptosis in infected cells

- Killing of infected CD4 T cells by CD8 cytotoxic lymphocytes

- Loss of cell-mediated immunity

- Infection with opportunistic infections (e.g. oral *Candida* sp., *M. tuberculosis*, Epstein–Barr virus-infected B-cell lymphoma, *P. carinii*, *M. avium* complex and cytomegalovirus).

Further reading

Cimaz R. Any increased risk of autoimmune disease? *Lupus* 2004;**13**:736–739.

Currie GP, Devereux GS, Lee DK, Ayres JG. Recent developments in asthma management. *British Medical Journal* 2005;**330**:585–589.

Demoly P, Romano A. Update on beta-lactam allergy diagnosis. *Current Allergy and Asthma Reports* 2005;**1**:9–14.

Lesho E. A pathophysiological approach to antiretroviral therapy. *Expert Review of Anti-infective Therapy* 2004;**4**:509–520.

Nielsen MH, Pedersen FS, Kjems J. Molecular strategies to inhibit HIV-1 replication. *Retrovirology* 2005;**2**:10–15.

Park MA, Li JT. Diagnosis and management of penicillin allergy. *Mayo Clinic Proceedings* 2005;**80**:405–410.

Petri M, Magder L. Classification criteria for systemic lupus erythematosus: a review. *Lupus* 2004;**13**:829–837.

Sawalha AH, Harley JB. Antinuclear autoantibodies in systemic lupus erythematosus. *Current Opinion in Rheumatology* 2004;**16**:534–540.

Waldman M, Madaio MP. Pathogenic autoantibodies in lupus nephritis. *Lupus* 2005;**14**:19–24.

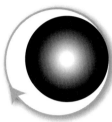# Recommended texts

The following textbooks are recommended for use in conjunction with this book.

Abbas AK, Lichtman AH (2003) *Cellular and Molecular Immunology*, 5th edn. New York: Saunders.

Ackermann U (2002) *PDQ Physiology*. Hamilton: BC Decker Inc.

Agur AMR, Lee MJ (2000) *Grant's Atlas of Anatomy*, 10th edn. Philadelphia, PA: Lippincott Williams & Wilkins.

Basmajian JV, Slonecker CE (1989) *Grant's Method of Anatomy*, 11th edn. Baltimore, MD: Williams & Wilkins.

Bennett PN, Brown MJ (2003) *Clinical Pharmacology*, 9th edn. Edinburgh: Churchill Livingstone.

Bhagavan NV (2002) *Medical Biochemistry*, 4th edn. San Diego, CA: Harcourt Academic Press.

Boron WF, Boulpaep EL (2003) *Medical Physiology*. Philadelphia, PA: Saunders.

Chandrasoma P, Taylor CR (1998) *Concise Pathology*, 3rd edn. Stamford, CA: Appleton & Lange.

Craig CR, Stitzel RE (2004) *Modern Pharmacology with Clinical Applications*, 6th edn. Philadelphia, PA: Lippincott Williams & Wilkins.

Damjanov I, Linder J (1996) Anderson's Pathology, 10th edn. St Louis, MO: Mosby.

Davis A, Blakeley AGH, Kidd C (2001) Human physiology. Edinburgh: Churchill Livingstone.

Drake RL, Vogl W, Mitchell AWM (2005) *Gray's Anatomy for Students*. Philadelphia, PA: Elsevier Churchill Livingstone.

Goldman L, Ausiello D (2004) *Cecil Textbook of Medicine*, 22nd edn. New York: Saunders.

Greenspan FS, Gardner DG (2001) *Basic and Clinical Endocrinology*, 6th edn. New York: Lange Medical Books/McGraw-Hill.

Guyton AC, Hall JE (2000) *Textbook of Medical Physiology*, 10th edn. Philadelphia, PA: Saunders.

Hardmann JG, Limbird LE (2001) *Goodman & Gilman's The Pharmacological Basis of Therapeutics*, 10th edn. New York: McGraw-Hill.

Hiatt JL, Gartner LP (1997) *Color Textbook of Histology*. New York: Saunders.

Johnson LR (1999) *Essential Medical Physiology*, 2nd edn. Philadelphia: Lippincott-Raven.

Jorde LB, Carey JC, Bamshad MJ, White RL (1999) Medical genetics. 2nd edn. St Louis: Mosby.

Junqueira LC, Carneiro J (2004) *Basic Histology: Text and atlas*. 10th edn. New York: Lange Medical Books/McGraw-Hill.

Kandel ER, Schwartz JH, Jessel TM (2000) *Principles of Neural Science*, 4th edn. New York, McGraw-Hill.

Katzung BG (2004) *Basic and Clinical Pharmacology*, 9th edn. New York, McGraw-Hill.

Kierszenbaum AL (2002) *Histology and Cell Biology*. St Louis, MO: Mosby.

Kumar P, Clark M (2002) *Clinical Medicine*, 5th edn. Edinburgh: Saunders.

Lilly LS (2003) *Pathophysiology of Heart Disease. A collaborative project of medical students and faculty*, 3rd edn. Philadelphia, PA: Lippincott Williams & Wilkins.

Mandell GL et al. (1998) *Principles and Practice of Infectious Diseases*, 5th edn. New York: Churchill Livingstone.

McPhee SJ, Lingappa VR, Ganong WF (2003) *Pathophysiology of Disease. An introduction to clinical medicine*. New York: Lange Medical Books/McGraw-Hill.

Mims C, Dockrell HM, Goering RV, Roitt I, Wakelin D, Zuckerman M (2004) *Medical Microbiology*, 3rd edn. New York: McGraw-Hill.

Moore KL, Dalley AF (1999) *Clinically Oriented Anatomy*, 4th edn. Baltimore, MD; Williams & Wilkins.

Murray RK, Granner DK, Mayer PA, Rodwell VW (2003) *Harper's Illustrated Biochemistry*, 26th edn. New York, McGraw-Hill.

Nolte J (1999) *The Human Brain: An introduction to its functional anatomy*, 4th edn. St Louis, MO: Mosby.

Page C, Curtis M, Sutter M, Walker M, Hoffman B (2002) *Integrated Pharmacology*, 2nd edn. Edinburgh: Mosby.

Pollard TD, Earnshaw WC (2004) *Cell Biology*. New York: Saunders.

Rubin E, Farber JL (1999) *Pathology*, 3rd edn. Philadelphia, PA: Lippincott.

Rudolph AM, Kamei RK, Overby KJ (2002) *Rudolph's Fundamentals of Pediatrics*, 3rd edn. New York: McGraw-Hill.

Souhami RL, Moxham J (2002) *Textbook of Medicine*, 4th edn. Edinburgh: Churchill Livingstone.

Underwood JCE (2000) *General and Systemic Pathology*, 3rd edn. Edinburgh: Churchill Livingstone.

Wilson JD, Larsen PR, Shlomo M (2002) *Williams' Textbook of Endocrinology*, 10th edn. Philadelphia, PA: WB Saunders.

Young B, Heath JW (2000) *Wheater's Functional Histology*, 4th edn. New York: Churchill Livingstone.

Young PA, Young PH (1997) *Basic Clinical Neuroanatomy*. Philadelphia, PA: Lippincott.

Williamson RCN, Waxman BP (1999) *Scott: An aid to clinical surgery*, 6th edn. Edinburgh: Churchill Livingstone.

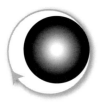

Index